Living

═ Low ═

Carb

Revised & Updated Edition

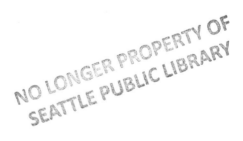

Living
Low
Carb

THE ESSENTIAL GUIDE TO CHOOSING THE
RIGHT LOW-CARB PLAN FOR YOU

REVISED & UPDATED EDITION

Jonny Bowden, PhD, CNS

FOREWORD BY Barry Sears, PhD, AUTHOR OF *The Zone*
INTRODUCTION BY Dr. Will Cole, AUTHOR OF *Ketotarian*

STERLING
New York

STERLING
New York

An Imprint of Sterling Publishing Co., Inc.
1166 Avenue of the Americas
New York, NY 10036

STERLING and the distinctive Sterling logo are
registered trademarks of Sterling Publishing Co., Inc.

Portions of this publication previously published as *Living Low Carb*.

ISBN 978-1-4549-3504-9

Distributed in Canada by Sterling Publishing Co., Inc.
c/o Canadian Manda Group, 664 Annette Street
Toronto, Ontario M6S 2C8, Canada
Distributed in the United Kingdom by GMC Distribution Services
Castle Place, 166 High Street, Lewes, East Sussex BN7 1XU, England
Distributed in Australia by NewSouth Books
University of New South Wales, Sydney, NSW 2052, Australia

For information about custom editions, special sales, and premium and corporate purchases,
please contact Sterling Special Sales at 800-805-5489 or specialsales@sterlingpublishing.com.

Manufactured in Canada

2 4 6 8 10 9 7 5 3 1

www.sterlingpublishing.com

Cover design by David Ter-Avanesyan

The low-fat–high-carbohydrate diet, promulgated vigorously by the National Cholesterol Education Program, National Institutes of Health, and American Heart Association since the Lipid Research Clinics-Primary Prevention Program in 1984, and earlier by the US Department of Agriculture food pyramid, may well have played an unintended role in the current epidemics of obesity, lipid abnormalities, type 2 diabetes, and metabolic syndromes.

This diet can no longer be defended by appeal to the authority of prestigious medical organizations or by rejecting clinical experience and a growing medical literature suggesting that the much-maligned low-carbohydrate–high-protein diet may have a salutary effect on the epidemics in question.

— "THE DIET-HEART HYPOTHESIS: A CRITIQUE" S. L. WEINBERG, *JOURNAL OF THE AMERICAN COLLEGE OF CARDIOLOGY* 43, NO. 5 (MARCH 3, 2004): 731–733.

"Never underestimate the convictions of the conventional, particularly in medicine."

—WILLIAM DAVIS, MD

═Contents═

≡ Introduction ≡

Rarely does one book perfectly amalgamate paradigm-shifting gravitas with actionable, easy-to-understand information. This powerfully updated edition of *Living Low Carb* artfully does just that. For decades, the word "fat" has been regarded as little more than a poison. We've been told to eat foods that keep it out of our bodies, take drugs that keep it out of our blood, and gauge our health by how much of it shows up on a lab test—no matter how healthy we are by any other metric.

But those tides—once held in place by outdated medical dogma—are finally turning. My esteemed colleague, functional nutritionist Jonny Bowden, stands out as a voice of both clarity and reason as the antiquated "low-fat" paradigm collapses and a new era of health arises.

In the time since this book's first publication in 2004, much has changed—and much has stayed the same. Mainstream medicine continues to hold fat and cholesterol as the main players in heart disease. Drug companies continue to fund studies to justify the use of statins for greater and greater portions of the population. The medical "authorities" continue to pontificate about the dangers of fat, particularly saturated fat. Why? Because it's believed to raise "bad" cholesterol.

But what if cholesterol doesn't cause heart disease, after all? Then the dietary guidelines of the last 5 decades crumbles like a house of cards. Meanwhile, doctors, however well intentioned, continue to unwittingly push dietary guidance more likely to prevent wellness than to cultivate it.

But the situation is far from grim. Outside the walls of the medical system, there is an awakening that is almost palpable. Patients are becoming more empowered—and better informed—than ever before. And, importantly, more curious. The democratization of health information is upon us and Dr. Jonny Bowden is leading the charge. Most people don't pick up a book on low-carb eating just for the fun of it (unless you're a super nerd like me), and chances are you found these pages because they hold some personal relevance. Maybe you were told your cholesterol is too high and want to know what to do next. Maybe you have not been able to lose weight on low-fat or low-calorie diets, no matter what you do. (You'll find in this book that you're not alone, and that it's not your fault!) Maybe you've watched a loved one try to navigate the weight-loss labyrinth from the inside and, after seeing what they've gone through, want to avoid the same fate.

No matter how you have ended up here, your curiosity will be rewarded: what you're about to read can change your life, and maybe even save it.

As a functional medicine practitioner who consults people around the world, I've too often seen the harm that comes from focusing on only one small aspect of health, like, for example "fat." Fear of fat and cholesterol has driven otherwise healthy individuals to cut back on fat, remove nutritious foods from their diet, and to pop statins to help move numbers in the right direction. Viewing obesity as inevitable—"it's just in my genes"—puts it outside our control, and fills us with anxiety and stress—itself a burden on our health.

But I've also seen deep and profound healing occur through changes that are simple, sustainable, and available to anyone. As much as this book exposes tragic misinformation about diet, it also offers hope. Instead of waging war against fat, we should be looking at the many ways our modern diets and environment are misaligned with our genetics and in turn the pursuit of health. We're surrounded by inflammatory foods rich in processed sugar and omega-6 fats, pushed into lifestyles that rob us of rest and sleep, born into a food landscape designed to addict us, and immersed in a culture focused on managing symptoms rather than digging for roots. *Living Low Carb* brilliantly walks us through all of these health traps and more, exposing their contribution to heart disease and teaching readers how to elevate their health from the inside out.

Of course, those seeking to understand why diets high in processed carbohydrates have to overcome more than just misinformation: they may also find themselves alienated from the conversation because of complex terminology and medical concepts.

It's here that this book truly shines. *Living Low Carb* makes the various low-carb eating plans—and the reasons behind them—accessible to anyone hungry to learn. In a world where readers are too often told by experts to just "take our word for it," Bowden never asks for your blind faith: he presents scientific evidence transparently and simply, so that any reader—even those who struggle with scientific language, or feel intimidated by the learning curve needed to understand health and diet—can walk away knowing what to do and why.

In my experience, the vast majority of us wield plenty of power to take back control of our health, have agency over our wellness, by pursuing the positive lifestyle changes contained in this book. Instead of doing the same things we always have, repeatedly, but expecting different results, we can start to enact positive changes today. Knowledge is power. This is not about shaming anyone about things they could have done differently in the past. But there's much we can do in the here and now.

My friends, whatever journey has led you here, the author warmly welcomes you. The words in this book were written with love and compassion for anyone who wants to reclaim their health. It was written for you. Dr. Jonny has been considered one of the clearest and most accessible writers on health for over two decades earning accolades (and achieving best-seller status) for his clear and entertaining way of making complex topics simple and accessible. Guided by the latest exciting research and gracious in its user-friendly language, this book takes power away from an opaque medical system and puts it back where it belongs: in your own hands.

—Dr. Will Cole
Leading functional medicine expert,
international best-selling author of
Ketotarian and *The Inflammation Spectrum*

Foreword

There are three things in life that induce powerful visceral responses—religion, politics, and nutrition. Each is based on assumptions, and the adherents of each want to believe in their hearts that they are right; and of course they refuse to be confused by the facts. In the world of nutrition, nothing has generated as much heartburn as lower-carbohydrate diets. To the nutrition establishment, they are the equivalent of devil worship. To the medical establishment, they will cause massive increases in chronic disease and death. But to the millions of people who have used them, they seem to work. Obviously, there appears to be a disconnect between reality and fantasy. Are lower-carbohydrate diets actually safe? And what really is a lower-carbohydrate diet? Is a lower-carbohydrate diet the same as a high-fat or high-protein diet? Are there any magical supplements that can make you lose excess body fat? Into this quagmire of controversy steps Jonny Bowden.

I first met Jonny nearly 13 years ago. I had just written my first book, *The Zone*, and I was speaking about it in New York City. At the time, Jonny was a very well-recognized nutritionist working with a wide variety of clients ranging from those seeking weight loss to fitness enthusiasts. Like any typical New Yorker, he was skeptical of anything new, especially when it concerned diets. His skepticism was on especially high alert since my book not only recommended lower-carbohydrate diets for patients with diabetes and heart disease, but also for world-class athletes. After all, he had been training athletes for years using high-carbohydrate diets, and here was some pointy-head scientist telling him that all of his nutritional advice for athletes was wrong. Needless to say, he was ready to rake me over the coals. That is, until he heard my lecture. For the first time, he was introduced to the nuances of hormonal control theory using food as a drug. Although there was a lot of endocrinology (the science of hormones) being thrown around in the lecture, there were enough key points that Jonny had to take notice. After the lecture, he asked if we could talk. And for the next 2 hours, I went into more detail (probably more than he ever wanted to know) on the intricate dance of hormones that are controlled by the diet. Jonny then asked me, "If you are right about this, then everyone in nutrition is probably wrong." My reply was "Yes."

While Jonny was intrigued, he still remained skeptical. Jonny was also trained as an academic with a background in psychology and statistics, which guaranteed that any references I gave him on lower-carbohydrate diets (there wasn't much) as well as the science behind them (of which there was a lot) would be read and analyzed to the nth degree. As a result, he has not only become exceptionally knowledgeable about the nutritional science behind lower-carbohydrate diets, but he has also become my friend.

It's been many years since that first meeting with Jonny. The science dealing with the molecular biology of obesity has become more complex, but the basic concept remains: if you lower the carbohydrate content of the diet, you get better weight loss and better health. The trick is doing it for a lifetime.

I have always considered Jonny to be one of the better science writers I have ever met. That's why this book is so important for the general public. He lays out the history of lower-carbohydrate diets, explains in clear and concise language the underlying hormonal principles of such diets, and addresses the common misunderstandings of such diets, all in an entertaining and lively style.

As Jonny correctly points out, there is no one correct diet for everyone, since we are all genetically different. However, the hormonal principles are invariant for choosing an appropriate diet for your genetics. Once you understand the hormonal rules that govern lower-carbohydrate diets, you are in a position to become the master of your future. This book should be considered the starting point of that journey.

—Barry Sears, PhD
Author of *The Zone*
March 2009

═ Preface ═
to the Revised Edition

When this book first came out, low-carb living was a novelty. (In fact, the original title of this book back in 2004 was *Living the Low-Carb Life!*) Now "keto-" is the new buzzword, and "paleo"-friendly items are cropping up on restaurant menus all over the country. I'm even seeing magazines devoted to ketogenic and paleo diets on the racks at supermarkets: you don't get much more mainstream than that.

Though things have definitely changed, not everyone is on board with a lower-carb way of life. Some people might be reading this book to find out what all the shouting is about. Some may be dyed-in-the-wool low-carb converts and are reading this book to get new ideas and stay up on the latest trends. Some folks may be somewhere in between.

I want this edition of *Living Low Carb* to serve as a living, breathing encyclopedia of what's going on in low-carb eating. I want high school students to use this book as a resource for writing papers on the history of a diet, and I want doctors to use it as a place to learn about the copious amount of research that's been favorable to low-carb approaches. (Two of the greatest letters I ever received were from a formerly anti-low-carb medical doctor who said I changed his practice, and from a scholarship-winning high school student who said my book inspired him to pursue a career in health.)

About thirty years ago, James and Phyllis Balch published a book called *Prescription for Nutritional Healing.* It went through at least five editions and is still available to this day. The book was continually updated throughout the years, and for a long time was considered a must-have book for the library of any health professional. I'd like *Living Low Carb* to have the same fate. I wanted to put as much information about controlled-carb eating as I could get into 100,000 or so words, and I want (and continue to want) to update it with any new information that's relevant for your diet and your health.

Getting sugar and processed carbs out of the diet has made an incalculable difference in many people's lives. I know, because I hear from them every day and I hear about the difference a lower-carb way of life has made for them. And I know from experience. My weight has stayed within a five-pound range for the better part of twenty years, I have no major health issues, my energy continues to be off the charts, and I just turned seventy-two.

I hope this book can, in some small way, help *you* to experience the low-carb difference.

Enjoy the journey.

Jonny Bowden
Los Angeles, 2019

Preface

to the First Edition

The high-carbohydrate, low-fat diet has been the longest uncontrolled nutritional experiment in history.

The results have not been good.

Perhaps you've noticed.

Perhaps you have been one of its victims. You're unable to lose weight—or, if you have lost, it certainly hasn't been easy. You found yourself constantly fighting cravings, you were hungry a lot of the time, and you suffered with feelings of deprivation. You felt fatigued, like you were running on empty, and you were still always battling the bulge, mostly unsuccessfully.

Maybe, like a lot of low-fat, high-carbohydrate dieters, you've noticed that your hair is dry, your nails brittle, your energy low, and your vitality sapped. And guess what? For all that, the weight *still* doesn't come off—or, if it does, it comes back on with a vengeance and you're right back where you started, except this time you feel even more discouraged.

Or maybe you're lucky enough to have never been on this delightful seesaw that I'm describing. Maybe you're just curious about all the fuss that's being made over low-carb diets and you want to learn more about how they work. Maybe you're thinking that you could stand to knock off a few pounds and are interested in low-carb dieting but don't know where to start. Or maybe you're already convinced that low-carb diets are for you but are concerned about some of the health implications that well-meaning people have warned you about.

Well, you've come to the right place.

Living Low Carb will help you understand three things:

1. What low-carb diets actually do to and for your body, and how they do it

2. Why some programs work for some people (and don't for others)

3. How you can adapt what you discover in this book to your own lifestyle

While I'd love to think that everyone who reads this book will devour it from cover to cover for its scintillating content and wealth of information, realistically I know that that's not going to happen. So I have designed *Living Low Carb* to be used like the I Ching: open it anywhere, and it will—hopefully—give you information you want.

I imagine that some of you may already be sold on the concept of a low-carb diet but are (understandably) confused about the distinctions between, say, "paleo" and "keto." You guys should go straight for chapter 9, find the plan or plans you are interested in, and dive right in. You may find that reading further will spark some questions, which you're likely to get answered in chapter 10, "Frequently Asked Questions." Maybe, as you dig deeper into the book, you'll find yourself wanting to know more about the hormonal mechanisms in the body that drive weight gain and weight loss; you will find those issues addressed in chapter 3, "Why Low-Carb Diets Work," as well as chapter 4, "The Major Culprits in a High-Carb Diet: Wheat and Fructose."

Some of you may have already been on one of the plans discussed in chapter 9 but want more in-depth information about the questions, concerns, and controversies you have been hearing about—for example, cholesterol or ketosis or bone loss or kidney problems. You might head straight for chapter 6, "The Biggest Myths About Low-Carb Diets." When you get those concerns addressed, you may want to go back to chapters 3 and 4 to read more about the science behind low-carb eating and how it actually does its good work in the body.

The permutations are endless.

I also expect that there will be some dyed-in-the-wool low-carbers who have already experienced myriad health benefits, including weight loss, and simply want some tips for staying motivated, not getting bored, finding new things to eat, or breaking plateaus. All that information will be found in chapter 10, "Frequently Asked Questions."

Wherever you start in this book, and wherever you wind up in your dietary journey, remember one thing, particularly when you read mainstream reporting on low-carb diets: Low-carb is not and never was a fad diet. It follows the way we've eaten for most of the time that humans have been on the planet. The agricultural experiment of the last ten to eleven thousand years is much more of a "fad" than low-carb is. The processed-food revolution, which is only about a hundred years old, is the true "fad" diet.

Low-carb diets do not work for everyone. No dietary plan does. But there are dietary options discussed here that have helped many thousands of people who, for some reason, did not "vibe" with the conventional dietary advice we've endured for the past forty years or so and have gotten heavier, sicker, more tired, and more depressed on standard high-carb, low-fat pro-cessed food products. Those people—and thousands more like them—are looking for solutions. Many people have found solutions in the programs you're about to read about. I hope you are one of them.

Enjoy!

CHAPTER 1

Low-Carb Redux: The Updated Truth About Low-Carbohydrate Diets

"Low-carb diets are dangerous!" "All that meat can't possibly be good for you!"

"What about the China Study?" "You can't cut out an entire food group!"

"You need carbs for energy!" "I tried that Atkins® diet once and it didn't work!"

"You lose weight on low-carb but then you gain it all back!"
"Isn't low-carb bad for the heart?"

Sound familiar?

Low-carb eating continues to be one of the most misunderstood dietary strategies on the planet. Despite the fact that some form of low-carb dieting has been around since 1850, despite the enormous popularity of the Atkins diet, and despite mounting research implicating sugar and high-carb foods as instrumental catalysts to just about every major disease, the myths about low-carb diets simply behave like a Buddy Holly lyric and "won't fade away."

Maybe it's time to take a fresh look at low-carb diets and see if we can separate myth from reality.

Back in 2004, it seemed low-carb diets were at the top of the popularity charts. The Atkins diet—long a "fan favorite" but widely panned as "dangerous" by the medical establishment—had just been shown to produce more weight loss than either a low-fat diet or a Mediterranean diet in two studies published in the prestigious *Annals of Internal Medicine*.[1] Several other studies published around the same time confirmed these results and went even further, showing that the weight loss produced by low-carb dieting was not accompanied by any increase in the risk for heart disease. Quite the contrary—many of the studies showed improvements in triglycerides (fats found in the blood and in the tissues), no significant change in cholesterol, improved body composition, and significant improvements in risk factors for diabetes.

Low-carb was on a roll. Programs like *Protein Power, the Zone Diet®*, and *the South Beach Diet®* were at the top of the diet-book charts, Atkins was back in fashion, low-carb groceries were springing up, and even mainstream supermarkets began featuring low-carb sections (right along with their low-sodium and low-fat departments).

And then . . . it fizzled.

Or at least low-carb's status as a *media darling* fizzled. Low-carb continues to be used successfully as both a weight-loss strategy and as a dietary plan for overall health by millions of people and in dozens of clinics and university programs around the country.[2]

The media had moved on to the latest bright and shiny object in the ever-changing diet-book landscape, but low-carb diets wouldn't go away, even if diet-book authors stayed away from the low-carb label. And why would it go away? It's effective, it's safe, and it has enormous health benefits that are obscured or played down by hopelessly out-of-date guidelines. Make no mistake—low-carb is alive and well, and, if you've been one of the folks who dismissed it, let's fast-forward to today.

Low-carb is no longer a fringe movement. Even the American Academy of Nutrition and Dietetics (formerly the American Dietetic Association) is slowly changing its opinion. (A position paper published in 2016[3] stated that "*there's an emerging body of evidence showing the benefits and safety of carbohydrate restriction in people with diabetes*," which, for an organization that traditionally saw low-carb diets as a dangerous fad, can be considered progress.) Meanwhile, dozens of everyday grocery products now proudly slap "keto" on their labels. (We'll get into that later on in the book.)

Outside the world of commercial food products, there is serious ongoing research being conducted on the keto diet by the Navy in conjunction with the University of Tampa. Keto diets are commonplace in hospitals across America due to their demonstrable effect on childhood epilepsy.

But it was not always so.

For years, low-carb suffered from bad publicity. Atkins—a superb nutritionist and very smart guy—couldn't shake the stigma of having "recommended" eating pork rinds (What he *actually* said was that pork rinds were probably better for you than sugar! And he was right.) People who didn't know any better also thought his diet forbade all carbohydrates, which it most certainly doesn't.

Then there was the ketosis confusion. Ketosis—a harmless metabolic state that the body goes into when carbohydrate intake is *very* low—became identified with low-carb diets largely because early editions of Atkins's books stressed ketosis as a desirable goal for the first stage of the Atkins diet (which limited carbs to 20 grams a day).

But not all low-carb diets put the body into ketosis. Unless one is specifically working to achieve nutritional ketosis, it may not happen, and for some people staying in ketosis is not easy. For many people, this matters a lot—for others, not so much.

The low-carb "movement" itself didn't help matters. Its supporters began to treat low-carb as something of a religion, becoming more focused on carb content than on the importance of good food. And many people forgot about the overarching, important message of controlled-carb eating—controlling blood sugar and eating whole foods—and instead replaced that message with a simple (and inaccurate) sound bite: *carbs are bad.*

This led to an explosion of junk-food products that had engineered out the carbs but were still junk food (echoes of the low-fat movement of the '80s and early '90s—remember SnackWell® cookies?). Junky low-carb processed foods now filled the shelves of the low-carb groceries and were also the reason those groceries are now out of business—they tasted terrible.

But that was then and this is now. A more twenty–first century controlled-carb approach requires more nuance.

First, we need some definitions. How exactly do we define low-carb, anyway?

What Exactly Is a Low-Carb Diet?

The American Academy of Nutrition and Dietetics designates "low-carbohydrate diets" as less than 130 grams a day (or 26% of calories from a 2,000-calorie diet). Though I hardly think this is "low," it seems to be a decent working definition, given that most Americans consume a whopping 300 grams of carbs a day! (Just for the record, carbohydrate consumption before the current obesity epidemic averaged 43% of daily calories, just about what is recommended by Dr. Sears in *The Zone.*)

Some low-carb diets for weight loss, such as the classic Atkins model, limit carbs to 20–30 grams a day, especially for the first couple of weeks, and then add them back gradually. It works very well for many people, as evidenced by the fact that the modern version of Atkins is still going strong. But many health professionals and weight-loss experts believe that you can get many of the benefits of controlled-carb eating while still consuming them.

Meanwhile, a copious amount of research supports the notion that even a *modest* reduction in carb intake is enough to stabilize blood sugar, reduce insulin, and, in the long run, facilitate weight loss. Gary Taubes, author of *Why We Get Fat* and three-time winner of the National Association of Science Writers' Science in Society Award, has postulated that mere calorie restriction can give you some of the benefits of carb reduction, even if you're not counting carbs specifically. Consider the math: let's say the average American (assuming that such a creature even exists in the first place) consumes about 3,600 calories per day.[4] Let's say that our mythical average American follows the conventional wisdom and 60% of his calories come from carbs. That means he's getting a whopping 2,160 calories a day from carbs (about 540 grams!).

Now let's say 60% of his diet still consists of carbs, but he consumes 1,800 calories instead of 3,600 per day. Just by decreasing calories, his carb intake has now dropped to 1,080 calories, or 270 grams of carbs, half the amount he was eating before, even though he has kept the proportions of carbs, protein, and fat the same. If Taubes is right about excess carbs being the real villain here—and I think he is—there's going to be a huge benefit just from decreasing your carbs by 50%. And all you've done, really, is to consciously change the amount of food you eat, not the proportions of carbs, fat, and protein.

Carb reduction seems to work for most people even if they don't think they're doing it—and even if, as in the example above, they are nowhere near "low-carb diet" territory. Merely *aiming* for a more Atkins- or keto-friendly eating plan is enough to bring at least *some* benefits—as we'll see now when we examine the famous A–Z diet study at Stanford.

The A–Z Diet Study: Atkins Wins, but the Good Part Was Left Out!

Back in March 2007, it seemed you couldn't swing a bat without seeing a headline proclaiming that the Atkins diet was finally vindicated. "Atkins beats Zone, Ornish, and U.S. diet advice," proclaimed CNN. "Atkins Diet Tops Others in Study," said the Washington Post.

Good news for low-carb diets—but, as usual, the headlines did not tell the whole story.

First, some background. Researchers at Stanford University[5] took 311 premenopausal women, all of them overweight or obese, and assigned them to four diet groups: Atkins, Ornish, the Zone, and the LEARN plan, a conventional eating program based on U.S. dietary guidelines. "We wanted a range of diets, from high-carbohydrate to low," explained lead researcher Christopher Gardner, PhD.[6] The Atkins® diet is famously low in carbohydrates (and can be high in either fat or protein, or both), the Ornish diet is extremely low in fat (about 10% of intake), and the Zone is right in the middle (technically 40% of the diet comes from carbs and 30% each from protein and fat). The LEARN diet is based on conventional recommendations of about 55–65% carbs and less than 10% saturated fat.

The researchers were interested primarily in weight loss, though other measures were taken as well (more on that in a moment). "In the weight-loss department, there was a modest advantage for the Atkins group," Dr. Gardner told me. Those in the Atkins group lost the most amount of weight (10 pounds on average).

But there were some problems. For one thing, the women in the study were far from meticulous about following the dietary regimen to which they were assigned. While the women in the Atkins group were aiming for between 20–50 grams of carbohydrate a day, by the end of the study they were eating well over 125 grams. The Ornish group, aiming for 10% fat, was eating almost 30%. Zone dieters shooting for 30% protein wound up eating 20%, and even the women attempting to follow the conventional LEARN diet had reduced their carbs to just over 47%. Critics—including the designers of the diets that bore their names—complained loudly that the study results were not valid because the diet strategies under investigation had not been followed to the letter.

Actually, this is the good part.

In real life, people rarely follow diets exactly as they're laid out in the diet books. So it's hardly a surprise that the folks in the Atkins group didn't achieve the target of 20–50 grams of carbs a day. What's worth noting—and what the media largely missed—is that merely *attempting* to reduce carbs resulted in vast improvements in weight and overall health. The folks in the study may have been aiming for 20–50 grams, but the 125 grams they wound up consuming was still well within the definition of low-carb, represented a huge reduction from their baseline consumption, and wound up giving them terrific results.

"So what we're seeing here in terms of deviation from the exact principles of each diet is a very real-world scenario," said Dr. Gardner. "It's what happens when even motivated people follow diet books. We think that's extremely relevant."

He has a great point. While the women may not have followed the diets to the letter, they *did* make changes in some important areas according to the principles of the respective plans. For example, the Atkins women had started the program consuming about 215 grams of carbohydrate a day (about 45% of their diet). By the end of the 12 months, they were down to about 34%. That's a big deal. At the end of the day they were eating a higher percentage of carbs than they were aiming for, sure, but they had *still* managed to reduce their carb intake substantially compared to where they started out. They may not have achieved perfection, but they did achieve results, and those results shouldn't be overlooked simply because the women didn't follow the diets perfectly. After all, who can?

It's worth mentioning that the women in the Atkins group also improved some of their risk factors. The HDL ("good") cholesterol at 12 months was *significantly* higher for the Atkins group than for the group on the low-fat Ornish diet, and triglycerides for the Atkins group went down by 29%, more than twice the percentage of any other group. The decrease in average blood pressure for the Atkins group was significantly greater than any other. The effect on LDL ("bad") cholesterol, the type that many health professionals warned would worsen on the Atkins diet, was the same among all of the diet groups after 12 months. These are important findings, particularly in view of the negative press low-carbohydrate diets have gotten for their supposed bad effects on cardiovascular health. In this study, at least in the short term, the opposite appeared to be the case.

So what's the takeaway? "I think one advantage that the Atkins diet had was the simplicity of the message," Dr. Gardner told me. "A lot of people say that the main Atkins message is to eat all the steak and brie that you want, but that's not it. The main message is this: you can't have any refined sugar. None. No soda, no white bread, no high-fructose corn syrup. It's simple and direct and easy to understand and I think it may turn out to be one of the most important messages of all."

Matching the Diet to the Person

Further analysis of the data from the A–Z diet study revealed something even more important. While the low-carb approach worked well for everyone, it worked *spectacularly* well for a certain subgroup in the population—the folks with *insulin resistance*. Folks with insulin resistance don't process carbs very well. When people with insulin resistance eat carbs—particularly grains, rice, cereal, bread, and sugar—their blood sugar goes up way more than it should; in response to that increased blood sugar, their pancreas secretes more insulin than is healthy. Now they have both elevated blood sugar and elevated insulin—which is a sign of pre-diabetes—and they have a fiendishly difficult time losing weight.

When Gardner analyzed the effects of the Atkins diet on this subgroup of people, he found that the results were even more impressive than they were in the population as a whole (more weight loss and even better blood tests). This finding gives credence to the notion that individual differences—genetic, enzymatic, hormonal, metabolic—may account for why some people do spectacularly well on certain diets and others fail miserably on the same routine.

The idea that low-carb diets are even more effective for those with metabolic conditions like insulin resistance was given another boost by a study involving 73 obese young adults aged 18–35. Half of the subjects were given a low-glycemic diet similar to the Zone (in this case, 40% carbs, 35% fat, 25% protein), and half were given a standard low-fat diet (55% carbs, 20% fat). Among those subjects whose bodies released the "normal" amount of insulin in response to food, the diets had an equally beneficial effect; but in those who had high levels of insulin secretion to begin with (insulin resistance), the low-carb diet was much the better performer, resulting in greater weight loss and reduction in body-fat percentage.[7] The researchers speculate that many of these diet studies produce different results for one simple reason: *individual differences*. Those with "high" insulin secretion do much better on low-carb diets than on low-fat ones, a finding exactly in accordance with what Gardner found in the A–Z diet study.

The takeaway: low-carb doesn't have to be extreme to be effective, a point that's been demonstrated numerous times in numerous studies.

As researcher Barbara Gower, PhD, once put it, "Over the long run, a *sustained modest reduction in carbohydrate intake* may help to reduce [calorie consumption] and facilitate weight loss."[8]

Will Low-Carb Diets Harm Your Health?

There isn't too much controversy anymore about the effectiveness of controlled-carbohydrate eating for weight loss, especially in the short term. The area of controversy concerns the question "At what cost?" Conventional wisdom—which is turning out to be far from wise on this subject—has held (at least until very recently) that only low-fat diets are effective for lowering the risk of heart disease. Even today, many conventional doctors recommend low-fat diets for diabetes, though emerging science suggests that this is precisely the wrong strategy.

Let's look at the evidence. An examination of data from the Nurses' Health Study involving over 85,000 women found that those consuming diets with the highest glycemic load (sugar, white rice, potatoes, low-fiber bread, and processed carbs) had a significantly higher risk of diabetes—more than *twice* the risk—than those consuming low-glycemic diets (fat, protein, vegetables, beans, fruits). Moreover, the women consuming diets rich in vegetable protein and fat had a modest *reduction* in the risk of diabetes.[9]

In a separate analysis, it was found that women in the study eating a low-carb diet with *higher* intake of animal fat and protein had a 6% *reduced* risk of cardiovascular disease! Considering that conventional wisdom would predict that the women eating the most animal fat and protein and the least carbs would have a vastly *higher* risk of heart disease, these results are pretty astonishing. When the researchers looked at women consuming a low-carb diet with higher rates of vegetable protein and fat, the reduction in risk went even higher, to a whopping 30%.[10]

Low-glycemic (low-carb) diets were also found to reduce the number of acne lesions.[11] They've been found to benefit women with polycystic ovary syndrome.[12] Low-carb diets were found to raise HDL ("good" cholesterol) by 10%.[13] And at least two different studies have shown that low-glycemic diets lower the risk for age-related macular degeneration.[14]

Add fiber to a low-carb diet, and your results are even better. In one study, researchers put 30 overweight or obese males on a carb-restricted diet. Half the subjects also got a soluble fiber supplement as well.

The carb-restricted diet reduced body weight, percentage of body fat, systolic blood pressure, triglycerides, and waist circumference—all risk factors for heart disease. Those consuming the fiber supplement along with their low-carb diet had a 14% reduction in LDL ("bad" cholesterol) as well as all the aforementioned benefits.[15]

In more recent years, studies have shown that even extremely low-carbohydrate, ketogenic diets don't promote heart disease in any way—in fact, quite the opposite. For more information on how keto diets impact the risk factors for heart disease (spoiler alert: they cause improvements across the board!), see page 240.

What About Deprivation?

Low-carb diets are always trashed in the mainstream media for being "restrictive" and leading to feelings of "deprivation," but the research—not to mention the daily experience of countless people—indicates the exact opposite. In one study involving 28 premenopausal overweight women, sticking to a low-carb/high-protein diet not only reduced these folks' body weight more than a high-carb/low-fat diet, it also reduced hunger.[16] The self-ratings of hunger for those on the low-carb diet went down over the course of the study, whereas hunger self-ratings remained essentially unchanged among the women eating high-carb/low-fat. It's always easier to stay on an eating plan if you're not starving, so this is an important consideration!

A separate study found that men and women put on a low-carb diet wound up consuming about ⅓ fewer calories without any special instructions to do so. In fact, these folks were told to limit their carbohydrates to a very low 21 grams per day (about the amount in the rigorous first stage of the Atkins diet), but were allowed to eat as much protein and fat as they wanted—they were even allowed limited amounts of cheese and cream cheese. Their insulin sensitivity improved by an incredible 75%, they lost weight, and they weren't hungry. Now there's a dietary trifecta![17]

What About Vegans?

Up until recently, conventional wisdom held that it's next to impossible to do a low-carb diet if you're a vegetarian or vegan. Once again, conventional wisdom turns out to be wrong, at least according to a study in the prestigious *Archives of Internal Medicine*, which investigated a diet that has since become known as "Eco-Atkins."[18]

The researchers wanted to see if they could design a low-carbohydrate diet that retained the proven weight-loss benefits of standard low-carb plans like Atkins but at the same time helped people improve their cholesterol. Remember that there is far from universal agreement in the medical profession that managing cholesterol is the most important thing to do to protect your heart. Nonetheless, lowering cholesterol was a stated goal of the researchers and remains a goal for the majority of conventionally trained doctors in this country. If you're interested in the other side of the cholesterol argument, please check out the book I co-wrote with cardiologist Stephen Sinatra, MD, *The Great Cholesterol Myth* (Fair Winds Press, 2012).

The researchers put one group of participants on a vegan diet that met their definition of low-carb and high-protein. The diet contained not a single animal product or by-product, including eggs.

Protein (31% of total calories) came mainly from gluten, soy, and nuts, with typical foods being soy burgers, veggie bacon, and breakfast links. Most of the fat (43% of total calories) came from nuts, vegetable oils, soy products, and avocado. The rest of the calories on this vegan low-carb diet were carbohydrates (26% of total calories), mostly from fruits and vegetables and some cereals; common starchy items like bread, rice, potatoes, and baked goods were eliminated.

The researchers tested the Eco-Atkins diet against a standard low-fat lacto-vegetarian diet, which contained 58% of calories from carbs, 16% from protein, and 25% from fat, and was designed to have both low saturated fat and low cholesterol; most of the protein on the "standard" diet came from low-fat or skim milk dairy products and egg whites. Both diets were calorie-reduced (60% of estimated caloric requirement, with allowance for exercise). All subjects in both groups were overweight at the start of the study, which lasted one month.

Both groups lost weight—not surprising, given the reduction in calories on both diets. And there were no significant differences between the two groups in weight loss—both groups lost about 4 kg (8.8 pounds), roughly the same amount of weight as would be expected on a more traditional low-carbohydrate Atkins diet. But there were some important differences between the two groups when it came to cholesterol.

The Eco-Atkins group saw their LDL (the so-called "bad" cholesterol) drop *significantly* more than the group on the low-fat vegetarian diet. As an added benefit, ApoB—a component of LDL that is related to heart disease—fell significantly more for the low-carb dieters than it did for the high-carbers.

Now you might easily argue that the Eco-Atkins diet—with its 130 grams of carbs a day—is very far from what we traditionally think of as a low-carb diet. And you might also argue that lowering cholesterol might not be nearly as important as the conventional medical establishment thinks it is (a position strongly taken by myself and an ever-growing field of experts). But, that said, this is a really valuable piece of research, and here's why:

It's been a long, uphill, and sometimes discouraging battle to get the conventional medical community to accept low-carb in any form. Fixated on cholesterol, they worry that conventional low-carb diets don't lower cholesterol (ignoring the fact that these same diets have been shown to not only produce weight loss, but also lower triglycerides and insulin resistance). And—not without some justification—many conventional docs continue to be worried about overconsumption of meat. (We'll talk much more about the meat controversy in the section on the Carnivore Diet, page 264.) So here's a legitimate study in one of the most prestigious and conservative journals that demonstrates that low-carb can be adapted to even the rigorous vegan eating pattern, producing not only the expected weight loss, lowered insulin resistance, and lowered triglycerides, but lowered cholesterol *as well*. This study convincingly showed that a low-carb diet performed *better* than the low-fat vegetarian diets so many of these docs seem to adore! The results went a long way toward reassuring conventional docs that low-carb is a viable alternative to standard recommendations of low-fat/high-carb diets, and can even "outperform" such diets on a number of variables. You can even find instructions on how to do a keto diet as a vegan! (Just search "keto vegan" online!)

Summing Up

Remember: as hard as it is to believe, your body has no physiological require-ment for carbohydrates—astonishing, but 100% true.[19] That's not to say you shouldn't eat carbs—you should!

But if you're looking to lose weight and improve your health, you've got to go for vegetables and fruits and beans, not for pasta, rice, bread, baked goods, cereal, and sugar-laden desserts.

Carbs from fruits and vegetables are loaded with vitamins, minerals, phytochemicals, fiber, and other good stuff that your body thrives on. And you can eat more vegetables and berries than you can imagine and still stay in a controlled carbohydrate range of under 100 or so grams of carbs a day! (For the record, I'd call the 130 grams of carbs used in the Eco-Atkins study a "relatively" low-carb diet, especially when compared to standard American fare. But it is by no means a *true* low-carb diet.)

We'll discuss how different dietary approaches, such as paleo and keto, handle carb restriction, and the role of carbs in non-low-carb diets, like the

Mediterranean Diet, in chapter 9. The point to take home here is that even a reasonably moderate reduction in starchy and processed carbohydrates can give you lots of benefits. And these benefits were not discovered yesterday. Researchers, scientists, doctors—and even patients—have known about them for a very long time.

CHAPTER 2

The History and Origins of Low-Carb Diets

I n the first few editions of this book, this chapter started by talking about the first actual low-carb diet book, which came out in the 1800's.

But I left out the cultural context in which low-carb diets arose.

You see, high-carb diets and processed foods *in general* have much deeper cultural, spiritual, political, and economic roots than you might imagine. Without an understanding of these forces, it's hard to understand why there was so much opposition to virtually every low-carb approach, opposition that is alive and well and endures up to the present day.

So let's take a short sojourn into the zeitgeist of the times so that we can understand the real roots of the current dietary orthodoxy—the almost fanatic opposition to everything low-carb which, in some corners of the dietary establishment, continues to this day. This opposition to low-carb eating runs deep with roots that date back more than 100 years and extend well beyond the field of nutrition.

Sex and the High-Carb Diet

Just as it's hard to talk honestly about the history of the United States without talking about slavery, it's hard to talk honestly about the dietary establishment and the roots of dietary orthodoxy without talking about sex.

To anyone born in the United States after 1970, what I'm about to say may seem unthinkable; but at the turn of the century—and for decades afterward—"self-abuse" was one of the "social issues" that evoked intense passion and profound division. According to many reformers of the time, masturbation was a gateway drug, leading to ill health for the self-abuser as well as the total breakdown of the social order.

This poster from 1890s eloquently expresses the prevailing attitude of the time toward "self abuse."

And it was the medical profession that led the crusade against "the heinous sin of self-pollution," with advocates like Dr. John Harvey Kellogg (1852–1943)—the inventor of corn flakes, a food specifically created as an anti-masturbatory aid—at the helm.

Kellogg was a devout follower of the Seventh-Day Adventist Church,

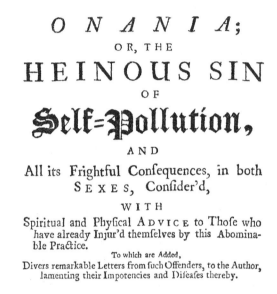

which strongly emphasized health and wellness and the belief that health was the foundation of a spiritual life. According to the Adventist text *Spirit of Prophecy* (written by a cofounder of the church, Ellen G. White), "A religious life can be more successfully gained and maintained if meat is discarded, for this diet stimulates into intense activities lustful propensities, and enfeebles the moral and spiritual nature."

In 1856, the entire Kellogg family moved to Battle Creek, Michigan, primarily so they could be close to the Church and to Ellen White. At the same time, the Whites were in need of a doctor to run their health programs, and John Harvey Kellogg perfectly fit the bill. For the Whites and Kellogg, the match was made in heaven, and the influence of that match on mainstream dietary thinking continues to this day, as we'll see throughout this book.

Keep in mind that both the Adventist Church led by Ellen White *and*

Kellogg—at his famous Battle Creek Sanatorium—believed in eliminating all stimulants and considered meat a prime example.

Kellogg was a great believer in sexual abstinence. The diet he recommended—and the one he fed patients at his sanatorium—was *specifically* designed to "reduce the sexual urges" of its adherents. He believed that the then-current rumors of "masturbation-related deaths" were true, and, along with many of his colleagues, believed that masturbation caused epilepsy, insanity, and even cancer of the womb.

Around 1880, Kellogg began his writing career and started churning out books that were little more than propaganda. In 1923, Kellogg published *The Proper Diet for Man,* which advocated "the diet chosen for us by our Creator." That diet was the strictly vegetarian diet that had been revealed to the young Ellen White so many years before.

Kellogg and White were aided and abetted in their campaign against meat (and sex) by the rise of the temperance movement in the 1860s, which, although it was focused on eliminating alcohol, was also against *all* stimulants, which, by their lights, included meat—an "undesirable" part of the diet.

The first Battle Creek Sanitarium dietitian, Lenna Frances Cooper (1875–1961) was the cofounder of the American Dietetics Association (now the American Academy of Nutrition and Dietetics) in August 1917, which ultimately advocated a vegetarian diet. The Seventh-Day Adventist Church established hundreds of hospitals, colleges, and secondary schools and tens of thousands of churches around the world, all promoting a vegetarian diet.

And remember, this was not for health reasons. No one had yet suggested that meat eating was related to cancer, or any other major disease. This was exclusively an attempt to remove sexually stimulating foods from the diet.

Please remember, this is not just ancient history. The legacy of John Kellogg and the Seventh-Day Adventist church influences nutritional policy to this day. The church owns twenty food industries worldwide, currently producing 2,475 products—all of which are meat and dairy substitutes, breakfast cereals, and soy products. Their food companies—such as Sanatarium Health and Wellbeing—are all tax-exempt, due to church ownership. One of their companies—Australian Health and Nutrition Association Limited—had, in 2012, an operating revenue of over 300 million dollars.[1] Gross annual sales for all of the Adventist-owned companies are hard to come by but are estimated to be in the billions.

In America, probably the most respected and cited nutritional researcher of our time—Walter Willett, MD, PhD, head of the nutrition department at the Harvard School of Public Health—has himself said: "From the beginning of the Adventist Health Studies, an important interaction has existed between the Department of Nutrition at Harvard School of Public Health and Loma Linda Adventist University."

Most people don't see the kind of behind-the-scenes influence that the anti-meat, anti-fat, pro-cereal forces exert. But from time to time a scandal erupts that exposes the influences of Big Food (and Big Pharma) on nutrition policy. (One such event happened when it was revealed that the sugar industry had paid important scientists, such as Mark Hegsted of Harvard, to write papers that would direct attention away from sugar as a cause of disease.[2] Hegsted went on to become the head of nutrition at the USDA, where he helped draft the early federal government dietary guidelines. And of course Big Sugar benefits greatly from the popularity of processed carbohydrate foods like cereals, which are virtually inedible without added sugar. It's also worth mentioning that sugar—along with wheat, corn, soy, and cotton—is one of the five biggest crops in American agriculture. And that the USDA—from its very inception in 1862 to the present time—has had the stated mandate of promoting America's agricultural products.[3] It's certainly not their goal to get Americans to eat *less* of the wheat, soy, and sugar that are the backbone of American agriculture.

Am I suggesting some secret conspiracy at work here? Absolutely not. I'm suggesting that a confluence of interests—a powerful, informal alliance among groups and industries with overlapping interests—Big Food, Big Pharma, and Big Agriculture—has had, and continues to have, an inordinate influence on nutritional policy and recommendations. And going publicly against those interests can do serious damage to the career of anyone who questions its collective dogma.

For example: In South Africa, a dietitian filed a complaint with the Health Professions Council of South Africa against Dr. Timothy Noakes for giving what she called "unconventional advice" to a breastfeeding mother on Twitter. (The "unconventional advice" in question was to eventually get the baby on a low-carb high-fat diet using what he described as "real foods"). Noakes is one of the most decorated, respected, and revered scientists in South Africa, but the HPCSA argued that Noakes was indeed giving unconventional and "unscientific" advice, and they brought charges against him which could have resulted in the loss of his medical license. The trial lasted over three years, with huge numbers of research studies being presented and two international witnesses testifying (Dr. Zoë Harcombe from London and Nina Tiecholz—the investigative journalist who published *The Big Fat Surprise*—from New York). Dr. Noakes won his trial after four years and was found not guilty of misconduct. He wrote a fascinating book, *Lore of Nutrition*, detailing the entire sordid episode and referencing hundreds of scientific studies that support the low-carb diets he recommended.

In the remote city of Launceston, Tasmania, a much-liked orthopedic surgeon named Dr. Gary Fettke was investigated and subsequently silenced by the Tasmanian Medical Board for merely recommending that his patients reduce sugar and include more healthy fat in their diets. (Again, the complaint was initiated by a mainstream dietitian, clearly with the support of the dietary and food establishment.) Dr. Fettke's wife—Bettina Fettke—started a website (isupportgary.com, #isupportgary) which is, in her words, dedicated to shining a light on "vested interests and medical evangelism." Her extraordinary research—along with that of the aforementioned Nina Tiecholz and Zoë Harcombe—has exposed many of the far-from-holy alliances that have influenced and shaped dietary policy in the Western world for over half a century. She writes: "*The legacy of the Temperance Movement, in an attempt to stop us from consuming alcohol and meat, created the processed food industry. Now the cereal industry and (the sugar industry) are dictating health policy and shaping dietary and health guidelines.*"[4]

And now, for those who are interested, here are the stories of some of the pioneers who "pushed back" throughout the years against the dietetic establishment.

The First Low Carb Diet Book

The first bona fide low-carb diet book came out in 1864, and it happened only because William Banting thought he was going deaf.

Banting was a prosperous London undertaker of sixty-six who was so overweight that he couldn't tie his own shoelaces. At 5 feet 5 inches in his stocking feet, he weighed in at 202 pounds and was so fat that he had to walk downstairs backward. On top of that, his eyesight was failing and he was having problems with his hearing. In August 1862, Banting took himself to an ear, nose, and throat surgeon named Dr. William Harvey, who examined him and promptly decided that Banting's problem wasn't deafness; it was obesity. His fat was pressing on his inner ear.

Here's what Banting was eating: "bread and milk for breakfast, *or* a pint of tea, with plenty of milk and sugar, and buttered toast; meat, beer, and much bread and pastry for dinner; more bread and milk at tea time; and a fruit tart *or* bread and milk for supper."

Harvey promptly put Banting on a diet, and by December 1862, Banting had lost 18 pounds. By August 1863, he was down to 156 pounds. In a little less than a year, he had dropped almost 50 pounds and 12½ inches from his waistline. Banting also reported feeling better than he had at any time in the previous 26 years. His sight and hearing were normal for his age, and his other bodily ailments had become "mere matters of history."

Here's what he ate on the new plan.

Breakfast (9 A.M.): 5 or 6 ounces of either beef, mutton, kidneys, broiled fish, bacon, or cold meat of any kind except pork or veal. A small biscuit or an ounce of dry toast. Large cup of tea or coffee without milk or sugar.

Dinner (2 P.M.): 5 or 6 ounces of fish, poultry, game, or meat, and any vegetable except potatoes, parsnips, beets, turnips, or carrots. An ounce of dry toast. Fruit. Two or three glasses of good claret, sherry, or Madeira (no champagne, port, or beer).

Tea (6 P.M.): 2 or 3 ounces of fruit. Toast and tea with no milk or sugar.

Supper (9 P.M.): 3 or 4 ounces of meat or fish as for dinner. A glass or two of claret or sherry.

Nightcap (if required): a tumbler of gin, whisky, or brandy with water but no sugar, or a glass or two of claret or sherry.

The man did like to drink.

Here's what he did *not* eat: milk, sugar, beer, potatoes, or pastry. And what he ate *way* less of: bread (3 ounces total, about a slice).

The calorie as a measurement was unknown at that time, but we know now that Banting was eating about 2,800 calories a day—not exactly a low-calorie diet. Banting may not have known much about the science and chemistry of food and weight, but he knew enough to observe that the *amount* of food he was eating didn't seem to be the determining factor in his weight loss. In Banting's words, "I can now confidently say that *quantity* of diet may be safely left to the natural appetite; and that it is the *quality* only which is essential to abate and cure corpulence."

In other words: it's *what* you eat, not how much, an idea that even then flew in the face of conventional wisdom. (It's worth noting that Banting was not completely right—as it turns out, it's *both* what you eat *and* how much. But he opened the door to the discussion that *quality* mattered as much as quantity, and that was a significant change from conventional thinking. Still is. Even as of this writing, there are "health authorities" all over America who continue to claim that calories in/calories out is all that matters, ignoring a couple of decades' worth of research into the hormonal effects of food.)

Banting became a man on a mission. Excited and inspired by his results on this high-calorie, low-carbohydrate diet—which was made up almost entirely of protein, fat, alcohol, and what was then called "roughage"—he published, at his own expense, the first commercial low-carb diet book, *Letter on Corpulence*.[5] (Interesting factoid: in many countries, such as South Africa, low-carb diets are known as "Banting diets," and there are still websites devoted to how to "do" Banting. Even the mainstream magazine *Good Housekeeping South Africa* has featured an article called "Banting for Beginners."[6]

Banting himself identified sugar as the main cause of his own obesity, and his physician, Dr. Harvey, promptly put both flour and sugar on the forbidden list.

It worked.

The book eventually went into 4 editions, with the first 3 selling 63,000 copies in England alone, and it was translated into French and German and sold heavily in those countries, as well as in the United States. The fourth edition included letters of testimony from at least 1,800 readers who had written to Banting to support his assertions and praise the diet.

Banting, by the way, kept the weight off and lived comfortably until the age of 81.

With Banting's book, the nascent debate—is it *what* you eat or *how much* you eat that makes you fat?—was born, and it continues, alive and kicking, to this day. But the controversy didn't gather its full steam until Wilbur Atwater figured out how to measure calories.

> *Once I did some reading, I realized that low-carb diets aren't brand new—they've been advocated by some forward-thinking scientists for more than a century.*
>
> *—Gary S.*

It's the Calories, Stupid! The Dominating Hypothesis in Weight Loss Is Born

Sometime between 1890 and 1900, an agricultural chemist named Wilbur O. Atwater got the bright idea that if you stuck some food in a mini-oven called a calorimeter and burned the food to ash, you could *measure* the amount of heat it produced. He called the unit of measurement a calorie (technically, the amount of heat it takes to raise the temperature of 1 gram of water from 14.5 to 15.5 degrees Celcius). He went to town. He constructed vast tables of the caloric content of various foods. (It's important to remember that calories are not actually found *in* food; they're a measure of how much heat or energy can be *produced* by food.) The idea that the human body behaves exactly like the chamber used in Atwater's experiments—that we all "burn" calories exactly the same way and our bodies behave like calorimeters—has been the dominating hypothesis in weight loss to this day.

And man, is it wrong. (More coming—stay tuned.)

Later, some enterprising scientists extended the calorie theory even further. They began to measure how much heat was produced (read: how many calories were "burned") in the course of daily activities, from resting to vigorous exercise, from sleeping to digesting food to running marathons.

It was now possible to form an equation: calories in versus calories out. The guiding concept of weight management was officially born.

That theory is called the *energy balance theory*, and it goes something like this: if you take in more calories than you burn up, you'll gain weight. If you burn up more calories than you take in, you'll lose weight. It doesn't matter where those calories come from. It's as simple as balancing a checkbook: spend more than you make, and you're calorically in the red (and dipping into your fat stores to make up the difference); make more than you spend, and you're in the black (and buying bigger jeans).

It was the first law of thermodynamics in action. What goes in must either come out in some other form (like heat) or stay in (in the form of fat or muscle). What it *can't* do is simply disappear.

Yet Banting, unscientific though he was, had made an interesting observation, which was that *what* he ate made more of a difference to his fat cells than *how much* he ate. This notion was heresy to the calorie theorists who believed, to paraphrase Gertrude Stein, that a calorie is a calorie is a calorie. It wasn't until much later that the idea surfaced that calories from certain kinds of food (or combinations of food) might have a greater tendency to be stored in the body than others, or that people might vary widely in their metabolic ability to "burn" calories as opposed to "saving" them, or that the type of food eaten might actually trigger bodily responses that say "stay" or "go."

Meanwhile, calorie counting had taken off with a vengeance. In 1917 (the same year, coincidentally, in which the ultraconservative American Dietetic Association was founded), an LA physician named Dr. Lulu Hunt Peters published what had to be the first calorie-counting book ever, *Diet and Health, with Key to the Calories*. She sold 2 million books, making it the first best-selling diet book in America. And here's the thing: by making calorie-counting equivalent to weight control, she also injected her own view of morality into the equation. People who couldn't control their calories (and therefore their weight) just lacked self-discipline. We can thank Dr. Peters for popularizing the concept that being overweight is a sign of moral weakness. And the idea that people are fat simply because they lack self-control is still very much alive and well today—witness, for example, the last decade of the Dr. Phil McGraw Show.[7]

In fact, calories in/calories out remains the dominant view of most mainstream weight-loss experts to this day, and it is even embraced to a degree by some of the gurus of the low-carb movement, albeit not nearly to the same extent as the mainstreamers, who have made it a virtual religion. All of the low-carb theorists have to be seen against the backdrop of this calorie-counting orthodoxy. But throughout the twentieth century and into the twenty-first, observations have indeed been made—and experiments performed—that have cast huge doubts on whether the calories in/calories out theory was the whole story or even the most important part of the story. No one claims it is not *part* of the story—the argument is whether or not it is the *whole* story. Answer: It's not.

And let's be clear about something else. We in the low-carb movement made a mistake with our collective response to the "calories are king" thinking. You see, there was a huge backlash in the early days of the low-carb movement, a backlash against the rigid (and incorrect) belief that calories are the only thing that matters when it comes to weight loss. We were so eager to convince people that the *composition* of the food we ate—not just its calorie count—was what was driving weight gain, that we may have gone too far and implied that calories don't count at all.

That was wrong. Calories *do* count—they're just very far from the whole picture, and ignoring the hormonal effect of food is what got us into this mess in the first place. We'll explore this distinction—and the whole notion of food having a hormonal effect—throughout this book.

Eat and Grow Thin: Low-Carbing Reappears on the Scene

In 1914, Vance Thompson, a nonscientist and the husband of a famous actress of the day, published a book called *Eat and Grow Thin*,[8] which touted the virtues of a low-carb diet. It suggested that corpulence was caused by eating the wrong *kinds* of food, not merely the wrong amounts, and singled out "starches, sugars, and oils" as particular culprits—pretty much what you'd expect from a guy whose most famous saying was "To the scientist there is nothing so tragic on earth as the sight of a fat man eating a potato." His list of forbidden foods included the fattiest meats (like bacon); bread, biscuits, crackers, macaroni, and anything else made from the flour of wheat, corn, rye, barley, or oats, which included all breakfast foods and cereals; rice; potatoes, corn, dried beans, and lentils; milk, cream, butter, and cheese; oils and grease of any kind; pies, cakes, puddings, pastries, custards, ice cream, sodas, candies, bonbons, and sweets; and wines, beers, ales, and spirits.

One can only imagine how many times he was asked the question we hear so often today: so, *what's left to eat?*

As it turns out, a lot. According to Thompson, the only things that had really been taken away were sugar, starch, oil, and alcohol. The rest of his book consisted of menus that included:

- All kinds of meat (except pig in any form)
- All kinds of game
- All kinds of seafood—fish, lobsters, oysters, etc.
- All kinds of fruit (except bananas and grapes)
- All kinds of salad
- Virtually all vegetables

The low-carb gurus of today would have loved this, except they would have added some good fat to the mix.

The book also contained this little caveat: "Never, under any circumstances—even when you have reduced to the desired weight and have, to some degree, discontinued the diet—*eat potatoes, rice, white bread, macaroni, or sweets.*"

Calories were never once mentioned in Thompson's book, which went through 113 printings by 1931 and was still in circulation when a little problem arose at the DuPont company.

The Problem at the DuPont Company: The Work of Alfred Pennington, MD

DuPont executives were getting fat.

Really fat. No kidding.

Shortly after World War I, the medical department of E.I. DuPont, a large American chemical firm, became concerned about the growing obesity problem among the staff. The company hired Dr. Alfred Pennington and entrusted him with the job of finding out why the traditional low-calorie diets of the time were bombing when it came to losing weight. Pennington applied his considerable brain power to an analysis of the scientific literature and came to the conclusion that our old friend—the formerly fat undertaker William Banting—was right all along: obesity was due not to overeating, but instead to the body's inability to use carbohydrates for anything other than making fat.

Pennington put the DuPont executives on a high-fat, high-protein, low-carbohydrate, *unrestricted-calorie* diet. He limited their carb intake to 60 grams a day, allowed them at least 24 ounces of meat and fat (more if they wanted it), and restricted them to one portion a day of any one of the following: potatoes, rice, grapefruit, grapes, melon, bananas, pears, raspberries, or blueberries.

Pennington published a number of articles in prestigious journals such as *The New England Journal of Medicine*,[9] but he summed up his results with the fat executives best in an interview he gave to *Holiday Magazine*. I've added the italics for emphasis.

Of the twenty men and women taking part in the test, all lost weight on a diet in which the total calorie intake was unrestricted. The basic diet totaled about 3,000 calories per day, *but meat and fat in any desired amount were allowed those who wanted to eat still more.* The dieters reported that they felt well, enjoyed their meals and *were never hungry between meals.* Many said they felt more energetic than usual; none complained of fatigue. Those who had high blood pressure to begin with [no longer did]. The[se] twenty obese individuals lost an average of twenty-two pounds each, in an average time of three and a half months. The *range of weight loss was from nine pounds to fifty-four pounds,* and the range of time was from about one and a half months to six months.[10]

Chalk up another one for the low-carb approach to weight loss. And start to take note of what's going to become a running theme throughout this book: meat, fat, and vegetables almost always "work" when nothing else seems to. (Vegetarians, you can substitute the "impossible burger" for meat, although—full disclosure—I'm not a fan of them myself.) If you're not a vegetarian, any good protein source that's essentially carb-free will do—eggs, chicken, tuna, and of course meat. And if you're wondering "How can meat possibly be good for you?" read on, my friends, read on.

In 1928, something really interesting happened at the dietetic ward of Bellevue Hospital in New York City. But to understand why it happened, you have to understand the experiences of a rugged young explorer named Vilhjalmur Stefansson.

Stefansson and the Inuit: All Meat, All Fat, All the Time

Kicked out of school at age 23 for inciting a protest within the student body, Vilhjalmur Stefansson picked up the pieces of his life and entered the world of his true love, anthropology. By 1906, at the age of 27, he had managed to get a master's degree at Harvard, where he became an assistant professor of anthropology and got really interested in the diets of other people. Not much for city life, Stefansson dumped Harvard and decided that it would be more fun to join the Anglo-American Polar Expedition, which was kicking off that year, and travel to the Arctic.

A couple of years after his first foray, he persuaded the American Museum of Natural History in New York to give him the money to do it again, and he departed on his second expedition in 1908; this time, he stayed 4 years. He discovered a previously isolated group of indigenous people called the Copper Inuit (so named because they used copper tools), and he lived with them for his entire stay. His third and final expedition began in 1913 and lasted for 5 years.

Later, he wrote: "In 1906 I went to the Arctic with the food tastes and beliefs of the average American. By 1918, after eleven years as an Eskimo among Eskimos, I had learned things which caused me to shed most of those beliefs."[11]

I've always found it easier to stay on a low-carb diet than on any other kind of diet. I just never feel as hungry so I don't really feel like I'm dieting.

—Doug M.

One of the beliefs Stefansson took to the Arctic was the prevailing notion that the less meat you ate, the better off you'd be. The view then—as now—was that if you ate a lot of meat, you would develop, among other things, hardening of the arteries, high blood pressure, and, very likely, a breakdown of the kidneys.

But this is what he found: the Inuit he lived with ate a diet that consisted almost exclusively of meat (or fish) and fat. And they were as healthy and robust as a bunch of wild horses. High blood pressure, coronary infarctions, and strokes were virtually unknown. The women rarely suffered from breast-feeding problems, complications in pregnancy, or difficult births. And prior to their contact with mainstream civilization, the Inuit seldom suffered from cancer. (Today, about a century after their contact with "civilization" and the modern diet, they routinely suffer from all of the above.)

Ever the anthropologist, Stefansson lived with an Inuit family for much of his time in the Arctic and adopted all their eating habits. Though he had hated fish all his life, he ate it night and day. He ate it raw, baked, and boiled. He ate the heads and the tails. He even came to like the Inuit delicacy of rotten fish, which he likened to his first taste of Camembert. It was the beginning of an aggregate of 5 years on a diet that consisted almost exclusively of protein, fat, and water.

According to the prevailing dietary wisdom of the times, he should've been dead.

He wasn't. And, by the way, he never gained weight. He also never saw a fat "Eskimo."

He wrote:

> Eskimos, when still on their home meats, are never corpulent—at least, I have seen none who were. Eskimos in their native garments do give the impression of fat, round faces on fat, round bodies, but the roundness of face is a racial peculiarity and the rest of the effect is produced by loose and puffy garments. See them stripped, and one does not find the abdominal protuberances and folds which are so in evidence on Coney Island beaches and so persuasive an argument against nudism.[12]

The guy did have a sense of humor.

By the way, lest anyone think that Inuit were somehow genetically or racially immune to getting fat, Stefansson was quick to point out how quickly they fattened up when they ate mainstream American or European diets. In other words, they stay nice and slim on a high-fat diet, but as soon as they start eating starch and sugar, guess what happens?

Stefansson was genuinely curious to see if this strange diet had produced any ill effects that he perhaps hadn't noticed. And there were plenty of doctors who were just as curious as he. A committee was convened, and Stefansson was put through as rigorous an examination as a potential astronaut would get today. The findings were published in the *Journal of the American Medical Association* on July 3, 1926, in an article titled "The Effects of an Exclusive Long-Continued Meat Diet." The result? The committee had failed to find even *one trace of evidence* of all the supposed harmful effects of the diet.

This brings us to the dietetic ward of Bellevue Hospital in 1928. Stefansson and Dr. Karsten Anderson, a colleague who had been on one of the expeditions with Stefansson, agreed to act as human guinea pigs in a two-person experiment. Stefansson had not only survived but thrived on a diet that was supposed to have killed him, but this experience had never really been verified under scientific conditions. So Stefansson and Anderson agreed to live in the dietetic ward of Bellevue Hospital under the strictest of medical supervision, eating an exclusive diet of meat, for a solid year. The aim of the project was not to "prove" something, but merely to get at the facts and answer the prevailing questions of the time: Would the men get scurvy? Would they suffer from other deficiency diseases? What would be the effect on the circulatory system? On calcium levels? On the kidneys? On their weight?

Lest anyone think this was a quaint little "experiment" supervised by a couple of country quacks, let's look at the committee assembled to supervise this dietetic experiment: from Harvard University, Dr. Lawrence Henderson, Dr. Ernest Hooton, and Dr. Percy Howe; from Cornell University Medical College, Dr. Walter Niles; from the American Museum of Natural History, Dr. Clark Wissler; from Johns Hopkins University, Dr. William McCallum and Dr. Raymond Pearl; from the Russell Sage Institute of Pathology, Dr. Eugene DuBois and Dr. Graham Lusk; from the University of Chicago, Dr. Edwin O. Jordan; from the Institute of American Meat Packers, Dr. C. Robert Moulton; and a physician in private practice, Dr. Clarence W. Lieb.

Not exactly "The Gang That Couldn't Shoot Straight."

This is how the experiment went: For the first 3 weeks, Stefansson and Anderson were fed the standard diet of the time: fruits, cereals, bacon and eggs, and vegetables. (Notice that there were no fast foods, no snacks, and no vending-machine fare available then, so by today's standards, the "ordinary" diet was already light-years better than what we eat now.) During those first 3 weeks, the two guys were given preliminary checkups and were basically free to come and go as they pleased. After the first 3 weeks, they went on the all-meat diet and were more or less under house arrest. Neither of them was permitted at any time, day or night, to be out of sight of a supervising doctor or a nurse.

One interesting sidebar: Anderson was able to eat anything he liked as often as he wanted, provided that it came under the experimental definition of meat: steaks, chops, brains fried in bacon fat, boiled short ribs, chicken, fish, liver, and bacon. But because Stefansson had reported in one of his books, *My Life with the Eskimo,* that he had become very ill when he had to go 2 or 3 weeks on just *lean* meat ("caribou so skinny that there was no appreciable fat"), DuBois, who headed the experiment, suggested that for a while they try a *lean-meat-only* diet on Stefansson to contrast the results with those of Anderson, who was eating whatever mix of fat and meat he felt like. They continued to give Anderson as much fat as he liked, but Stefansson was limited to chopped fatless meat.

Stefansson wrote:

> The symptoms brought on at Bellevue by an incomplete meat diet (lean without fat) were exactly the same as in the Arctic, except that they came on faster—diarrhea and a feeling of general baffling discomfort. Up north the Eskimos and I had been cured immediately when we got some fat. DuBois now cured me the same way, by giving me fat sirloin steaks, brains fried in bacon fat, and things of that sort. In two or three days I was all right, but I had lost considerable weight. If yours is a meat diet then you simply must have fat with your lean; otherwise you would sicken and die.[13]

I can't help but be pessimistic about what would happen if a study like that were done in today's poisoned atmosphere of partisan nutritional politics. Let's say researchers created two randomized groups of subjects and had one of them eat only lean meat and the other eat meat plus fat. And let's say the results mirrored what happened in the Stefansson experiment—the meat-plus-fat eaters did great, the lean-meat eaters did terrible. You can be sure there'd be anti-meat groups proclaiming that the results—people eating nothing but lean meat did badly—"proved their point" that meat is terrible for you. They would conveniently ignore the fact that it was *not* meat that was the problem but the *absence* of *fat.* That kind of agenda-driven thinking, sadly, continues to inform many of today's "interpretations" of research.

Back to Stefansson and Anderson and the original "study of two." For the rest of the year, both men were kept on a diet of meat and fat in whatever proportion they liked, and the experiment went off without a hitch. Every few weeks, with DuBois supervising, they would run around the reservoir in Central Park, then run up to DuBois's house, going up the stairs two or three at a time, after which they would plop down on cots and have their breathing, pulse rate, and other measurements taken. These tests showed that their stamina increased the longer they stayed on the meat diet.

In 1930, DuBois and associates published the results of the study in the *American Journal of Biological Chemistry*. (Keep this significant study in mind when later we discuss the all-meat Carnivore Diet of Dr. Shawn Baker on page 264.) The title of the paper was "Prolonged Meat Diets with Study of Kidney Functions and Ketosis." Here's a summary of what they wrote: Stefansson, who was about 10 pounds overweight at the beginning, lost his excess weight in the first few weeks on the all-meat diet. His total caloric intake ranged from 2,000 to 3,100 calories per day. His metabolic rate rose—from 60.96 to 66.38 calories per hour during the period of the weight loss, indicating an increase of almost 9%. His blood cholesterol at the end of the year was 51 milligrams lower than it had been at the start. He wound up choosing a ratio of somewhere around 3:1 (in grams) of lean meat to fat. He continued the diet a full year, with no apparent ill effects.

Everyone warned me that if I went on a high-protein diet my cholesterol and triglycerides would go through the roof. Meanwhile, the exact opposite happened.
—Pamela R.

Stefansson wrote about his experiences in a fascinating and very long three-part piece called "Adventures in Diet" in *Harper's Monthly Magazine* between November 1935 and January 1936. His conclusions were surprisingly moderate: "So you *could* live on meat if you wanted to; but there is no driving reason why you *should*. Apparently you can eat healthy on meat without vegetables, on vegetables without meat, or on a mixed diet."

What he did not say, but undoubtedly would have had he been alive today, was this: you *cannot* eat "healthy" if most of your food comes from a convenience store.

The low-carbers of today would've loved him.

A postscript: it seems that in the twenty-or-so-year interim between his days in the Bellevue dietetic ward and his life in the 1950s as a scholarly (and relatively sedentary) academic, Stefansson suffered a mild cerebral thrombosis, put on a few pounds, and became quite a grump. According to Mrs. Stefansson, her husband had mostly recovered from the thrombosis but couldn't dump the extra weight. Her words: "By will power and near starvation, he had now and then lost a few [pounds] but [they] always came back when his will power broke down." Mrs. Stef also noted that he had become a real pain in the butt. As she delicately put it, "Stef had grown a bit unhappy, at times grouchy."[14]

Stef then asked Mrs. Stef if she wouldn't mind if he went on the "Stone-Age Eskimo sort of all-meat diet" he had thrived on during the most active part of his Arctic career. Mrs. Stef was not exactly a stay-at-home wife. She lectured, she wrote books about the Arctic, she was the director of a course called the Arctic Seminar, and she sang in madrigal groups. She had better things to do with her time than to prepare two different menus. But she bit her tongue and said "Of course, dear. That will be fine."

So back it was to *all meat, all fat, all the time* in the Stefansson household. Mrs. Stef wrote:

> When you eat as a primitive Eskimo does, you live on lean and fat meats. A typical Stefansson dinner is a rare or medium sirloin steak and coffee. The coffee is freshly ground. If there is enough fat on the steak we take the coffee black, otherwise heavy cream is added. Sometimes we have a bottle of wine. We have no bread, no starchy vegetables, no desserts. Rather often we eat half a grapefruit. We eat eggs for breakfast, two for Stef, one for me, with lots of butter.
>
> Startling improvements in health came to Stef after several weeks on the new diet. He began to lose his overweight almost at once, and lost steadily, eating as much as he pleased and feeling satisfied the while. He lost seventeen pounds; then his weight remained stationary, although the amount he ate was the same. From being slightly irritable and depressed, he became once more his old ebullient, optimistic self.
>
> An unlooked-for and remarkable change was the disappearance of his arthritis, which had troubled him for years and which he thought of as a natural result of aging. One of his knees was so stiff he walked up and down stairs a step at a time, and he always sat on the aisle in a theatre so he could extend his stiff leg comfortably. Several times a night he would be awakened by pain in his hip and shoulder when he lay too long on one side; then he had to turn over and lie on the other side. Without noticing the change at first, Stef was one day startled to find himself walking up and down stairs, using both legs equally. He stopped in the middle of our stairs; then walked down again and up again. He could not remember which knee had been stiff!
>
> Conclusion: The Stone-Age all-meat diet is wholesome. It is an eat-all-you-want reducing diet that permits you to forget you are dieting—no hunger pains remind you. Best of all, it improves the temperament. It somehow makes one feel optimistic, mildly euphoric.[15]

A post-postscript: Stefansson remained married to the former Evelyn Schwartz Baird (Mrs. Stef) for 21 years; continued his research, writing, and public speaking at Dartmouth College; and died, by all accounts happy, on August 26, 1962, at the age of 83.

Meanwhile, back at the ranch . . .

In 1944, cases of obesity were being treated at New York City Hospital by a cardiologist named Blake Donaldson. After a year of unsuccessful results with traditional low-calorie diets, he decided to investigate alternative methods. He took himself to the American Museum of Natural History, where, using teeth as an indicator of both body condition in general and diet specifically, he hit the mother lode when he looked at skeletons dug from Inuit burial grounds. Looking further into Inuit diets, he consulted with Vilhjalmur Stefansson and became convinced that a meat-only diet was the answer for his obese patients. Donaldson allowed his patients to eat as much as they liked, but the *minimum* was one 8-ounce porterhouse steak *3 times a day*, with a cooked weight of 6 ounces lean meat and 2 ounces fat, the same 3:1 ratio of lean to fat that had worked so well in the Stefansson–Anderson experiment (and the same one that Pennington had used with his DuPont execs).

Foreshadowing many of the low-carb diets of the 1990s, Donaldson kept his patients on a strict version of the diet until they reached their target weight, at which point they could add back certain "prohibited" foods, unless they began to put on weight again. Donaldson treated some 15,000 patients and claimed a 70% success rate using this diet. He also claimed that the 30% who were unsuccessful failed to lose weight not because of any fault in the diet but because they couldn't stay on it. He wrote a book in 1960 called *Strong Medicine*,[16] so named because Donaldson knew that his diet was not for the faint of heart—it took a lot of willpower and dedication to stick with it, and he knew that not everybody would be up for the challenge.

Then came a seminal moment in the history of low-carb theory, one that served as an acknowledged inspiration to the main guru of the low-carb movement of the late twentieth century, Robert Atkins. It happened in the 1950s and 1960s, and it happened in London.

Inspiration for Atkins

Professor Alan Kekwick was director of the Institute of Clinical Research and Experimental Medicine at London's Middlesex Hospital, and Dr. Gaston L. S. Pawan was senior research biochemist of the hospital's medical unit. These two researchers joined forces in the middle of the twentieth century to perform some visionary experiments.[17] They wanted to test the theory that different proportions of carbs, fat, and protein might have different effects on weight loss *even if the calories were kept the same.*

In one study, they put obese subjects on a 1,000-calorie diet but varied the percentages of protein, carbs, and fat. Some subjects were on a diet of 90% protein, some 90% fat, and some 90% carbs. The subjects on the 90% protein diet lost 0.6 pounds per day, the ones on the 90% fat diet lost 0.9 pounds per day, and the ones on 90% carbs actually gained a bit.

In another study, subjects didn't lose anything on a so-called "balanced" diet of 2,000 calories; but when these same subjects were put on a diet of primarily fat with very low carbohydrate, they were able to lose even when the calories went as high as 2,600 per day. The February 1957 issue of the American journal *Antibiotic Medicine and Clinical Therapy* reported: "If . . . calorie intake was kept constant . . . at 1,000 per day, the most rapid weight loss was noted with *high-fat diets* . . . But when the calorie intake was raised to 2,600 daily in these patients, *weight loss would still occur provided that this intake was given mainly in the form of fat and protein.*" [Emphasis mine.]

Still, the criticism from the medical establishment was enormous—this work contradicted the mantra that a calorie is a calorie is a calorie. One of the criticisms leveled at the two researchers was that the weight their patients lost was "just water weight." So Kekwick and Pawan did water-balance studies that showed water loss to be only a small part of the total weight lost. Interestingly, as recently as 2002, a very well-designed study done at the University of Cincinnati and Children's Hospital Medical Center[18] compared weight loss on a very low-carbohydrate diet to weight loss on a calorie-restricted low-fat diet, and found again that the greater weight loss experienced by the low-carb dieters was *not* due to water loss. The exact words: "We think it is very unlikely that differences in weight between the two groups . . . are a result of [water loss] in the very low-carb dieters." Yet to this day, the myth persists that the majority of weight lost on low-carbohydrate diets is mainly from water.

Eat Fat and Grow Slim and the Theory of Metabolic Disorder

The dietary establishment remained firmly convinced, as it does to this day, that the only thing that mattered when it came to weight reduction was calories; but there were pockets of dissent popping up throughout the

1950s, '60s, and '70s. One of the leaders of this dissent was Dr. Richard Mackarness, who ran Britain's first obesity and food allergy clinic and who in 1958 wrote *Eat Fat and Grow Slim* (which was revised and expanded in 1975).[19] He argued that it was c*arbohydrates*, not calories, that were the culprit in weight gain. The following lines, from the foreword to the book, give the reader some idea of what's coming. They were written by Sir Heneage Ogilvie—a consultant surgeon at Guy's Hospital in London, the editor of *The Practitioner*, and a former vice president of the Royal College of Surgeons, England.

> There are three kinds of foods—fats, proteins, and carbohydrates. All of these provide calories. *But the carbohydrates provide calories and nothing else.* They have none of the essential elements to build up or to repair the tissues of the body. *A man given carbohydrates alone, however liberally, would starve to death on calories.* The body must have proteins and animal fats. *It has no need for carbohydrates,* and, given the two essential foodstuffs, it can get all the calories it needs from them.

You heard it here first, folks. And you'll be hearing it again throughout this book: *the body has no physiological need for carbohydrates.* You cannot live without protein. You cannot live without fat. But you can survive perfectly well without carbohydrates. No one is saying you *ought* to, or that you *have* to—just that you *can.* This is simple, basic human biochemistry. There is no "minimum daily requirement" for carbohydrates—which raises the question worth keeping in the back of your mind as you read through the rest of the book: why would the dietary establishment—including the American Academy of Nutrition and Dietetics*—continue to insist that the only healthful diet consists of one in which the *majority* of the calories come from the *one macronutrient for which we have no physiological need?*

But I digress.

Sentiments similar to those of Ogilvie were echoed in the Mackarness book's introduction, written by Dr. Franklin Bicknell:

---

*The American Dietetic Association recently renamed itself the "American Academy of Nutrition and Dietetics," in an ill-fated attempt to rebrand itself as something other than the handmaiden of mainstream medicine and the protector of the Food Pyramid. In my opinion, it'll take a lot more than a name change to undo the impression that the organization exists to act as a rubber stamp for the Big Food/Big Pharma medical-industrial complex.

The cure of obesity . . . can be, of course, achieved by simple starvation, but as Dr. Mackarness explains, this is both an illogical and an injurious treatment, while [a treatment] based on eating as much of everything one likes except starches and sugars and foods rich in these, is both logical and actively good for one's health, quite apart from the effect on one's weight. *The sugars and starches of our diet form the least valuable part and contribute nothing which cannot better be gained from fat and protein foods like meat and fish, eggs and cheese, supplemented by green vegetables and some fruit.* Such a diet provides an abundance . . . of vitamins, trace elements, and essential amino acids—an abundance of all those subtle, yet essential, nutrients which are often lacking in diets based largely on the fat-forming carbohydrates.

A little context: ever since 1829, when William Wadd, surgeon-extraordinaire to the prince regent, proclaimed that the cause of obesity was "an over-indulgence at the table" (i.e., eating too darn much!), the conventional wisdom was that fat people are fat because they eat too much food. Period. This view, that only the quantity and not the quality of food that people eat makes a difference, had a stranglehold on mainstream medicine—a stranglehold that continued through the twentieth century with the cooperation of the sycophantic American Academy of Nutrition and Dietetics (formerly the American Dietetic Association) and is only now, in the twenty-first century, beginning to loosen.

To give you a sense of the spirit of the era, the medical correspondent of the *London Times*, on March 11, 1957, wrote at the time of Mackarness's book: "It is no use saying as so many women do: 'But I eat practically nothing.' The only answer to this is: 'No matter how little *you imagine* you eat, *if you wish to lose weight you must eat less.'*" [Emphasis mine.]

Mackarness comes out swinging, right in his author's introduction, leaving no doubt what "side" of the quality-versus-quantity argument he's on: "Starch and sugar are the causes of obesity. Particularly modern refined and processed starches and sugars, the ever ready, highly publicized carbohydrate foods of twentieth-century urban man." He puts forth the interesting argument—foreshadowing much of what we hear today in the discussions of metabolic type—that there are two kinds of people, whom he characterizes as Mr. Constant-Weight and Mr. Fatten-Easily.

According to Mackarness, if you give both types the same exercise and feed them the same food, one will stay the same weight while the other will gain. When Mr. (or Ms.) Constant-Weight—people we hate who seem to be able to eat anything and not gain an ounce—take in too much carbohy-drate, the extra food simply causes a revving-up in their metabolism that burns the extra calories consumed, and they stay the same weight. Nothing is left over for laying down fat. "But," Mackarness writes, "when Mr. Fatten-Easily eats too much bread, cake, and potatoes, the picture is entirely differ-ent: his metabolic rate does not increase. Why does he fail to burn up the excess? The answer is the real reason for his obesity: Because he has a defective capacity for dealing with carbohydrates."

Mackarness was suggesting a metabolic disorder, and he was on to something. He was really the first diet-book author to postulate some sort of metabolic defect in the way some people process food (especially carbohy-drates) that causes them to send much of what they eat to their fat stores. Dr. Alfred Pennington (of the DuPont-execs study) had come to the same conclusion. Summing up a 1953 paper called "Obesity: Over-nutrition or Disease of Metabolism?" published in the *American Journal of Digestive Dis-eases*, Pennington wrote: "Analysis of the results . . . appear[s] to necessitate an explanation of obesity on the basis of some intrinsic metabolic defect."

Writing for the general public, Mackarness had a simpler way of putting it. He came up with a great analogy: the steam engine.

The orthodox view is that a fat man's engine is stoked by a robot fireman, who swings his shovel at the same pace whether fat, protein, or carbohydrate is in the tender. This is true for Mr. Constant-Weight, but as he does not get fat anyway, it is only of academic interest to us. It is certainly not true for Mr. Fatten-Easily, with whom we are concerned. Mr. Constant-Weight has a robot stoker in his engine. The more he eats—of whatever food—the harder his stoker works until any excess is consumed, so he never gets fat. Recent research has shown that Mr. Fatten-Easily's stoker is profoundly influenced by the kind of fuel he has to shovel. On fat fuel he shovels fast. On protein slightly less fast *but on carbohydrate he becomes tired, scarcely moving his shovel at all.* His fire then burns low and his engine gets fat from its inability to use the carbohydrate, which is still being loaded into the tender. *Mr. Fatten-Easily's stoker suffers from an inability to deal with carbohydrate.*

At the back of his book, Mackarness lists foods that can be eaten with-out reservation, which are meat, poultry, game, fish and other seafood, dairy products, fats and oils, most vegetables, and some fruits; foods that can be eaten in moderation with some caution, including nuts and higher-carb vegetables and fruits; and foods that could be eaten once a day, such as beans, beets, corn, potatoes, and bananas. While some low-carb theorists of today might quibble with the inclusion of dairy, what's more interesting is the Mackarness list of "never eat" foods. Are you ready? Don't shoot the messenger.

- breakfast cereals
- bread and rolls
- biscuits and crackers
- macaroni products, noodles, spaghetti, and other pastas
- rice
- jellies, jams, and preserves
- ice cream, cakes, pies, and candy
- sauces and gravies thickened with flour or cornstarch
- beer
- sweet wines and liqueurs
- sodas (and all "sweetened fizzy drinks")
- sugar

The Mackarness diet suggests that carbs be kept as low as possible—no more than 60 grams a day for most people (and in some cases 50 grams or fewer a day). This figure is in the ballpark of the recommendations of many low-carb diet books of today. (*Life Without Bread*[20] recommends a maximum of 72 grams a day, and the ongoing weight loss and maintenance programs of the Atkins diet and Protein Power are in the Mackarness range, as is the beginning program for overweight sedentary people adhering to the Schwarzbein Principle. It is also practically identical to the generic program for beginners that I recommend in chapter 10.)

We should not leave Mackarness without mentioning that he was one of the first to note the emotional and psychological component of overeating. Here's what he said, in words that will undoubtedly ring true for thousands of people today. [Emphasis mine.]

So far, then, two big factors in the production of obesity have emerged.

A *defect in dealing with carbohydrates* which makes a person fatten easily on an ordinary mixed diet;

Overeating, especially of sugars and starches as a result of *loneliness, fear or emotional dissatisfaction.*

When the two factors are present, weight is gained very rapidly. *So anyone who finds himself tempted to overeat for emotional reasons and who shows a tendency to get fat, should be careful to choose low-carbohydrate foods.*[21]

Overeaters Anonymous

Mackarness was not the only one to notice the emotional component of overeating. Interestingly, on the other side of the ocean, in 1959—less than a year after the publication of Mackarness's book and 24 years after the founding of Alcoholics Anonymous—two women in Los Angeles began the fellowship now known as Overeaters Anonymous. A spiritual program to address compulsive overeating, it was based on the same 12-step principles as its predecessor, but with one significant difference. While alcoholics and drug addicts could conceivably abstain from their drug of choice, compulsive overeaters could not. They had to eat to survive.

This presented an entirely different set of issues, since for overeaters, complete "abstinence" from their "drug" (food) was not possible. Many of the original participants in OA attended because they were terribly overweight, but most understood that there was a compulsive emotional component to their overeating that could not be addressed by simple diets or by the prescription drug of the day, *dextroamphetamine*, sold under the brand name *Dexedrine*. What's especially interesting for our purposes is a particular subgroup of OA that developed in Los Angeles in the early '60s. This group had noticed that, even though many people lost weight in Overeaters Anonymous, many were nibbling their way back to obesity and that certain foods seemed to feed the compulsion to eat more than others.

Can you guess what the culprits were? Yup.

By 1963, there was a very vocal minority of OA members who were convinced that carbohydrates sabotaged any weight-loss plan because they produced cravings and addictive eating behavior. The OA contingent called them "binge foods." One of the founders of this faction—which later came to be known as the Grey Sheet Group—wrote "I wonder if we have an *allergy of the body* too. Are we going to help the Doctors understand obesity just as the alcoholic had to educate the medical profession?"[22]

From that time on—although it is little known—there has always been a faction of OA that believes strongly that "abstaining" from carbohydrates (with a very low-carbohydrate diet) is a necessary component of emotional sobriety when it comes to food, just as it is a necessary strategy for weight loss in carbohydrate-sensitive individuals. Could this be another case of the patient profoundly understanding the disease far in advance of the medical professionals?

Calories, Carbs, or Just Plain Fat?
The Roaring '60s

In the 1960s, two books came out in favor of the low-carb approach, both of which got a lot of attention. One of them deserved it; the other did not. The one that did was a thoughtful, if somewhat misguided, treatise called *Calories Don't Count* by a New York doctor named Herman Taller. Taller had been a fat man all his life, at one time almost 100 pounds over his ideal weight. He described himself as one of those who "only had to look at a platter of spaghetti to gain [weight]." He struggled with every version of the low-calorie diet available with virtually no results. A physician friend of his was sure that Taller had to be lying about how much he was eating, so Taller hatched a plan. Reading his experience will no doubt produce quite a number of nodding, sympathetic heads.

> I proposed an interesting vacation test [to the physician who was certain I was cheating]. We would go away together for ten days, stay in each other's company continually, eat and drink the same things, and check the results. He accepted, and we went off to a resort. I followed what was then the accepted method of weight control: a low-calorie diet. I concentrated on salads, which I now know was a mistake, ate fat sparingly, another mistake, and, since this was a vacation, drank a cocktail each night before dinner. My physician friend, who was slim, did the same. At the end of the vacation, he had lost a pound or two and I had gained nine pounds. "I don't understand it," he said as we drove back to New York. Neither did I.[23]

Taller didn't reject the calorie theory at all. On the contrary, he wrote: "No one, least of all myself, would dispute the concept that led to the calorie fad. Any person will lose weight when he burns up more energy than he eats. This is a simple chemical law. Why, then, didn't a low-calorie diet work? Why did people lose weight on high-calorie, high-fat diets?" Taller postulated that all calories are not the same and that carbohydrates present a different problem to the body, *at least for some people*. He rightly pointed out that low-fat diets were by nature high in carbohydrates, thus stimulating insulin and creating more fat, particularly in people who were sensitive to carbohydrates. (It is noteworthy that, almost four decades later, Eleftheria Maratos-Flier, director of obesity research at Harvard's prestigious Joslin Diabetes Center, said, "For a large percentage of the population, perhaps 30 to 40 percent, low-fat diets are counterproductive. They have the paradoxical effect of making people gain weight.") Taller completely agreed that the underlying reason people get fat is an imbalance between calories taken in and calories burned. But he suggested that for some people there is a disturbance in the metabolism, with three results, none of them good: (1) the body forms fat at a rate that is faster than normal; (2) the body stores fat at a rate that is faster than normal; and (3) the body disposes of stored fat at a rate that is slower than normal. Taller summed up: "The crux of the matter is not how many calories [we] take in, but what [our bodies do] with those calories."[24]

Taller did not recommend a diet devoid of carbohydrates—in fact, a typical day's menu contained up to three slices of "gluten bread," something no low-carb advocate today, including myself, would recommend (there are far more healthful starchy carbs to choose from, including sprouted-grain or gluten-free breads). The rest of the day's food came from meat, poultry, seafood, and plenty of vegetables as well as some oils. There was no counting of calories.

Now here's where it gets interesting.

In the '50s and '60s, when Taller was writing, a scientist named Ancel Keys had begun studying heart disease and diet—research that culminated in what has come to be known as the diet-heart hypothesis. Keys concluded that cholesterol is a cause of heart disease, saturated fat causes a rise in cholesterol, and therefore saturated fat causes heart disease. Keys's seven-country study[25] became the basis for dietary policy for more than three decades, indirectly birthed the fat phobia of the '90s, and directly spawned an entire bureaucracy devoted to lowering cholesterol (the National Cholesterol Education Program) and also to producing some of the most profitable pharmaceutical drugs in history. Note for now that there are serious problems with this theory, and it is finally being reexamined.[26] (Between the third and fourth editions of this book, cardiologist Dr. Stephen Sinatra and I published *The Great Cholesterol Myth*, a thorough investigation of the evidence that fat and cholesterol cause heart disease. Spoiler alert: we concluded that the evidence is awfully weak.)

Taller, a product of the time, accepted the demonization of cholesterol and believed that if you could reduce it in the diet, you could significantly lower heart-disease rates. He was very concerned about the saturated fat in the low-carb diets of the past, so he came up with what he thought was a perfect solution: his version of the diet would incorporate tons of polyunsaturated fats. Problem was, he lumped all unsaturated fats together. He was correct in pointing out how healthy marine fats are (the famous omega-3s from fish and flaxseed), but he was dead wrong in advocating excessive amounts of man-made refined vegetable oils like safflower, sunflower, and corn oils, which we now know are associated with a host of diseases, inflammatory conditions, and cancers.[27]

Taller's book went through eighteen printings and ultimately had more than a million copies in circulation, but his career came to an unfortunate end when he was convicted of six counts of mail fraud for using the book to promote a particular brand of safflower capsules, which the court called "a worthless scheme foisted on a gullible public."[28] Too bad. By all reports, he was a good guy and very sincere in his efforts to bring healthy low-carb living to the masses.

The other low-carb book published in the '60s—also against a backdrop of the fledgling no-fat madness started by the flawed Keys research—was one that didn't deserve much attention, though that little detail didn't stop it from selling 5½ million copies. *The Doctor's Quick Weight Loss Diet*,[29] otherwise known as the Stillman diet, put forth a high-protein solution that attempted, at the same time, to satisfy the low-fat contingent. On the Stillman diet, you ate nothing—and I mean nothing—but protein with every drop of fat trimmed from it. You could eat all you wanted from the following selection: lean meats with all possible fat trimmed; chicken and turkey without skin; all nonfatty fish; eggs made in nonstick pans without butter, margarine, oil, or other fat; cottage cheese and other soft cheeses made only from skim milk; and at least eight glasses of water a day. We know from the Stefansson experiment that this diet, if followed for any length of time, would make you very sick precisely because of the *absence* of fat.

The Stillman diet was a dumb idea and should not be followed for any reason. Although the Stillman all-protein plan was in fact a low-carb diet, it's important to remember that not all low-carb diets are *high-protein* diets. Even the Atkins diet, which will be discussed at greater length in chapter 9, is not necessarily high-protein. In fact, the average protein content of all three major phases of the Atkins diet is only 31% (the average *fat* content is 56%); and during the Atkins maintenance phase, the average protein content is only 5% higher than Weight Watchers (25% versus 20%)![30] Some of the diets discussed in this book don't even approach high-protein: for example, Barry Sears's Zone diet (see chapter 9) has often been called a high-protein diet by magazine writers who have either not read his books or not understood them, and by members of the American Dietetic Association, who have frequently done neither. The point is that *low-carb does not necessarily equal high-protein*, and the Stillman diet is Exhibit A in making the case that all low-carb diets are not the same.

Atkins, Yudkin, and the Question of Sugar

By 1970, the Keys research had been published and was being picked up by the media; the low- or no-cholesterol brigade was gearing up for an assault on the consciousness of the American public. In 1972, Robert Atkins published the first edition of the *New Diet Revolution*, the Cadillac of low-carb diet plans, which became the de facto poster child for the low-carb movement two decades later.

Atkins was the first popular diet-book author to seriously focus on insulin as a determinant in weight gain. He preached the virtues of something he called "the metabolic advantage": benign dietary ketosis (a process that, because it is so central to the discussion of low-carb diets and so misunderstood, will receive much further attention in chapter 9). Because his high-fat, high-protein, low-carb diet went so dramatically against the conventional "wisdom" of the times, Atkins was attacked mercilessly in the press and vilified by the medical mainstream, who turned him into a pariah in the medical community. His voice was drowned out by the low-fat, no-cholesterol, calorie-counting establishment, and although he remained active, he didn't catch on big-time until the early 1990s, when an updated edition of the *New Diet Revolution* was published.

The public, with their rapidly expanding waistlines, was growing weary of the low-fat dogma and beginning to realize that their low-fat diets were accomplishing very little in the way of weight loss; people were finally ready to look elsewhere for a solution.

In the same year in which Atkins published the first edition of his book, which firmly took the position that the problem in obesity was carbohydrates, not fat, a brilliant English doctor named John Yudkin was making waves by politely and reasonably suggesting to the medical establishment that perhaps their emperor, while indeed cholesterol-free and low-fat, was nonetheless as naked as a jaybird. A professor of nutrition at Queen Elizabeth College, London University, and the surgeon-captain of the British Royal Navy, Yudkin was a highly respected scientist and nutritionist and the possessor of both an MD and a PhD, with dozens of published papers in such august peer-reviewed journals as *The Lancet, Cardiovascular Review, British Medical Journal, The Archives of Internal Medicine, The American Journal of Clinical Nutrition*, and *Nature* to his credit.

Yudkin was typically portrayed by his detractors as a wild-eyed fanatic who blamed sugar as the cause of heart disease, but in fact he was nothing of the sort. In his 1972 book, *Sweet and Dangerous*, he was the embodiment of reason when he called for a reexamination of the data—which he considered highly flawed—that led to the hypothesis that fat causes heart disease. (These data, as you will recall, came originally from a study of seven countries published by Ancel Keys, a study that conveniently omitted a substantial amount of data that did not fit his hypothesis.)[31]

Yudkin pointed out that statistics for heart disease and fat consumption existed for many more countries than those referred to by Keys, and that these other figures didn't fit into the "more fat, more heart disease" relationship that was evident when only the seven selected countries were considered. He also pointed out that there was a better and truer relationship between *sugar consumption* and heart disease, and he said that "there is a sizable minority—of which I am one—that believes that coronary disease is *not* largely due to fat in the diet." (Three decades later, Dr. George Mann, an associate director of the Framingham Study, arrived at the same conclusion and assembled a distinguished group of scientists and doctors to study the evidence that fat and cholesterol cause heart disease, a concept he later called "the greatest health scam of the century."[32] Around the same time, the brilliant Danish scholar Uffe Ravnskov, MD, PhD, reanalyzed the original Keys data and came to the identical conclusion. His exemplary scholarship is supported by hundreds of referenced citations and studies from prestigious, peer-reviewed medical journals and can be found in book form[33] and at the website http://www.ravnskov.nu/cm/.

While Yudkin did not write a low-carb diet book per se, he was one of the most influential voices of the time to put forth the position that sugar was responsible for far more health problems than fat was. His book called attention to countries in which the correlation between heart disease and sugar intake was far more striking than the correlation between heart disease and *fat*. And he pointed to a number of studies—most dramatically of the Masai in Kenya and Tanzania—where people consumed copious amounts of milk and fat and yet had virtually no heart disease. Interestingly, these people also consumed almost no sugar.[34]

Yudkin patiently explained that sugar consumption is *one* of a *number* of indices of health. Heart disease is associated with many of these indices, including fat consumption, overweight, cigarette smoking, a sedentary lifestyle, and television viewing. It is *definitely* associated with a high intake of sugar. He never said that sugar *causes* the diseases of modern civilization, just that a case could easily be made that it deserved attention and study— certainly as much as, if not more than, fat consumption. (Yudkin himself performed several interesting studies on sugar consumption and coronary heart disease. In one, he found that the median sugar intake of a group of coronary patients was 147 grams, twice as much as it was in two different groups of control subjects who didn't have coronary disease; these groups consumed only 67 and 74 grams, respectively).[35]

As Yudkin put it, "It may turn out that [many factors including sugar] ultimately have the same effect on metabolism and so produce coronary disease by the same mechanism." What is that mechanism? Fingers are beginning to point suspiciously to an *overload of insulin* as a common culprit at the root of at least some of these metabolic and negative health effects like heart disease; controlling insulin was the main purpose of the original Atkins diet and has become the raison d'être of the low-carb approach to living. (In the next chapter, we will explore some of the connections between high levels of insulin and heart disease, hypertension, obesity, and diabetes.)

Cholesterol Madness

Yudkin's warnings against sugar and Atkins's early low-carb approach to weight loss were mere whispers lost in the roar of anti-fat mania. By the mid-1980s, fat had been utterly and completely demonized, and fat phobia was in full bloom, with hundreds of no-cholesterol foods being foisted on a gullible public (despite the findings that dietary cholesterol had little or no effect on serum cholesterol, a fact acknowledged even by Ancel Keys himself, who, in 1991, said that dietary cholesterol only mattered if you happened to be a rabbit!).[36] In November 1985, the National Heart, Lung, and Blood Institute launched the National Cholesterol Education Program with the stated goal of "reducing illness and death from coronary heart disease in the United States by *reducing the percent of Americans with high blood cholesterol.*"[37] [Emphasis mine.]

Though high cholesterol *doesn't* cause heart disease and, in fact, has turned out to be a relatively poor predictor of it, the juggernaut was already in full swing, and the cry of "hold the butter" was heard all over America. Fat-free foods were everywhere. SnackWells replaced Oreos as the best-selling cookie in America. In 1976, Nathan Pritikin opened his Pritikin Longevity Center in Santa Barbara, California, and for the next decade he preached the super-low-fat dogma to all who would listen, which included most of the country. Jane Fonda ushered in a new generation of aerobicized exercise fanatics whose motto was "no pain, no gain" and who looked upon fat of any kind as a Tootsie Roll in the punch bowl. (Later, Apex, a supplement company based in California, got a strong foothold in health clubs as nutrition "experts" largely by being the handmaiden of the American Dietetic Association, and Apex's people taught gullible trainers and their clients the dogma of high-carbohydrate diets for weight loss while they railed against the "dangers" of high protein and ketosis.)[38] It became a point of pride to exorcise any hint of fat from the diet: egg-white omelets became de rigueur on every urban menu, and waiters across America became accustomed to orders without butter, oil, or fat of any kind.

Pritikin died in 1985, but his mantle was quickly taken up by Dr. Dean Ornish. Ornish's reputation—and much of the public's faith in the low-fat diet approach—was fueled by his famous 5-year intervention study (the Lifestyle Heart Trial), which demonstrated that intensive lifestyle changes may lead to regression of coronary heart disease.[39] Ornish took 48 middle-aged white men with moderate to severe coronary heart disease and assigned them to two groups. One group received "usual care," and the other group received a special, intensive 5-part lifestyle intervention consisting of (1) aerobic exercise, (2) stress management training, (3) smoking cessation, (4) group psychological support, and (5) a strict vegetarian, high-fiber diet with 10% of the calories coming from fat.

When Ornish's study showed some reversal of atherosclerosis and fewer cardiac events in the 20 men who completed the 5-year study, the public perception—reinforced by Ornish himself—was that the results were largely due to the low-fat diet. This is an incredible leap that is in no way supported by his research. The fact is that *there's no way to know* whether the results were due to the low-fat diet portion of the experiment (highly unlikely in the view of many), the high fiber, the whole foods, the lack of sugar, or some combination of the interventions. It is entirely possible that Ornish would have gotten the same or better results with a program of exercise, stress management, smoking cessation, and group therapy plus a whole foods diet of high protein, good fats, high fiber, and low sugar. (Interestingly, critics of low-carb diets frequently proclaim with great righteousness that the only reason a low-carb diet works is because it is a low-calorie diet in disguise. They never level that criticism at Ornish, whose diet, in a scientific analysis, turned out to be *lower* in calories [1,273 calories] than the Atkins ongoing weight-loss phase [1,627 calories], the Atkins maintenance phase [1,990 calories], the Carbohydrate Addict's Diet [1,476 calories], Sugar Busters! [1,521 calories], the Zone [approximately 1,500 calories], and even Weight Watchers [1,462 calories].)[40]

The Tide Turns: A Reexamination of the Low-Carb Solution

By the 1990s, it was pretty obvious that low-fat dieting wasn't getting results. The country was fatter than ever, diabetes was becoming epidemic, and people were getting more and more frustrated and confused. The time was right for another look at the low-carb wisdom that had been around in one form or another since Banting's day in the 1800s. To the chagrin of the medical establishment and the American Dietetic Association, Atkins resurfaced with a vengeance with his newly updated *New Diet Revolution* in 1992, followed by perhaps the most influential nutrition book of the 1990s, Barry Sears's *The Zone*, in 1995, a year that also saw the publication of the brilliant *Protein Power* by Drs. Michael and Mary Dan Eades.

After massive resistance by the establishment, serious research was finally comparing low-carb diets to traditional diets, and the results were impressive. While it would be incorrect to say that low-carb diets always produced greater weight loss than the traditional kind, they *often* did; they frequently produced it faster (a huge motivating force for many people); and they almost always produced better health outcomes such as blood-lipid profiles, precisely the measures that the anti-low-carb forces had predicted would be disastrous on these regimens (see chapter 3). In 2004, in what will probably turn out to be a signal event for the death of the high-carb dictatorship, Dr. Walter Willett—chairman of the Department of Nutrition at Harvard University's School of Public Health and one of the most respected mainstream researchers in the country—recently came out publicly against the 1992 USDA Food Guide Pyramid, which for a decade had promoted 6 to 11 servings a day of grains, breads, and pastas.[41]

Internecine battles among advocates of different diets were hardly something new. What was different this time was that the arguments were finally taken public. On February 24, 2000, the U.S. Department of Agriculture hosted a major symposium, "The Great Nutrition Debate," which featured, among others, Dr. Robert Atkins (the Atkins diet), Dr. Barry Sears (the Zone diet), low-fat advocates Dr. Dean Ornish and Dr. John McDougall, and various representatives of the dietary establishment.[42]

Then, on July 7, 2002, the *New York Times* published a cover story in its Sunday magazine section titled "What If It's All Been a Big Fat Lie?" in which Gary Taubes, a brilliant science journalist and three-time winner of the National Association of Science Writers' Science in Society Award, brought to the table massive evidence that the low-fat diet had been the dumbest experiment in dietary history. The article created a predictable uproar, with defenders of the faith rallying to discredit Taubes—not an easy task, I might add—and the low-carbers beaming ear to ear with I-told-you-so grins.

An interesting side note: on the Dietitian Central website (a dietitian Internet community), the following post was found on July 14, a week after the Taubes article appeared: "Please, dietitians, download from the NY Times Magazine section from last Sunday, July 7, the article 'What If It's All Been a Big Fat Lie?' by Gary Taubes. *It is full of information that could rock our world.* As dietitians, we need to be prepared and informed re: changes that may be completely different from what we have learned and have been educating people about." (Taubes has since published a superb full-length book based on that article called *Good Calories, Bad Calories*—highly recommended.)

Low-carbing had come back, but this time with a clarity and a scientific validation that had simply not been present in previous decades. It's time now for a reassessment of the twin sacred cows of dietary commandments—*high carbohydrates* and *low fat*—and for a clearer look at just what could be gained in terms of health and weight loss by following a diet more like the one that sustained the human genus for 2.4 million years and sustained modern man for at least 50,000 years.

It's time to revisit the low-carb wisdom of the past, evaluate the wisdom of the present, and see what they have to teach us about living healthy in the twenty-first century.

CHAPTER 3

Why Low-Carb Diets Work

In other fields, when bridges do not stand, when aircraft do not fly, when machines do not work, when treatments do not cure, despite all the conscientious efforts on the part of many persons to make them do so, one begins to question the basic assumptions, principles, theories, and hypotheses that guide one's efforts.

—Arthur R. Jensen, PhD Professor of psychology at the University of California at Berkeley, in *Harvard Educational Review*, winter 1969

On November 1, 1999, Woody Merrell—the Muhammad Ali of doctors, loved, respected, and admired across the entire political spectrum of medicine and nutrition—wrote an article in *Time* magazine about weight loss. This is how it started:

"In my 25 years of medical training and practice in Manhattan, I've seen a wide range of diets come and go. *Virtually none of them work.*"

A few paragraphs later, Merrell wrote: "For most of my professional career, I adhered to the generally recognized dictum of weight management. *I advised my patients to count their calories and follow a low-fat diet.*"

He then talks about his experience with a few patients who weren't getting anywhere, no matter what they tried. Skeptically, he put them on a low-carb diet.

Finally he wrote: "I have become a convert. Carbohydrates . . . are often prime saboteurs of our weight. [O]f all the diets I've seen over the past few decades, the moderate-fat, lower-carbohydrate ones are the most successful.

They stress not how much food you eat but what kinds. Calorie counting is not as important as carbo counting." [All emphases mine.]

The article is titled "How I Became a Low-Carb Believer."[1]

What convinced Merrell—and what is convincing more and more of his colleagues—is the fact that lower-carbohydrate diets *really work* for many, many people. The evidence of the senses is hard to argue with. People lose weight, feel better, and, equally important, have major improvements in their health. Chronic complaints and ailments have been known to disappear. Some of these people had tried every possible diet, had adhered to every conventional cholesterol-lowering, fat-reducing program, and wound up in exactly the same place as when they started—and sometimes were even worse. Yet on lower-carb diets, they do great.

GENIUS AND ANTIAGING GURU CHOOSES LOW-CARB DIET!

Ray Kurzweil is a scientist, inventor, and recipient of the National Medal of Technology. Largely considered a genius (the *Wall Street Journal* called him "the restless genius," and Forbes called him "the ultimate thinking machine"), his fans range from Bill Gates to Bill Clayton.

Recently Kurzweil teamed up with Terry Grossman, MD, the founder and medical director of the Frontier Medical Institute in Denver and the author of *The Baby Boomers' Guide to Living Forever*. The two turned their not-inconsiderable brain power and experience to studying the science of life extension.

In their seminal book, *Fantastic Voyage: The Science Behind Radical Life Extension*, they discuss genes, diet, exercise, stress, genomics, and cutting-edge research on gene manipulation.

They also discuss their personal dietary programs, arrived at after consuming and digesting hundreds—if not thousands—of research papers related to even the most obscure areas of health and longevity.

These guys are serious about health and life extension.

Would you like to know what they personally eat?

Low-carb diets. Both men consume no more than 80 grams a day of carbs, or ⅙ (about 16%) of their total calories from carbohydrates on a daily basis.

Food for thought.

My doctor kept telling me not to try a low-carb diet because he thought it was so dangerous. Then his wife lost 50 pounds on Protein Power and now he's really done a 180.
—Adele P.

How can something that is so counterintuitive work? (And it *is* counterintuitive for most of us—after all, even Gary Taubes, in his seminal article "What If It's All Been a Big Fat Lie?"[2] said he couldn't quite get over the feeling that the bacon and eggs on his plate were going to somehow jump up and kill him.) We need to remember that low-carb eating is counterintuitive precisely *because* we have all been taught a number of "truths" that we have internalized as nutritional gospel but which may in fact be nutritional hogwash.

We "know" low-carb diets can't work because they are often high in fat or cholesterol (which we "know" causes heart disease), are often high in protein (which we "know" causes heart disease, bone loss, and possibly cancer), and may be higher in calories (which we "know" causes weight gain). Yet people eating the low-carb way are losing weight and lowering their risk for heart disease, hypertension, diabetes, and obesity. There is even some indication that they may be lowering their risk for some cancers.[3] How do we explain this? It is as though all three of Christopher Columbus's ships returned home with great bounty from the New World, but the people back in Spain shook their heads in disbelief, saying "How can this be? It must be a trick. The ships had to have fallen off the earth because we *know* the earth is flat!"

I've got news for you: low-fat is the flat-earth theory of human nutrition.

See, all theories of weight loss fit into one of two major categories of thought—*all of them*. There is no exception to this rule. If you understand the two categories, you're immediately better informed than half the population on the subject of dieting and weight loss.

Let's call category one the Checkbook Theory. This is the idea that when it comes to calories and weight loss, the human body is like a checking account. You eat a certain number of calories, and you burn up a certain number of calories. If you eat *more* than what you need, you *gain* weight. If you eat *less* than what you need, you *lose* weight. Much like a checking account: if I deposit (take in) more money than I write checks for, I have some extra cash (i.e., I gain weight). If I spend (put out) more than I take in, I have to dip into that cash (i.e., I lose weight). If what I *deposit* exactly equals what I *spend*, I have a zero balance (i.e., my weight stays the same).

Let's call category two the Telephone Theory of weight loss, based on the game of Telephone you may have played as a child. You line ten people up, and then whisper something in the ear of the first person. That person whispers it to the second person, and so on down the line, until the words are repeated to the last person, who then says them out loud. What usually happens is that you start out with something like "A rose is a rose is a rose" and you wind up with "Gardenias don't grow on the planet Mars." Applied to weight loss, the theory goes something like this: the stuff that goes on *in between* the calories coming in and the calories going out is *much* more important than the actual number of calories involved. There are so many enzymes, cofactors, energy cycles, hormones, neurotransmitters, eicosanoids, genes, and other variables in the human body that determine the fate of the food coming in, that it is impossible to predict what's going to happen to someone's weight just by knowing the number of calories that go in. It would be like predicting the outcome of Telephone simply by knowing the phrase that was originally said. Sure, if everything goes perfectly, "A rose is a rose is a rose" comes out as "A rose is a rose is a rose." More often, though, it comes out as something like "Game of Thrones is the *bomb.*" No. Sorry. Every comedian—and public speaker—knows that the specific is more effective AND funnier. If you're telling a joke and you say "all of a sudden a big car comes out of nowhere," it is nowhere near as "funny" as "all of a sudden here comes this humongous F-150 barreling down the 405."

The checking-account model, known as the *energy-balance theory*, has been the dominant theory of weight loss for years. The entire low-fat movement has been built on it: take in fewer calories and burn more, and you will lose weight. You have probably been hearing this advice for years. While this view is not entirely without merit, it's so far from the whole picture as to almost constitute dietary malpractice.

The thinking behind low-carbing belongs to the second category of theories about weight loss, the Telephone Theory. This view asks a critical question: What goes on inside the body once those calories are taken in? What happens that directs some folks' bodies to store everything as fat while others seem to get a free pass and burn up everything they eat? In other words, what determines whether what you eat goes on your hips or is burned up as energy and disappears as heat into the atmosphere?

The answer is one word: hormones.

Hormones control just about every metabolic event that goes on in your body, and you control hormones via your lifestyle. Food—along with several key lifestyle factors such as stress—is the drug that stimulates hormones, and those hormones direct the body to store or burn fat, just as they direct the body to perform a gazillion other metabolic operations. (Dr. Barry Sears has said that "food may be the most powerful drug you will ever encounter because it causes dramatic changes in your hormones that are hundreds of times more powerful than any pharmaceutical.") Hormones are the air-traffic controllers determining the fate of whatever flies in. *If your food is stimulating the wrong hormones or creating a hormonally unbalanced state, you will find it extremely difficult, if not impossible, to lose weight and keep it off.*

In this chapter, you will learn why it is so vitally important to balance your hormones if you want to lose weight. It is probably as important as—or more important than—counting calories, and it is *certainly* more important than reducing dietary fat. But managing our hormones has even bigger consequences. Insulin—the hormone most targeted by the low-carb diet plans discussed in this book—is at the hub of a significant number of diseases of civilization. When you control insulin, you hugely increase the odds that you will be able to control your weight. But, as you will see, you *also* reduce the risks for heart disease, hypertension, diabetes, polycystic ovary syndrome, inflammatory diseases, and even, possibly, cancer.

So let's get to know the players in our hormonal dance. If I've done my job, at the end of this chapter you'll have a much better understanding of what has now come to be popularly known as "Endocrinology 101": how the body *makes* fat, *stores* fat, and, finally, *says good-bye* to fat. You'll also understand why the same eating plan that helps you lose weight *also* has the positive "side effect" of preventing you from becoming a medical statistic.

THE STAR OF THE SHOW: EXPERTS WEIGH IN ON INSULIN

"Insulin is the key to the vast majority of chronic illness."
—Joe Mercola, DO

"There is an epidemic of insulin resistance in the world at large."
—Gerald Reaven, MD

"When you have excess levels of insulin, it's like a loose cannon on the deck of a hormonal ship." —Barry Sears, PhD

"Insulin sensitivity is going to determine, for the most part, how long you are going to live and how healthy you are going to be. It determines the rate of aging more so than anything else we know right now." —Ron Rosedale, MD

The Good, the Bad, and the Ugly: Insulin and Its Discontents

Insulin, a hormone first discovered in 1921, is the star actor in our little hormonal play. It is an anabolic hormone, which means it is responsible for building things up—putting compounds (like glucose and amino acids) inside storage units (like cells). Its sister hormone, glucagon, is responsible for breaking things down—opening those storage units and releasing their contents as needed. Insulin is responsible for *saving*; glucagon is responsible for *spending*. Together, their main job is to maintain blood sugar within the tightly regulated range it needs to be in, to keep your metabolic machinery running smoothly.

And to keep you from dying. Without insulin, blood sugar would sky-rocket and the result would be metabolic acidosis, coma, and death, the fate of virtually every type 1 diabetic in the early part of the twentieth century prior to the discovery of insulin. On the other hand, without glucagon, blood sugar would plummet and the result would be brain dysfunction, coma, and death. So the body knows what it's doing. This little dance between the forces that keep blood sugar from soaring too high and those that prevent it from going too low is essential for survival. It's interesting to note that while insulin is the only hormone responsible for preventing blood sugar from rising too high, there are several other hormones besides glucagon—cortisol, adrenaline, noradrenaline, and human growth hormone—that prevent it from going too low. Insulin is such a powerful hormone that five other hormones counterbalance its effects.

How a High-Carbohydrate Diet Raises Triglycerides

Let's follow the nutrients you eat on their journey through the body. When you eat food—any food—it mixes with acids and enzymes from the stomach, pancreas, and liver that break it down into smaller molecules. The nutrients are then absorbed through the intestinal walls, while the indigestible parts of the food pass through the digestive system as waste. Proteins break down into amino acids, carbohydrates into glucose, and fats into fatty acids. These pass through the intestinal walls into the portal vein, which is like their private passageway into the liver, the central processing plant of the body. After the liver works its magic, often repackaging these compounds into different forms, the new forms are released into the general circulation of the bloodstream, where they are transported to cells and tissues to be either used or saved for a rainy day.

As these smaller units pass through the portal vein en route to the liver, the pancreas immediately takes notice of the parade and responds by secreting our star player, insulin. It secretes *some* insulin in response to protein; but when it sees carbohydrates in the passageway, its eyes light up, and it brings out the big guns and goes to town. (Fat doesn't even rate a "hello" from the pancreas and has no impact on insulin.)

Under the influence of this incoming insulin, the liver does a number of things. First, it decides how much of the sugar coming in is excess. It makes that decision based largely on how much insulin the pancreas has decided to send along to accompany the payload. If there's a lot of insulin, the liver says, "*Woo-hoo, we've got a truckload of sugar on our hands; let's get busy.*" Some of the incoming sugar will pass right through (as glucose) to the bloodstream to be transported to muscle cells—which can use a hit of sugar now and then for energy—and to the brain, which needs sugar (or ketones, which we'll discuss in detail later) to think and do all the other good things that brains like to do. Part of the excess sugar will be converted to the storage form of glucose, called glycogen, much of which will stay right there in the liver. (Glycogen is also stored in the muscles, but muscle glycogen is like a private bank account that can be used only by the muscle in which it is stored.) The liver doesn't hold a lot of glycogen, so if there is still excess sugar, which there almost always is after a high-carbohydrate meal, it is packaged into triglycerides (fats found in the blood and in the tissues). This is how a high-carbohydrate diet raises triglycerides—a known risk factor for heart disease.

Which Is Worse, Sugar or Fat? No Contest!

Why, you may ask, does the liver feel this compelling need to get rid of the excess sugar, anyway? Why doesn't it just give it a pass and let it go into the bloodstream as is? Why create all this work for itself? Why bother to turn it into triglycerides in the first place?

That's a very good question, and the answer is central to understanding the health effects of a lower-carbohydrate diet: *sugar is far more damaging to the body than fat.* In a very real sense, what the liver is doing is *detoxifying* sugar into triglycerides.

At this point, it may start to occur to you that since sugar is made into triglycerides, then maybe one of the reasons that blood levels of triglycerides are lowered on a low-carb diet is because there's less excess sugar coming in to require packaging into triglycerides in the first place. And you'd be absolutely, 100% right. (Cholesterol sometimes comes down as well, but as you'll see later, that doesn't matter nearly as much.) This lowering of triglycerides is one of the major health benefits of a low-carb diet—high triglycerides are far more of a danger sign for heart disease than high cholesterol ever was.

You may also be thinking that the higher levels of fat that are frequently (though not always) part of low-carb diet plans may not be so bad after all, if they're not accompanied by the high insulin levels that go with high-carb diets. You'd be right on that count as well.

Insulin Prevents Fat Loss

An important thing to remember just from a weight-loss point of view is that insulin isn't only responsible for getting sugar into the cells and out of the bloodstream: it's also responsible for getting *fat* into the fat cells *and keeping it there*. Insulin actually prevents fat burning. That's why a low-carb diet usually produces more weight loss than a high-carb, low-fat diet with the same calorie count. By lowering insulin, you open the doors of the fat cells and allow the body to release fat.

One of the ways insulin interferes with fat burning is by inhibiting carnitine, an amino acid–like compound in the body that is responsible for escorting fatty acids into the little central processing units of the muscle cells, where those fats can be burned for energy. By inhibiting carnitine, insulin inhibits fat-burning. That's one reason you shouldn't eat a big meal before going to bed—the resulting high levels of insulin virtually ensure that your body will not be breaking down fat as you sleep but instead will be busy storing whatever is around in the bloodstream.

Many years ago, an American health magazine decided to run a weight-loss story on sumo wrestlers. The writers reasoned that the wrestlers knew everything there was to know about putting on weight, so if we could just learn what it was they did, we'd know what not to do if we wanted to slim down. One of the major rituals of the sumo wrestlers was eating a huge meal and then going right to bed.

So on a high-carbohydrate diet, you've got all this sugar coming into your system—because all carbs eventually break down into sugar—and your liver can basically do one of three things with it:

1. Pass it right through and send it into the bloodstream

2. Transform it into glycogen and store it (in the liver or the muscles)

3. Use it to make triglycerides

Remember, as far as your body is concerned, the most important thing is to prevent blood sugar from getting too high. Your insulin may very well be able to keep your blood sugar in the normal range, but the high level of insulin needed to do the job—plus the high levels of triglycerides and VLDLs* being created at the same time—are silently laying the foundation for future damage: you are slowly on your way to becoming overweight and/or insulin-resistant.

Insulin Resistance: The Worst Enemy of a Lean Body

Insulin resistance makes losing weight incredibly difficult and is a risk factor for heart disease and diabetes. It is not something you want, and you *can* do something about it. Here's how insulin resistance develops: the muscle cells don't want to accept any more sugar (this is especially true if you have been living a sedentary life). They say "Sorry, pal, we're full, we don't need any more, we gave at the office, see ya." Muscle cells become *resistant* to the effects of insulin. But the fat cells are still listening to insulin's song. They hear it knocking on their doors, and they say "Come on in; the water's fine!" The fat cells fill up and you begin to put on weight.

Meanwhile, back in the bloodstream, those little packages called VLDLs that we talked about earlier are carrying triglycerides around, trying to dump them. After the VLDL molecules drop off their triglyceride passengers to the tissues and the ever-expanding fat cells, most of them turn into LDL ("bad") cholesterol. (See Figure 1.)

Now you're overweight, with high triglycerides, high LDL cholesterol, and *definitely* high levels of insulin, which the pancreas keeps valiantly pumping out in order to get that sugar out of the bloodstream. From here, two scenarios are possible, neither of them good.

In one scenario, your body will continue to deposit fat where it's "intended" to go and your hardworking pancreas will keep your blood sugar from getting high enough for you to be classified as diabetic. But you will be paying the price for that with rising numbers on the scale, high levels of insulin, and the increased risk factors for heart disease that go with them. In another scenario, fat cells will "max out" their capacity to store new fat, which the body then deposits in unintended places—particularly the internal organs and skeletal muscle. (Non-alcoholic fatty liver disease—about 25% of

---

*VLDL's (very low-density lipoproteins) are another type of lipoprotein—like HDL and LDL— that traffic cholesterol through the bloodstream. VLDL's are part of the community of lipoproteins that is commonly referred to as "bad" cholesterol.

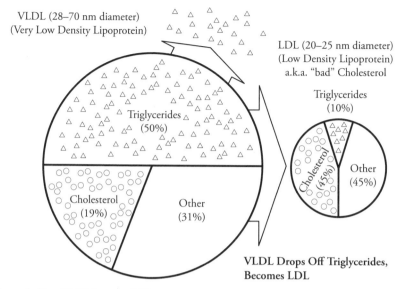

Figure 1: How VLDL becomes LDL

Americans have it—is nothing if not excess fat stored in the liver, due to too much sugar in the diet!) Once fat infiltrates the liver and muscle, it's *game on* for insulin resistance: your poor pancreas will keep chugging along for a while, secreting more and more insulin to try to compensate for the fact that the insulin in the bloodstream just isn't getting the job done anymore.

But this is an unsustainable strategy. Eventually, fat invades the pancreas as well, leading to *lipotoxicity* for insulin-secreting beta-cells—literally, poisoning them with renegade fatty acids.

When the fat-clogged pancreas can no longer keep up, sugar will rise. Now you'll have elevated insulin *and* elevated blood sugar, plus, of course, high triglycerides and abdominal obesity. If your blood sugar continues to rise even more, beyond the capacity of your insulin to reduce it, you'll eventually have full-blown type 2 diabetes.

Welcome to fast-food nation.

What's So Bad About a Little Sugar?

Obviously, the body knows how important it is to protect the tissues, the brain, and the bloodstream from excess sugar. So what exactly does sugar do that's so damaging to the body that the body is willing to risk the effects of large amounts of insulin and dangerously high levels of triglycerides just to prevent it?

Well, for one thing, excess sugar is sticky (think cotton candy and maple syrup). Proteins, on the other hand, are smooth and slippery (think oysters, which are pure protein). The slippery nature of proteins lets them slide around easily in the cells and do their jobs effectively. But when excess sugar keeps bumping into proteins, the sugar eventually gums up the works and gets stuck to the protein molecules. Such proteins are now said to have become *glycated*. The glycated proteins are too big and sticky to get through small blood vessels and capillaries, including the small vessels in the kidneys, eyes, and feet, which is why so many diabetics are at risk for kidney disease, vision problems, and amputations of toes, feet, and even legs. The sugar-coated proteins become toxic, make the cell machinery run less efficiently, damage the body, and exhaust the immune system.[4] Scientists gave these sticky proteins the acronym AGEs—which stands for advanced glycolated end-products—partially because these proteins are so involved in aging the body.

For another thing, high blood sugar is also a risk factor for cancer—cancer cells consume more glucose than normal cells do.[5] Researchers at the Harvard Medical School suggested in the early 1990s that high levels of a sugar called *galactose*, which is released by the digestion of lactose in milk, might damage the ovaries and even lead to ovarian cancer. While further study is necessary to definitively establish this link, Walter Willett, MD, DrP.H.,—chairman of the Department of Nutrition at the Harvard School of Public Health and one of the most respected researchers in the world—says: "I believe that a positive link between galactose and ovarian cancer shows up too many times to ignore the possibility that it may be harmful."[6]

Sugar depresses the immune system. A blood-sugar level of 120 reduces the phagocytic index—a measure of how well immune-system cells gobble up bacteria—by 75%.[7] Since refined sugar comes with no nutrients of its own, it uses up certain vitamin and mineral reserves of the body that are needed to metabolize it, which, in turn, throws off micronutrient balances and results in nutrient depletions.[8] (One of the minerals that refined sugar depletes is chromium, which is needed for insulin to do its job effectively! It also suppresses vitamin D levels,[9] increasing the risk of obesity and insulin resistance.[10]) Since minerals are needed for dozens of metabolic operations, these mineral deficiencies can wind up slowing down your metabolism and creating havoc with your energy level. Finally, sugar reduces HDL, the helpful, "good" cholesterol, adding yet another risk factor for heart disease to its résumé.[11]

Is it any wonder that people drastically improve their health when they switch to a diet lower in sugar?

Why Should We Care About High Levels of Insulin?

Now you understand the problems caused by high levels of sugar in the blood. But what problems are associated with high levels of *insulin?* See, insulin doesn't just bring blood sugar down and then call it a day and go home: it affects many other systems as well. Bringing in a huge amount of insulin to fix the sugar problem is like importing twenty thousand workers to fix a broken power plant in a city. The city can't run efficiently without electricity—hospitals are in danger, computers shut down, there's no public transportation, and you can't cook. So the prime order of business is to fix the emergency. At first, city officials aren't thinking about the effect of that influx of workers on the *rest* of the city's business; they just want to get the immediate problem fixed. Yet all those workers are going to have a major impact: the roads will be overcrowded, pollution will increase, crime may go up, and there will be additional demands for housing and food. But the city is faced with a life-and-death situation, so it imports however many people are needed to fix the problem. The same thing happens when the body produces high levels of insulin to cope with high blood sugar: damn the torpedoes, full steam ahead—the body will worry about the consequences later.

Insulin and Heart Disease

One of insulin's many effects on the body is to make the walls of the arteries thicker. It does this by encouraging growth and proliferation of the muscle cells that line those artery walls. Insulin also makes the walls stiffer, reducing the "flow space" inside and increasing blood pressure. Smaller arteries are also more prone to plaque.

Numerous studies have shown a hand-in-hand relationship between elevated insulin and high LDL cholesterol (the so-called "bad" cholesterol) in the blood. But despite what you may have heard, we don't really care about that until that LDL becomes damaged (oxidized) and then gets deposited on the lining of the artery walls. *Now* we have something to worry about. Damaged LDL attracts cells called macrophages, little Pac-Man–like creatures that come out to feast on the LDL like sharks on a bleeding carcass. When LDL is not damaged, the macrophages leave it alone, but as soon as damage occurs, the macrophages zoom in and feed, gorging themselves until they're full, at which point they're called "foam cells."

These foam cells group together and make a fatty streak, the first step in the formation of plaque.

How does the LDL get damaged in the first place? By two processes—*oxidation,* the interaction with oxygen that produces the same kind of "rusting" damage you see when you leave a cut apple out in the air; and *glycation,* bumping into sticky sugar. We just discussed how glycosylated proteins cause all sorts of damage in the body. This same process of glycation damages LDL, and damaged LDL attracts macrophages like red flags attract bulls.

So insulin increases the amount of LDL in the system, and excess sugar damages the LDL, leading ultimately to plaque. If this were not enough to increase your risk for heart disease, you're also going to have lowered levels of magnesium, a mineral that is absolutely essential for the health of the heart. Why is your magnesium level lowered? Because insulin, in addition to storing sugar and fat in the cells, is also responsible for storing magnesium, so when your cells become resistant to insulin, you lose the ability to store some of that magnesium. Magnesium relaxes muscles, including those in the arterial walls. When you can't store magnesium, you lose it and your blood vessels constrict, causing a further increase in blood pressure. The loss of magnesium can also lead to heart arrhythmia and other cardiac problems.[12] And because magnesium is required for virtually all energy production that takes place in the cells, you may also find yourself with lower energy to boot.

How Does a Low-Carb Diet Lower Your Risk of Heart Disease?

There are numerous ways in which a low-carb diet can significantly lower your risk for heart disease. Lowering your insulin levels is certainly one of the most important. Raising your HDL ("good" cholesterol) is another. A third—the importance of which it is difficult to overstate—is by lowering triglycerides. Researchers from the cardiovascular divisions of Brigham and Women's Hospital and Harvard Medical School, in a study led by J. Michael Gaziano, looked at various predictors for heart disease and found that the ratio of triglycerides to HDL was a better predictor for heart disease than anything else, *including* cholesterol levels. They divided the subjects into four groups according to their ratio of triglycerides to HDL and found that those with the highest ratio (i.e., high triglycerides to low HDL) had *a sixteen times greater risk of heart attack* than those with the lowest ratio (low triglycerides to high HDL).[13]

There's more. Most of us are familiar with "good" cholesterol (HDL) and "bad" cholesterol (LDL), but what is not as well known is that both types of cholesterol have subparts that behave very differently from one another. What *kind* of LDL you have, and—even more significantly—the actual number of LDL particles in your blood, turns out to be much more important metric than total LDL levels or even LDL particle size. (Several LDL-"particle tests" are now widely available. These tests tell you and your doctor your *total particle number*, and also identify a number of other factors that go way beyond the simple "good" and "bad" cholesterol test.)

For example, LDL cholesterol comes in two basic flavors: it can be a big, fluffy, cotton ball–like molecule (LDL-A type), carrying lots of cholesterol per particle; or it can be more like a dense, tight, BB-gun pellet (LDL-B type), carrying less cholesterol per particle. Think of it like two different ways to transport cargo (aka cholesterol): you can stack that cargo in a couple of semi-trucks (LDL-A type), or stuff it into a whole fleet of passenger cars (LDL-B type). Both vehicles will get the job done, but you'll need quite a few passenger cars to accomplish what a single semi can do.

When it comes to cholesterol tests, there are two ways of looking at this whole cargo–vehicle situation: we can calculate how much total cargo is coasting down the road at a given moment (standard LDL-C tests); or we can count how many vehicles—and what kind—are out there shuttling that cargo around (LDL-particle count and particle size tests).

Standard LDL-C tests—the kind that have been used for decades by scientists studying cholesterol and heart disease—tell us nothing about the vehicle, only the total cargo. And, as it turns out, the total cargo is the *least* important part of the puzzle!

Here's why. For one, the big, fluffy LDL-A's are associated with much lower heart-disease risk than their little LDL-B brethren. The science is still fuzzy about whether this is due to their larger size (which seems to reduce their likelihood of becoming oxidized or damaged and causing problems), or due to the fact that the larger the LDL particle, the fewer there tend to be in the blood (which means there are fewer "vehicles" to crash through the endothelium and begin the process of atherosclerosis). But for now, one thing's for sure: if big LDL-A's dominate your lipid profile, you're most likely stationed at the lower end of the risk curve. Go ahead and breathe a well-earned sigh of relief. (And keep in mind, a high number of predominantly small LDL particles or a lower number of predominantly large LDL particles can both yield the *same results* on a standard LDL-C test, since only their "total cargo" is calculated. As a result, these tests can easily scare someone with lots of cargo from large

LDL-semis into thinking they're about to keel over, and give a false sense of security to someone with less cargo but lots of little LDL passenger sedans cruising around and causing trouble.)

At any rate, the little LDL-B's are the ones that cause problems, and those are the ones you should be concerned about. The Gaziano study found that high triglycerides correlate strongly with high levels of the dangerous LDL-B particles, and low levels of triglycerides correlate with higher levels of the larger LDL-A's. In other words, the higher your triglycerides, the greater the chance that your LDL cholesterol is made up of the B-particles (the kind that is more strongly associated with heart disease). The take-home point: reduce your triglycerides (and raise your HDL), and you reduce your risk of heart disease.

Insulin and Hypertension

As you saw in the previous paragraphs on heart disease, high levels of insulin can narrow the arterial walls which, in turn, will raise blood pressure, since a more forceful pumping action is required to get the blood through the narrower passageways. But there's an even more insidious way in which insulin raises blood pressure.

It talks to the kidneys.

Insulin's message to the kidneys is this: *hold on to salt.* Insulin makes the kidneys do this even if the kidneys would much prefer not to. Since sodium, like sugar, is controlled by the body within a very tight range, the kidneys figure "Listen, if we have to hold on to all this salt, we'd better bring on more water to dilute it so that it stays in the safe range." And that's exactly what they do. Increased sodium retention results in increased water retention. More fluid means more blood volume, and more blood volume means higher blood pressure. Fully 50% of people with hypertension have insulin resistance.[14]

Insulin will also ultimately raise adrenaline, and adrenaline will raise both blood pressure and heart rate. We'll discuss the insulin–adrenaline axis a little more under the topic of obesity in the next section.

How Does a Low-Carb Diet Lower Your Risk of Hypertension?

Lowering insulin levels will intercept the message to the kidneys to hold on to salt. You will almost immediately lose water weight, and bloat and blood pressure will go down. Lowering insulin is actually such an effective strategy for lowering blood pressure that it sometimes works too well too fast. In rare cases, your blood pressure might dip too low, and you may experience lightheadedness or dizziness upon standing up. This is why some clinicians recommend increasing salty foods or adding a teaspoon of salt to your food on a daily basis if you find this happening to you.[14]

When the kidneys dump excess sodium, potassium sometimes gets caught in the crossfire and you wind up dumping potassium as well. This is even truer if you exercise and sweat a lot. You don't want to lose too much potassium, because that can cause muscle cramps, fatigue, and breathlessness. This is why I always recommend potassium supplements, especially during the first week of a low-carb diet, and particularly when you are on one of the very restricted carbohydrate plans such as the induction phase of Atkins or the first 2 weeks of Protein Power. Potassium supplements come in 99-milligram tablets, and you can get them at any drugstore or health-food store. Take one or two at each meal. Foods rich in potassium, such as liver, broccoli, and avocados, are also a good idea, as is using over-the-counter salt substitutes like Morton's Lite Salt or No Salt, which are both potassium salts.

Insulin and Obesity

The connection between a high-sugar diet, high levels of insulin, and becoming overweight or obese should be painfully obvious by now. The more sugar—i.e., carbohydrates—you take in, the more sugar you need to store and the more your insulin levels rise. The more your insulin levels rise, the less fat you burn and the more sugar you store in fat cells, along with those extra triglycerides that the liver made from excess sugar. The more you store, the fatter you get. The fatter you get, the more insulin-resistant you become.

When there are consistently high levels of insulin floating around, the body will put out more cortisol and adrenaline (the "breakdown" hormones) to counteract the "building-up" effects of insulin and attempt to bring the body back into balance. Cortisol in part breaks down muscle, further reducing your metabolic rate. Too much adrenaline can eventually lead to even *more* insulin, as insulin will eventually be secreted to combat the effects of too much adrenaline!

Even if you don't remember the basic biochemistry discussed here, tattoo the following on the inside of your eyelids: *insulin is the fat-storage hormone*. It is also the hunger hormone. When it finally does its job of lowering blood sugar, it causes blood sugar to go really low, setting you up for a cycle of craving (and eating) more high-carb foods. Result: higher blood sugar, more insulin, and more fat storage as the cycle continues.

How Does a Low-Carb Diet Help You Lose Weight?

When you eat a lower-carb diet, you stimulate less insulin, but you also stimulate more glucagon, its sister hormone, which responds more to protein (remember that neither hormone is stimulated by fat). Glucagon liberates the fat from storage sites and gets it ready to burn for energy. Meanwhile, since you no longer have elevated levels of insulin, you are not suppressing carnitine, which, you may remember, is the compound in the body responsible for escorting fat into the central furnaces of the cells, where it can be burned for fuel.

Along with insulin and glucagon, a pair of enzymes plays a major role in the whole fat-storage/fat-release equation: *lipoprotein lipase* and *hormone-sensitive lipase*. Lipoprotein lipase is responsible for storing fats: it breaks down triglycerides in the bloodstream and shoves the fatty-acid parts into fat cells. People who are trying to lose weight are not fond of this enzyme. It's very persistent; in fact, when people lose weight, the activity of lipoprotein lipase is ramped up, almost as if the body is fighting to hold on to fat. This is one of the reasons it's so difficult to keep weight off. (Lipoprotein lipase is also suppressed when you smoke and increases when you stop smoking, one of the reasons people usually put on a few pounds when they first give up cigarettes.)

Hormone-sensitive lipase, on the other hand, reaches into fat cells and releases fatty acids into the bloodstream when they are needed—for example, if you're doing a long aerobic exercise session and your legs need some fuel. Its ability to liberate fat is really intense. Consider this: there's a protein called *perilipin* that shields fat from the fat-burning effects of hormone-sensitive lipase. Mice that don't have any perilipin to protect their fat from hormone-sensitive lipase don't get fat, no matter what they eat![16] The fat-burning effect of hormone-sensitive lipase is that intense.

Insulin and glucagon have profound effects on both lipoprotein lipase and hormone-sensitive lipase. Can you guess what effects they have? By now, it should come as no surprise: insulin *stimulates* lipoprotein lipase (the fat-storing enzyme) and *inhibits* hormone-sensitive lipase (the fat-releasing enzyme). If you want your fat cells to let go of fat, you want all the hormone-sensitive lipase activity you can scrounge up—you certainly don't need high levels of insulin turning down the volume. Glucagon, on the other hand, has exactly the opposite effect on these enzymes. It *inhibits* the fat-storing enzyme and *stimulates* the fat-releasing one. This is just one more way that restoring a healthy balance between insulin and glucagon helps you to lose weight.

Fat Cells Know How to Protect Their Existence!

When you do lose weight, you stack the hormonal deck in your favor even more. We used to believe that fat cells were these inert little sacks of blubber that basically didn't do anything metabolically—they just took up space and held on to a gazillion calories' worth of energy that never got burned up fast enough. We now know that fat cells are anything *but* inactive. They are actually endocrine glands that releases a host of hormones—including estrogen—and other substances that can have a profound effect on our weight.

Many of the hormones that are released by the fat cells have one major purpose—to keep those fat cells in business! In this way, you might say that fat actually perpetuates its own existence by releasing hormones that make it harder for the body to get rid of it.

One of the hormones released by fat cells is *resistin*. The more fat cells you have, the more resistin gets released into your body. Mice given extra dosages of resistin develop insulin resistance in 2 days;[17] and, as we've just seen, insulin resistance is a major obstacle to fat loss. Another substance released by the fat cells is TNF-alpha 1, also known as tumor necrosis factor. This is a good guy, at least some of the time: it's part of the immune system's arsenal, and, as you can tell by the name, it's involved in destroying tumors. But TNF-alpha 1 is also found in fat tissue, and in the circulatory system it appears to act like a hormone. In low amounts, it *inhibits* the ability of insulin to lower blood sugar, essentially making insulin's job harder to accomplish and thereby forcing the pancreas to put out even more insulin to get the job done.[18] Once again, a hormone-like compound released by the fat cells raises insulin and makes fat loss difficult. As you can see, the fat cells *themselves* contribute to the difficulty in losing weight by releasing substances that offer "fat-protection insurance"— chemicals that, in essence, help your fat cells stay in business. By lowering your fat stores with a low-carbohydrate diet, you will also lower the amounts of these fat-protecting substances in the bloodstream.

A Low-Carb Diet Helps Reduce Insulin Resistance

When you are insulin-resistant, your cells stop making insulin receptors to import sugar and fat into the cells. This process is called down-regulation.

Receptors are like job recruiters. When the market is flooded with unemployed workers, companies don't have to go hunting for job applicants, because there are so many knocking at the door. When you're insulin-resistant, you've got a hell of a lot of insulin—applicants—knocking at the cell door. The cells figure there's enough insulin hanging around, beating on the doors, so they stop sending "recruiters" to the surface of the cells. When you bring your insulin down with a low-carb diet, suddenly there's not so much insulin banging at the doors of the cells. Now you begin to lose weight. Eventually, the cells start to send up more receptors to bring in the fuel, a process called up-regulation. The cells are now gradually becoming more insulin-*sensitive*—a condition you most decidedly want. Insulin sensitivity always improves when you lose weight.

There are other ways in which a low-carb lifestyle will help you lose weight. One way has to do specifically with protein itself, which is usually more plentiful on lower-carb diets. Protein has less of an effect on insulin, has a greater effect on glucagon, and increases metabolic rate considerably more than carbohydrates do. Specific amino acids found in protein may also play a role in weight loss. Several papers by D.K. Layman demonstrated greater body-fat loss on a high-protein diet than on a high-carb diet,[19] and in one paper he argued that *leucine*—an amino acid—may be one of the reasons.[20] Other studies have also suggested the possible role of specific amino acids in weight loss. In one animal study, a diet deficient in the amino acid lysine resulted in the accumulation of larger amounts of fat both in the bodies of the animals and in their livers.[21] Increasing the proportion of protein to carbohydrates appears to be more *satiating* during weight loss—it makes you feel fuller.[22] And metabolic rate, technically called thermogenesis—the heat production in our bodies from burning calories—is turned up after eating protein. In one study, thermogenesis was 100% higher with high-protein meals—even 2½ hours after eating—in young, healthy women.[23]

You may have heard that it is easier to stay on a low-carb diet than it is to stay on a traditional high-carb, low-fat diet. Let me say one word about that: *appetite*. A low-carb diet contains built-in appetite controls—it's like having your own little diet pill built into the meals. Here's how it works. One of the major hormones involved in telling the brain that you are full is *cholecystokinin* (CCK), which is secreted in the intestines in response to a meal. (You may also have heard, correctly, that it takes about 20 minutes for this hormone to reach your brain and tell you you've had enough—another reason to listen to your grandmother and eat slowly if you want to lose weight!) But here's the thing: CCK, being part of our ancient digestive system, recognizes protein and fat very well because they've been the mainstay of our diet for as long as the human genus has been on the planet. But CCK does *not* respond very well to carbohydrates. It barely recognizes them! That's why it is so easy to overeat carbs—you really have no idea when you've had enough.

Insulin Resistance and Diabetes

Insulin resistance is a huge risk factor for the development of both heart disease and diabetes.[24] Eighty percent of the 30 million Americans who have diabetes are insulin-resistant.[25] Dr. David Leonardi, founder of the Leonardi Medical Institute for Vitality and Longevity in Denver, insists that insulin resistance is reversible and that many type 2 diabetics can be cured. He says: "Diabetics die from *diabetes complications, all of which are a direct or indirect result of high blood sugar.* Normalizing the blood sugar prevents disease, normalizes life expectancy, and profoundly enhances quality of life. Cured or not, they're winners either way."

In case you hadn't noticed by now, low-carb diets are all about normalizing blood sugar. Insulin resistance *is* reversible. And it's hardly a rare phenomenon. According to the CDC,[26] more than 100 million Americans now have diabetes or pre-diabetes—insulin resistance is a central feature of both. The prevalence of insulin resistance among adolescents is an astonishing 52%,[27] with obesity being the primary driver. And let's remember that roughly 25% of the 30 million or so diabetics in America are walking around undiagnosed. According to the findings of the National Diabetes Statistics Report, nearly one in four adults living with diabetes—7.2 million Americans—didn't know they had the condition. Only 11.6 percent of adults with prediabetes knew they had it.[28]

In fact, the prevalence of insulin resistance has probably been underestimated from the beginning. Gerald Reaven of Stanford University did the original work on insulin resistance in the 1980s. Here's how he approximated the number of people who were insulin-resistant: he divided his test population—nondiabetic, healthy adults—into quartiles and tested their ability to metabolize sugar and carbohydrates. He found that while the top 25% of the population could handle sugar just fine, the bottom 25% could not—they had insulin resistance (or, in the parlance of researchers, impaired glucose metabolism). So for a long time, it was thought that the number of people with insulin resistance was one in four.

But there's a problem.

What happened to the 50% of the people *between* those two extremes? It turns out they had neither the terrific glucose metabolism of the top

DIABETES AND COMPLICATIONS

- *1.5 million people are newly diagnosed with diabetes every year.* *
- *The overwhelming majority of type 2 diabetics are insulin-resistant.*
- *Diabetes is the seventh leading cause of death in the United States.* [†]
- *About half of all diabetics have nerve damage.* [‡]
- *Vascular disease—including diabetes— is the leading cause of lower-extremity amputations in the United States.* [§]
- *In the United States, about 73,000 amputations a year are related to complications from diabetes.* **
- *Adults with diabetes are nearly twice as likely to die of heart disease or stroke.* [††]
- *Diabetes and high blood pressure are the leading causes of kidney failure, representing 3 out of 4 new cases.* [‡‡]
- *Diabetic retinopathy is a leading cause of new cases of blindness in adults.* [§§]

*http://www.diabetes.org/diabetes-basics/statistics/

† https://www.healthline.com/health/leading-causes-of-death

‡ http://www.diabetes.org/living-with-diabetes/complications/neuropathy/

§ https://www.amputee-coalition.org/resources/limb-loss-statistics/

**https://www.azuravascularcare.com/infopad/diabetic-foot-amputation-stats/

†† https://www.niddk.nih.gov/health-information/diabetes/overview/preventing
-problems/heart-disease-stroke

‡‡https://www.cdc.gov/kidneydisease/basics.html

§§https://www.preventblindness.org/millions-diabetes-and-prediabetes-risk
-vision-loss-and-blindness

25% nor the full-blown insulin resistance of the bottom 25%; instead, they fell somewhere in between. One could easily argue that since only 25% of the population had flawless glucose metabolism, the rest of us—up to 75% of the population—have *some* degree of insulin resistance! Remember, too, that Reaven used young, healthy adults as subjects, and their numbers are obviously not representative of the population as a whole: the fact is, insulin sensitivity actually decreases as you get older.

The take-home point: insulin resistance isn't something that just happens to other people. Recently, the American Association of Clinical Endocrinologists estimated that one in three Americans is insulin-resistant.[29]

As of 2015, there were approximately 30 million diabetics in the United States, of which 7 million are not yet diagnosed.[30] Approximately 80% of them are insulin-resistant. Even if you are insulin-resistant and somehow manage to dodge the diabetes bullet, you are still at serious risk for heart disease. Being overweight (having a body mass index of greater than 25 or a waistline of greater than 40 inches for men and 35 inches for women) is a risk factor for insulin resistance—a big one. So are hypertension (high blood pressure), elevated triglycerides, and low-HDL cholesterol.[31] It's estimated that 47 million Americans have some combination of these risk factors.[32] As you have seen in this chapter, all of them are related to insulin, and virtually *all of them improve substantially on a low-carbohydrate diet.*

How a Low-Carb Diet May Help Prevent— or Even Reverse—Diabetes

Dietary treatment for diabetes is currently one of the hottest topics of debate in the diabetes community.[33] Some factions are passionately holding on to the old recommendations of a high-carb diet, while other clinicians are making strenuous arguments for lower-carb, higher-fat, higher-protein diets.[34] The precise dietary treatment for full-blown type 2 diabetes is beyond the scope of this book, though it is a fascinating subject and in my opinion has great relevance for nondiabetics as well. What can we say for sure? A number of studies have shown that people on low-carbohydrate diets experience increased glucose control, reduced insulin resistance, weight reduction, lowered triglycerides, and improved cholesterol.

Excess Insulin and PCOS

One in ten women has polycystic ovary syndrome (PCOS), the most common reproductive abnormality in premenopausal women, which puts them at high risk for both cardiovascular disease and diabetes.[35] One of the major biochemical features of PCOS is the combination of insulin resistance and hyperinsulinemia (elevated insulin levels). The ability of obese women with PCOS to use glucose is significantly impaired, and they have a marked reduction in insulin sensitivity.[36]

When we talk about insulin resistance, we often forget that not all tissues and cells become resistant at the same time, and some do not become resistant at all. For example, overweight people may—at least in the begin-ning—have very nonresistant fat cells. Their muscle cells refuse to take any more sugar, but the fat cells still have open arms. These cells are said to be insulin-sensitive. The ovaries also tend to remain insulin-sensitive.

If there's a genetic predisposition for these glands to overproduce androgen hormones—as there is with women who have PCOS—the excess insulin that's sent into the bloodstream to deal with the excess sugar bathes these nonresistant tissues in an ocean of insulin that is way too much for their needs. One of the responses to all that insulin hitting the ovaries is that they produce even more testosterone and androstene, which leads to hair loss, acne, obesity, infertility, and other symptoms of PCOS.

Interestingly, those affected with PCOS often have relatives with adult onset diabetes, obesity, elevated triglycerides, and high blood pressure.[37] Sound familiar? This is why a low-carb diet is the dietary treatment of choice for PCOS.

Excess Insulin and Inflammation

Essential fatty acids, notably omega-6 and omega-3, are the parent molecules for an entirely different group of fascinating hormones called *eicosanoids*. Eicosanoids, also known as *prostaglandins*, live in the body for only seconds and act on the cells that are in their immediate vicinity—they don't travel in the bloodstream. They are very, very powerful modulators of human health. Like many other systems in the body, they need to be in balance. Sometimes, as a shorthand, we'll talk about "good" eicosanoids (the prosta-glandin 1 series, or PG1), which inhibit clotting, promote vasodilation (the relaxing of the blood vessels), stimulate the immune response, and are anti-inflammatory, versus the "bad" eicosanoids (the prostaglandin 2 series, or PG2), which have the opposite effects, promoting clotting, constriction, and inflammation. But this shorthand is not completely accurate, as you need a *balance* of the two. For example, if you clot too much and too easily, you can have a stroke, but if you didn't clot at all, you'd bleed to death from a hemorrhage!

Here, too, insulin leaves its mighty footprint. Insulin inhibits a critical enzyme called *delta-6-desaturase*, which is responsible for directing traffic into the production line for the "good," anti-inflammatory eicosanoids. Inflammation has been implicated in a host of conditions, from heart disease to Alzheimer's to arthritis to food allergies. In fact, the modulation of insulin for the purpose of controlling eicosanoid production and

LOW-GLYCEMIC DIET AND DIABETES

Low-glycemic foods—beans, peas, lentils, pasta, rice boiled briefly, and breads like pumpernickel and flaxseed—do a better job of managing glycemic control for type 2 diabetes and risk factors for coronary heart disease than diets based around the "traditional" high-fiber foods such as whole-grain breads, crackers, and breakfast cereals.

That's the finding of a 2008 study published in the *Journal of the American Medical Association.*[*]

Although the American Dietetic Association continues to mindlessly parrot the "conventional" wisdom about whole-grain breads and cereals, the truth is that most of these whole-grain products are fiber lightweights. (Read the label—whole grains typically offer 1–2 grams of fiber at best, compared to 11–17 in a cup of beans.) And if you check the glycemic index/glycemic load tables, you find that the difference between a processed grain like white rice and its whole-grain counterpart (brown rice) is—from a *blood-sugar* point of view—almost negligible.

Obviously, whole grains are better than white junk, but only because they contain slightly more vitamins and other nutrients. From a blood-sugar—and from a food-sensitivity or allergy—standpoint, they're not that much of an improvement. If you've got a gluten sensitivity—which is way more common than you might think—whole grains will be just as much a problem for you as the processed kind.

In the JAMA study, researchers found that hemoglobin A1c—a very important marker for diabetes—decreased *significantly* more in subjects on the low-glycemic group than it did for people eating the "traditional high-fiber" choices with cereal fiber. The low-glycemic group also saw a significant *increase* in HDL (the so-called "good" cholesterol) as well as a significant *reduction* in LDL (the so-called "bad" cholesterol).

The low-glycemic group did eat some breads—like pumpernickel, rye pita, and quinoa bread with flaxseed—and some cereals—like real oatmeal—but they were all low-glycemic.

Bottom line: just because a cereal or bread product says "made with whole grains" *doesn't* mean it's the best food for you. Many of these products raise your blood sugar to a level that is way too high,

---

[*] David J. Jenkins, Cyril W. Kendall, Gail McKeown-Eyssen, et al., "Effect of a low-glycemic index or a high-cereal fiber diet on type 2 diabetes." *Journal of the American Medical Association* 300 (2008): 2742–2753.

and manufacturers are notorious at trading on the "whole grain" buzz to create ridiculous products like "whole grain Cocoa Captain Sugar Krispies" (I made that one up, but you get the point).

Glycemic impact is very important and should be paid attention to by anyone interested in his or her health. And you don't have to walk around with a bunch of scientific formulas to figure out whether a food has high or low glycemic impact: just look for foods that have minimal processing, maximum color (the exceptions are oatmeal, cauliflower, and chicken), and as much fiber as possible.

reducing the risk of heart disease was the major reason for the development of the Zone diet by Barry Sears. If you're interested in learning more about this diet, be sure to read about it in chapter 9.

Excess Insulin and Aging

"If there is a single marker for life span," asserts Dr. Ron Rosedale, creator of the Rosedale Diet (see chapter 9), "it's insulin sensitivity."[38] He's right. In 1992, researchers collected data on people who were both mentally and physically fit and were at least 100 years old. The researchers looked carefully to find the factors these folks might have in common, the ones that could be predictors for a long and healthy life. They came up with three. The first was low triglycerides. The second was high HDL cholesterol. Can you guess the third? A low level of fasting insulin![39] You've learned in this chapter how a lower-carbohydrate diet almost always improves all three of these variables. Since this kind of diet is what our ancestors ate for eons, it makes sense that we would live the longest and stay the healthiest by adhering to it.

By the way, the only dietary strategy shown to actually *increase* life span in laboratory animals has been calorie restriction. When we humans try calorie restriction on a standard high-carb, low-fat diet, we generally hate it—we're hungry all the time. With a diet higher in protein, higher in fat, and lower in carbohydrates—and high in fiber—we're more satiated and our appetite is much more under control. Insulin—the hunger hormone—is no longer out of control, blood sugar is manageable, and weight becomes stabilized. We can actually wind up eating fewer calories and feeling more satisfied in the bargain. That's a recipe for an anti-aging, health-producing diet *without* creating cravings or hunger pangs.

How a Low-Carb Diet Keeps You Healthy and Slim

We've talked about what sugar does to the body and why eliminating it is such a good idea. Obviously, a low-carb diet removes a great deal, if not all, of the refined sugar you've probably been eating. The health benefits of this reduction are enormous. But a low-carb diet can also remove three other substances

> After learning of the dangers of trans-fats, I began avoiding fast-food lunches—it's better for me and my kids.
> —Gina D.

that are a huge problem, albeit for very different reasons. One is trans-fats. The other two are wheat and fructose. (The latter two are discussed at length in chapter 4).

The subject of trans-fatty acids has been the center of a great deal of debate in the area of public policy regarding food and food labeling. It has been discussed extensively elsewhere, particularly in the writings of Dr. Mary Enig, a lipid biochemist who, before passing away in 2014, was widely considered to be the leading authority on trans-fats in the country, if not the world. For now, let's just say that, in the opinion of many experts, saturated fats have gotten a raw deal and have in fact been blamed for damage done, for the most part, by trans-fats. We know that trans-fats raise LDL cholesterol, probably way more than saturated fats do, and that these damaged trans-fats actually *increase* the risk for type 2 diabetes.[40] They also lower HDL cholesterol and raise the risk for heart disease. A prediction was made in the prestigious medical journal *Lancet* as far back as 1994 that trans-fats would turn out to be a major factor in insulin resistance;[41] that was the same year that the Center for Science in the Public Interest petitioned the FDA to require that Nutrition Facts labels disclose amounts of trans-fat. On July 10, 2002, the National Academy of Science's Institute of Medicine issued a report that concluded that "the only safe intake of trans-fats is *zero*." After much hemming, hawing, and stalling, the FDA finally mandated that trans-fat content be listed on food nutrition labels, a ruling that went into effect in 2006.

The intelligent low-carb diet is almost *always* naturally low in trans-fats, which may be one of the many reasons it can impart such health benefits. Consider this: the top sources of trans-fats are baked goods, muffins, cakes, cookies, doughnuts, granolas, crackers, pies, fast food, French fries, anything deep-fried, partially hydrogenated vegetable oils,

SENIOR MOMENT?
MAYBE IT'S YOUR BLOOD SUGAR!

Is the phrase "I'm having one of those senior moments" becoming an increasingly common utterance?

Research suggests that it might be related to your sugar levels.

The research, published in the December 2008 *Annals of Neurology*,[*] focused on a particular section of the hippocampus—an area of the brain associated with memory and learning. This section—the *dentate gyrus*—is typically affected by changes seen with aging.

"In this study, we were able to show the specific area of the brain that is impacted by rising blood sugar," said Scott Small, MD, the lead researcher on the study, which was partly funded by the National Institute on Aging. Using special high-resolution brain imaging, Small and his team found that rising blood sugar was directly associated with decreased activity in the dentate gyrus.

The result: you forget where you put your keys!

The important point here is that the research strongly suggests that keeping blood sugar under control could be the key to preventing "senior moments" and lapses in memory, even in healthy individuals with no hint of diabetes!

"Our findings suggest that maintaining blood sugar levels, even in the absence of diabetes, could help maintain aspects of cognitive health," said Small.

Two of the most effective measures to manage blood sugar are exercise and a controlled-carb diet!

[*] S. A. Small, *Annals of Neurology*, December 2008; online edition.

and most margarines. The intelligent low-carb diet naturally contains almost none of these foods—or, it does, they are present in extraordinarily low amounts. The health benefits of this restriction alone are incalculable.

The other ingredient that is either missing in action or has an extremely low profile on the low-carb diet is wheat. Now, most people are probably under the impression that wheat and grains are "good" for you. Maybe; maybe not. Certainly, foods made with whole grains—which are far harder to find than you might think and most certainly do *not* include most commercially available "wheat breads"—are better than foods made with the refined grains that constitute the vast majority of the grains we eat. But grains, particularly wheat, have a high propensity for turning into sugar quickly, and wheat is also one of the foods most likely to be implicated in food sensitivities.[42] At one point, it was believed that celiac disease—an intolerance of gluten, which is found in most grains—was fairly rare, affecting only 1 in 1,700 people. Estimates are now running closer to 1 in 133; for those who have a parent, sibling, or child with celiac, the estimates are 1 in 22![43] And this doesn't include the hard-to-estimate number of people who have delayed food sensitivities, very often to grains in general or, at the very least, to wheat. A 2002 book by clinician James Braly, MD, suggests that gluten insensitivity may affect tens of millions of Americans.[44]

Dr. Joseph Mercola, medical director of the Optimal Wellness Center in Illinois, contends that grains—along with starches and sweets—trigger a "hormonal cycle of grain and sugar addiction, weight gain, and diabetes."[45] And numerous studies link carbohydrates that have a high glycemic load—the tendency to turn into sugar quickly—with increased risk of coronary heart disease[46] and with risk of type 2 diabetes.[47] Most high-glycemic processed grains fall into this category, but these grains are virtually eliminated on low-carbohydrate diets.

Insulin: The Smoking Gun

Controlling insulin is the number one priority of all low-carb diets. The dietary approaches discussed in chapter 5 differ only in how they go about accomplishing this—what degree of carbohydrate restriction they believe is necessary to successfully control insulin, whether they emphasize protein or fat (or both) in the diet, what kinds of fat they recommend, other aspects of metabolism they stress, and whether they include a component on emotional eating and holistic self-care.

Once you understand what runaway insulin levels and unregulated sugar metabolism in general can do to your health, it's easy to understand why correcting those imbalances brings about not only weight loss but a myriad of wonderful health benefits.

In chapter 9, we'll explore exactly how a number of popular diet plans approach the issue of insulin control, and you'll be able to determine which one is best for you. But first, let's talk a little more about wheat and fructose. Then we'll dispel a few myths about fat, cholesterol, and health.

HORMONES AND WEIGHT:
A SHORT GUIDE TO THE PLAYERS

Insulin: *lowers blood sugar*

Also known as "the fat-storage hormone," insulin is secreted by the pancreas in response to elevated blood sugar. Its job is to escort the excess sugar into the muscles, where it can be burned for fuel. High levels of insulin effectively "lock" the doors to the fat cells by blocking glucagon (described next), whose job it is to open the fat cells and allow fatty acids to enter the bloodstream.

Glucagon: *raises blood sugar*

Like insulin, glucagon is secreted by the pancreas. But, unlike insulin, it's secreted in response to low blood sugar, and it has an opposite effect—it raises blood sugar instead of lowering it. Sensing that blood sugar is low, glucagon prompts the release of sugar (glucose) from the liver as well as the release of free fatty acids from fat stores. Glucagon is stimulated by decreased blood sugar (hunger); it's inhibited by high levels of insulin.

Leptin: *tells the brain you're full*

Leptin is a hormone produced by the fat cells in the body. When things are working as they should, leptin travels to the brain while you are finishing up your meal, where it sends a message that the body is full and it's time to stop eating. In this way, it's essential to appetite regulation and plays a major part in minimizing the desire for food. Scientists originally believed that obese people simply didn't produce enough leptin, but research in the '90s showed that this wasn't the case at all. Obese people make plenty of leptin, but their brains aren't getting the message to stop eating. The leptin is there, but the brain cells are simply not "listening." In a very real sense, they have become leptin-resistant. High-carb diets, fructose, high triglycerides, and inflammation all contribute to leptin resistance.

Cortisol: *puts fat around the middle*

Cortisol is the main "stress" hormone produced by the body. It's a crucial hormone and necessary for survival. But high levels of cortisol—

produced by chronic stress, intense physical activity, and sleep deprivation—prompt the body to store fat around the middle, even in relatively lean people. Cortisol also breaks down muscle, raises blood sugar, and increases insulin-resistance.

Resistin: *makes you more insulin-resistant*

Resistin is a hormone produced by the fat cells. It gets its name from the fact that it helps cause the condition known as "insulin resistance," which is a key player in obesity and diabetes. Insulin resistance is the name for the condition in which the cells have stopped "listening" to insulin, resulting in higher levels of blood sugar and insulin (both very bad news if you're trying to lose weight). Resistin is one of the ways fat cells protect their own existence. The more fat cells you have, the more resistin is produced, the more insulin-resistant you become, and the harder it is to lose weight.

Adiponectin: *makes you less insulin-resistant*

Adiponectin makes the cells more sensitive to insulin (i.e., it reduces insulin resistance). It's secreted by the fat cells. Low levels of it are found in people who are obese; high levels are associated with a reduced risk of heart attack and type 2 diabetes.

Ghrelin: *makes you hungry*

Ghrelin, also known as "the hunger hormone," is an appetite stimulant. When we're hungry, ghrelin levels go up. They also go up when we're stressed or sleep-deprived. This is one reason why sleep disturbance often leads to overeating and why you'll eat anything in sight after pulling an all-nighter.

Neuropeptide Y (NPY): *makes you hungry*

Neuropeptide Y stimulates appetite, especially for carbohydrates, and is elevated by chronic stress, low protein intake, and high-carb diets.

Peptide YY (PYY): *makes you stop eating*

This hormone sends a message to the brain that says "stop eating." Protein stimulates a lot of PYY; carbs release very little. (This is why your bagel breakfast leaves you starving at 11 A.M.) PYY also improves sensitivity to leptin.

Glucagon-like peptide-1 (GLP-1): *makes you stop eating*

This hormone's message is similar to that of leptin (see earlier entry): it sends a message to the brain that says "stop eating." It is released by the small intestine after you eat. GLP-1 levels are inversely correlated with body mass, meaning higher levels are associated with less body fat. Meals with a lower glycemic index (fewer carbs, more fat and protein) seem to increase GLP-1.

Cholecystokinin (CCK): *makes you stop eating*

A gut hormone that tells the brain you're full. Levels go much higher after a high-fat meal than after a low-fat, high-carb meal, one reason why it's so easy to eat six bowls of cereal and not so easy to eat six marbled steaks.

CHAPTER 4

The Major Culprits in a High-Carb Diet: Wheat and Fructose

I f you're like most people, you've come to investigate low-carb diets because of a noticeable and visible concern: your body. You've read—or seen for yourself—that low-carb diets are effective for weight loss. That's probably the reason you picked up this book in the first place: to find a solution to a problem that's causing you pain. It's a problem you'd understandably like to solve.

When I first got involved in low-carb—certainly when I wrote the original edition of this book—that was really all I was concerned about as well. My mission was to debunk the myths about low-carbing and to show people how low-carb could be an effective and safe weight-loss strategy.

Which it is.

But over the years, the evidence has mounted that low-carb diets offer a heck of a lot more than that.

Lucky to Be Fat?

So many people are attracted to a low-carb approach because of a concern with their weight. Or they have some visible, noticeable health issue that they'd like to address immediately. If this sounds like you, you've come to the right place. I'd like to suggest that if you're reading this book to solve an immediate, pressing problem like being overweight, you are "lucky," and here's why.

You're lucky that in the sense that your problem has caused you to seek out a solution, and that *very solution* may actually help you avoid an awful lot of problems down the road that may have flown under the radar for you. These problems—like high blood pressure, high triglycerides, and insulin resistance—might very well have *remained* under the radar right up until the point at which they began to cause serious (and perhaps even fatal) damage.

See, unlike being overweight, most of the conditions mentioned above don't have any real noticeable symptoms. High blood pressure certainly doesn't. Nor, really, does diabetes, at least not at first. An overabundance of triglycerides is another condition that produces exactly zero symptoms or discomfort, even though it puts you at serious risk for heart disease. (Triglycerides drop like a rock on a low-carb diet.) You can walk around with full-blown heart disease without a single clue. Sadly, for many people, the first symptom of heart disease is sudden death. (Many risk markers for heart disease improve dramatically on a low-carb diet.)

You can't, however, be unaware of your own fat.

It's pretty easy to ignore some very important indicators of health, especially when they don't hurt and they're not "in our face" all the time. We're not constantly reminded of our triglycerides or blood pressure every time we look in the mirror. After trying to put on a pair of too-tight pants, we don't often find ourselves saying "Note to self: today I *really* need to start doing something about my HDL cholesterol levels."

But we *do* look in the mirror and say "I've *got* to do something about my weight."

Which is why I made the statement that being overweight makes you— in a very real sense—lucky.

You're lucky in the same way that a person who has a fire in her basement is lucky she has a smoke detector. Without the smoke alarm, the fire would burn unnoticed and, left alone, might actually incinerate the house. The alarm is a loud, annoying, pressing reminder that something is wrong and that someone had better do something about it. The smoke alarm won't put out the fire, but it *will* call your attention to it in time for you to prevent your whole house from turning into a pile of smoldering ash.

Your fat is your smoke detector. It got you to pay attention. Which got you to this book. Congratulations on your new life!

Everything Is Related

Even a cursory glance at the copious amount of research on obesity shows that a number of diseases of civilization, including heart disease and diabetes, all overlap, so much so that it is almost difficult to talk about them as discrete entities. Hundreds of research papers that discuss obesity *also* touch on risk factors like high blood pressure, high triglycerides, abdominal fat, and uncontrolled blood sugar—all factors that are usually shared with heart disease and diabetes. Some of these risk factors cluster together so often that they have their own name: *metabolic syndrome*, also known as prediabetes.

Being overweight or obese puts you at much higher risk for metabolic syndrome, which is one of the fastest growing obesity-related health concerns in the United States.[1] According to the National Heart, Lung, and Blood Institute, a person who has metabolic syndrome is twice as likely to develop heart disease and a whopping six times as likely to develop diabetes than someone who doesn't have metabolic syndrome.[2] Having metabolic syndrome increases the risk of *dying* from heart disease by an incredible 74%![3]

Then there's diabetes. Almost 80% of diabetics are also overweight or obese,[4] and while being overweight or obese doesn't *always* lead to diabetes, it certainly puts you much more at risk. And diabetes and heart disease themselves are hardly strangers. Diabetics are twice as likely as nondiabetics to have heart disease or strokes,[5] and, as of 2017, more than 30 million people in the United States alone have it, with an additional 86 million having prediabetes.[6] Hypertension (high blood pressure) is twice as common in adults who are obese,[7] and hypertension is a major risk for heart disease[8] as well as one of the hallmarks of metabolic syndrome.

Then there's the connection between weight and heart disease. A 2007 study in the *Archives of Internal Medicine* found that—completely independent of other risk factors like high blood pressure—being overweight increases the risk for cardiovascular disease by 17%, while being obese increases the risk by a whopping 40%![9]

Beginning to get the picture? These "diseases of civilization"—obesity, diabetes, hypertension, metabolic syndrome—are so intimately connected that it's almost hard to talk about one without referencing the others. Living low-carb may be the solution to your extra padding, but it may *also* turn out to be the solution to heart disease and diabetes. The foods you wind up eliminating from your diet when you go low-carb are turning out to be powerful promoters of these diseases of civilization in ways that are only now beginning to be discovered.

We'll take a closer look at two of those foods in particular—wheat and fructose—in just a moment. But first let's talk a little more about the connection between carbs, appetite, fat cells, and health.

Your Fat Cells Don't Just Sit There

One of the biggest discoveries in recent years, at least in the area of fat metabolism, is that fat cells don't just sit there on your hips annoying the heck out of you. We all thought fat cells were just these little inert sponges of greasy stuff accumulating in all the places you didn't want them to accumulate, staying fat and jolly and sedentary until you somehow figured out how to get rid of them.

Nope.

Fat cells are busy little beavers.

We now know that fat cells behave more like endocrine glands. They secrete hormones—lots of them. They have names like *leptin, resistin, adiponectin,* and *ghrelin.* Some of those hormones protect fat cells themselves from extinction (like resistin, for example). Some are involved in appetite (leptin, ghrelin). The fat cells also secrete inflammatory chemicals called *cytokines,* which include *interleukin-6* and *tumor necrosis factor-alpha,* both of which contribute to the inflammation increasingly seen in obesity, diabetes, heart disease, Alzheimer's disease, and virtually every degenerative disease known to humankind.[10]

So your fat—your "smoke detector," if you will—may have brought you to this book, and you may be reading it with one specific goal: to lose weight and keep it off. But the fact is that by addressing that pressing, obvious problem—the one that painfully calls attention to itself every time you glance in the mirror—you will *also* be decreasing your risk for heart disease, diabetes, metabolic syndrome, and hypertension. Not least of all, you'll be reducing inflammation, which is turning out to be a much greater contributor to disease than anyone ever suspected, and which is turbocharged by the very fat cells you're trying to get rid of.

For you, the most important part of low-carb may be that it gives you the best chance of looking decent in a bathing suit. But in fact, that lower-carb diet will provide you with a range of health benefits you probably didn't even think about, including a dramatic decrease in your risk of developing cancer and heart disease.

See, not all carbs are created equal. "Carbohydrate" is what they call in politics a "big tent"—a category that encompasses a huge range of foods (and food "products") ranging from cauliflower to Twinkies. Unless all your carbs are coming from vegetables (which, for the average American, would be pretty uncommon), the majority of your carbs are coming from foods like cereals, breads, pasta, potatoes, rice, and an assortment of highly sweetened processed foods. These foods are almost always "high-glycemic," meaning they raise blood sugar very quickly, a fact which has all sorts of metabolic consequences, none of them good.

Emerging research continues to implicate high-glycemic diets in a host of conditions, including cancer[11] (cancer cells, after all, feed on sugar). Consuming carbohydrates that have a high-glycemic index (meaning those that raise blood sugar quickly) is associated with an increased risk for coronary heart disease,[12] while *low*-glycemic diets have been reported to reduce measures of inflammation, aid in weight control, and lower the risk of diabetes and cardiovascular disease.[13] And, by definition, lower-carb diets are almost always low-glycemic diets, since most of the carbs in a low-carb diet will be coming from vegetables, fruits, and the occasional healthy grain (like oatmeal), all of which have very low glycemic indexes.

Betcha Can't Eat Just One

One thing you probably know from experience is the effect high-glycemic foods have on your appetite. Remember one of the most successful ad campaigns in recent decades, the "Betcha Can't Eat Just One" ad? They weren't kidding. There's a reason it's so easy to go through three bowls of Cap'n Crunch while watching reruns of *Friends*. High-glycemic carbs make you hungry. Low-carb diets don't.

And that may be one reason why people do so much better on lower-carb diets. A 2005 study from the Temple University School of Medicine found that the reason pounds melt off so quickly on low-carb diets is not at all related to water, metabolism, or boredom.[14] Nope. It's related to appetite. "When carbohydrates were restricted," lead researcher Guenther Boden, MD, told *Science Daily*, "study subjects spontaneously reduced their caloric intake to a level appropriate for their height, did not compensate by eating more protein or fat, and lost weight." Boden added: "We concluded that excessive overeating had been fueled by carbohydrates."[15]

The path from eating a high-carbohydrate diet to being overweight is a pretty clear one: It has to do primarily with the ability of carbohydrates to raise blood sugar, which, in turn, raises a fat-storing hormone called *insulin.* When insulin is constantly elevated, it's darn near impossible to burn fat. (See chapter 3 for a full explanation.) But there are a few other "side effects" of lower-carb diets that may also have a lot to do with why lower-carb diets make it so much easier to lose weight and get healthy.

One of those "side effects" has to do with wheat. Another has to do with fructose.

Let me explain.

The Wheat Connection

Since virtually all low-carb diets recommend that you keep carb intake to somewhere under 100 grams a day (as low as 20 grams on the first stage of Atkins), one of the first things that gets eliminated—at least in the beginning—is wheat.

You can eat a ton of vegetables and still manage to keep your carbs under 100 grams a day; you can even eat some fruit. But once you start including bread, bagels, pasta, rice, and all the rest of the starches and grains, your carb allowance is quickly used up. (A single slice of bread has between 20 and 25 grams of carbs.) Not only that: all wheat products are high-glycemic, meaning they raise blood sugar quickly and keep it up there for a while, stimulating a ton of insulin, which essentially locks the doors to your fat cells.

I first experimented with eliminating bread from a client's diet back in 1990. I was a personal trainer, working at Equinox, and my nutrition knowledge was still pretty limited. Like most personal trainers, I had received all my education in nutrition from American Dietetic Association–approved programs and instructors, so I totally bought into the low-fat, high-carb, lots-of-grains paradigm. But some of the other trainers had been experimenting with lower-starch diets for their clients, so I decided to try that approach with Lucy, a woman who came to me for the express purpose of losing some stubborn pounds she just couldn't seem to get rid of.

In a few short weeks, she dropped about 8 pounds.

But that's not the interesting part.

The interesting part was that Lucy had suffered from inexplicable headaches for most of her life. Not migraines, mind you, nor cluster headaches, but just regular, annoying, day-ruining garden-variety headaches that no doctor, naturopath, chiropractor, or nutritionist had ever been able to explain. When she came back to see me, she had some interesting news: "My headaches went away!" she exclaimed.

This was well before I knew much about gluten sensitivity, celiac disease, or delayed food reactions. I had taken bread out of her diet because I thought it would help her lose weight (which it did). I had no idea there would be a side effect like the elimination of a lifelong problem no one else had been able to fix.

As the years went by and my nutrition education continued, I did indeed learn all about celiac disease and gluten sensitivity. Gluten is a protein found in grains, particularly wheat, that triggers symptoms in a huge number of people; when your body responds to gluten with a full-blown autoimmune reaction, the condition is called *celiac disease*. But celiac disease, like many things, exists on a continuum. You don't have to have celiac disease to have a profound sensitivity to gluten, which is clearly what Lucy had. (Gluten sensitivity can lead to a host of symptoms like headache, bloating, weight gain, water retention, aches and pains, and digestive issues.) But, like most nutritionists at the time, I still thought the only problem with wheat was that it raised blood sugar—and insulin by extension—thus making it a good thing to avoid if you wanted to lose weight.

Most people still think the problem with wheat is limited to gluten, and gluten-free foods have taken off as a "niche" market that's growing like weeds. But the problems with wheat go a lot deeper than gluten. As you'll soon see, substances in wheat—particularly a type of starch called *amylopectin A*—can cause all sorts of problems in susceptible people. The most obvious problem is weight gain, but it's hardly limited to that.

Some Call It Fat, Some Call It "Wheat Belly"

In 2010, a brilliant cardiologist named William Davis, MD, published a book called *Wheat Belly*, which instantly (and deservedly) went to the top of the *New York Times* Best Seller list. Davis explains that the wheat we're consuming today is a genetically modified kind of wheat that had never been seen on earth before about 50 years ago. This wheat—called *dwarf wheat*— has replaced most of the other strains of wheat in the United States (and in much of the world). "Modern wheat, despite all the genetic alterations to modify hundreds, if not thousands, of its genetically determined characteristics, made its way to the worldwide human food supply with nary a question surrounding its suitability for human consumption," writes Davis.

In 2011, journalist/educator Tom Naughton interviewed Davis on the subject of wheat. (The interview is available on Naughton's website, www.fathead-movie.com.) One exchange was particularly telling:

Naughton: *You're a cardiologist by profession, yet you just wrote an in-depth book about the negative health effects of consuming wheat. How did wheat end up on your radar? What first made you suspect wheat might be behind many of our modern health problems?*

Davis: *If foods made from wheat raise blood sugar higher than nearly all other foods (due to its high-glycemic index), including table sugar, then removing wheat should reduce blood sugar. I was concerned about high blood sugar since around 80% of the people coming to my office had diabetes, pre-diabetes, or what I call "pre-pre-diabetes." In short, the vast majority of people showed abnormal metabolic markers.*

I provided patients with a simple two-page handout on how to do this, i.e., how to eliminate wheat and replace the lost calories with healthy foods like more vegetables, raw nuts, meats, eggs, avocados, olives, olive oil, etc. They'd come back three months later with lower fasting blood sugars, lower hemoglobin A1c (a reflection of the previous 60 days' blood sugar); some diabetics became non-diabetics, pre-diabetics became non-pre-diabetic. They'd also be around 30 pounds lighter.

Then they began to tell me about other experiences: Relief from arthritis and joint pains, chronic rashes disappearing, asthma improved sufficiently to stop inhalers, chronic sinus infections gone, leg swelling gone, migraine headaches gone for the first time in decades, acid reflux and irritable bowel symptoms relieved. At first, I told patients it was just an odd coincidence. But it happened so many times to so many people that it became clear this was no coincidence: this was a real and reproducible phenomenon.

That's when I began to systematically remove wheat from everyone's diet and continued to witness similar turnarounds in health across dozens of conditions. There has been no turning back since.

Removing wheat—or grains in general—from the diet is a hard sell. For decades we've been sold a bill of goods on how healthful grains are and how "necessary" they are in our diet. We've heard the phrase "fruits, vegetables, and healthy whole grains" so many times it sounds like a vaudeville act, and the pairing of "healthy whole grains" with two things that actually *are* good for us has convinced most of us that grains—especially whole grains—are as wholesome and nutritious as vegetables.

Actually, that's not the whole truth.

THE STRANGE CASE OF MY TENNIS-PLAYING BUDDY

Every Wednesday morning, I play a couple of sets of tennis with a guy I'll call Marty. He's in his late 60's and in great shape. Recently he told me that he had atrial fibrillation, the most common kind of irregular heartbeat, a condition that has symptoms like heart palpitations and shortness of breath.

Two years ago, Marty told me, he had a "procedure" that effectively stopped the problem. Except that now, all of a sudden, it was coming back.

In the course of discussing his health, Marty also mentioned that he had constant bloating, gas, and other digestive problems.

Going for the low-hanging fruit (the digestive problems), I asked him if he'd considered a gluten-free diet. "Worth a shot," I said.

About a week later, I met him on the court and was greeted with good news. "This gluten-free thing seems to be really working. My gas and bloating is gone and I'm not having any stomach pains!"

I asked him how the atrial fibrillation was and if he had seen his doctor about it yet.

"Oh," he said, almost as an afterthought. "It seems to be gone! I haven't had any problems with it in a week."

As Davis points out in his book, the species einkorn was the great-granddaddy of wheat, and has the simplest genetic code. But einkorn and other wild and cultivated strands of wheat are no longer what we're eating. They've been preempted by literally thousands of man-made offspring of *Triticum aestivum*, which are genetically quite different from the original einkorn wheat. Today's wheat has been bred for greater yield and hardiness. It even looks different. Those "amber waves of grain" we sang about as children hardly exist anymore. They've been replaced by wheat varieties that barely stand two feet tall. The name for that stuff is dwarf or semi-dwarf wheat, and unless you've got access to a time machine, that's exactly what you're eating when you eat today's cereals, pastas, and breads.

Why does that matter?

Pull up a chair.

Wheat: The Real Story

Wheat—like all starches—is made up of two fractions: amylose and *amylopectin*. They have somewhat different effects on the body, something that's been known since at least 1989 when researchers fed men a diet containing 34% of calories as either 70% amylose starch or 70% amylopectin starch and measured the results. What's interesting is that there were no major differences—for the first 4 weeks. But when the meals were given after 5 weeks on each starch, some significant differences showed up. Blood-sugar and insulin responses were significantly lower when the amylose meal was compared to the amylopectin meal. Fasting triglyceride levels were also lower during the period when amylose was consumed.[16]

The complex carbohydrate in wheat is actually 75% amylopectin and 25% amylose. But the problem isn't just the amylopectin—it's the *type* of amylopectin. Amylopectin actually comes in several "flavors." Amylopectin C is found in beans and legumes and is the least digestible of the three; amylopectin B is found in potatoes and bananas, and it's a little more digestible than amylopectin C. But when it comes to digestibility, amylopectin A—the kind found in wheat—is the clear winner. It breaks down quicker than you can say "blood sugar hell."

That's why it's no surprise that whole-wheat bread increases your blood sugar more than even pure sucrose (table sugar).[17] And—as you'll learn throughout this book—high blood sugar is quickly followed by a surge of the fat-storing hormone, insulin. This is exactly what you do *not* want if you're trying to control your weight. The higher your blood sugar, the higher your insulin, and the easier it is to store fat. Not only that: amylopectin A has a curious ability to keep that blood sugar/insulin surge going for about 2 hours.[18] That surge means there's going to be a big drop, and those drops in blood sugar—the aforementioned "blood sugar hell"—are largely responsible for cravings and hunger. That's why it's a breeze to binge on sugar-coated wheat cereal. Steak and broccoli? Not so much.

"Wheat is the Haight-Ashbury of foods, unparalleled for its potential to generate entirely different effects on the brain and nervous system," says Davis. Indeed. As anyone who recognized herself in the reference to the compulsive eating of cereal knows, wheat can stimulate addictive behavior. And there's a very good reason for that.

This Is Your Brain on Gluten

Gluten, you see, is broken down in the body to chains of amino acids called *polypeptides*. These polypeptides have a unique ability to get past the sentry who stands guard at the door of the brain, a structure called the *blood-brain barrier*. The blood-brain barrier functions like a bouncer at an exclusive night-club. The brain can't let just any old riffraff get in, or it would be severely damaged by some of the crap floating around in our bloodstream. The blood-brain barrier protects it from this riffraff by being very selective about what it opens the door for. But the polypeptides that result from the breaking down of gluten somehow get a free pass. And when they get in, guess what they do?

They bind to the brain's morphine receptors.

One researcher—Christine Zioudrou at the National Institutes of Health—termed these sneaky polypeptides exorphins, a contraction of exogenous morphine–like compounds. The dominant one is called *gluteo-morphin*. And if you doubt that it can exert a drug-like effect on your brain, consider the following. (Faint-hearted readers beware: you may never feel the same way about that "wholesome" wheat bread of yours again.)

Naloxone is a drug given to reverse the effects of narcotic drugs. It's frequently given to addicts, and if you're stoned it will make you immedi-ately *un*-stoned. Fine, you say, and what could that possibly have to do with me? Or, come to think of it, with wheat *or* with low-carb diets?

Well, in one ingenious study conducted at the University of South Caro-lina, two groups of healthy participants were let loose in the cafeteria, but one of them was first given a dose of naloxone. Those given the naloxone consumed ⅓ fewer calories at lunch and just under ¼ fewer calories at din-ner, averaging about 400 fewer calories for the day.[19] In another study at the University of Michigan, researchers put binge eaters in a room loaded with all kinds of food and left them there for an hour. Those given the naloxone beforehand consumed a whopping 28% fewer wheat crackers, pretzels, and bread sticks.[20]

As Davis puts it, "block the euphoric reward of wheat, and calorie intake goes down, since wheat *no longer generates the favorable feelings that encourage repetitive consumption.*" [Emphasis mine.]

Or, put another way: wheat is addictive. It's an appetite stimulant. Not only does it raise blood sugar more than any other carbohydrate—which alone would make it a disaster from a weight-control standpoint—but it also affects your brain in a way that makes overeating far more likely. "Just as the tobacco industry created and sustained its market with the addictive property of cigarettes, so does wheat in the diet make for a helpless, hungry consumer," says Davis. "From the perspective of the seller of food products, wheat is a perfect processed food ingredient: The more you eat, the more you want."

The Glyphosate-Gluten-Gut Connection

In recent years, research has churned up a brand-new strike against wheat. And it all starts with *glyphosate*, the active ingredient in the notorious herbicide Roundup®.

For decades, farmers have been using glyphosate to kill pesky weeds that interfere with crops like corn, soy, and canola. Throughout the U.S. and other countries, glyphosate is also used as a pre-harvest treatment for wheat, meaning it's sprayed on wheat crops a week or two before harvest time to assist with weed control and to hurry up the crop's dry-down.

For a long time, even expert scientists believed glyphosate was harmless for humans. After all, the whole reason glyphosate works is by inhibiting something called the *shikimate pathway*, a metabolic route that bacteria, fungi, and plants use to produce proteins necessary for their growth. When this pathway gets obstructed in plant cells, those plants can't stay alive. But when it comes to humans? Animal cells (including ours) don't have a shikimate pathway, so there's nothing for glyphosate to block! No harm, no foul, right?

If only it were so simple. As research continues to shine light on the gut microbiome (including its incredible role in health and disease), glyphosate is starting to look more and more suspect. The reason? While glyphosate can't kill human cells, it can kill bacteria cells. And that includes those trillions (yes, *trillions*) of bacteria residing in your gut. You know, the ones that shape your immune system, produce nutrients, regulate hormones, ferment fiber, communicate with your human genes, and—the kicker— have a major say in how much energy you store and expend.[21] That's right: the gut microbiota calls some shots when it comes to your metabolism— and, consequently, your waistline.

Like weeds in a wheat field, these hardworking little critters get blasted— sometimes fatally—with glyphosate when we eat foods with Roundup residue, wheat included. Starting to see the problem here?

The rabbit hole goes deep. It turns out that glyphosate exposure can absolutely disrupt the delicate balance of gut bacteria in animals, despite technically being "nontoxic" to the animals themselves (too often, this stuff is all about semantics). In fact, studies show that glyphosate can kill off "helpful" microbes like *Bifidobacteria* and *Lactobacillus*, creating a chance for the bad guys—including *Salmonella* and *E. coli* (which are resistant to glyphosate)—to run amok.[22] And we're not talking crazy-high exposures, either: this stuff happens even at doses deemed "safe" by regulatory agencies (including Acceptable Daily Intake levels in the U.S.[23]). Even more disturbing, glyphosate exposure causes gut bacteria composition to look eerily similar to what we see with obesity and metabolic diseases—including a rise in inflammatory microbes and an increased ratio of Firmicutes to Bacteroidetes,[24] which scientists deem a hallmark of "obese" microbiomes.[25]

And in case you're wondering, glyphosate *can't* be baked or fermented out of wheat once it's there—researchers have already tried that.[26] Nor can you do yourself any favors by buying only whole-wheat products: because glyphosate is incorporated into the outer hulls of wheat grains, whole-wheat products actually have *more* glyphosate than refined-wheat products. According to an analysis by Health Research Institute Laboratories, whole-wheat bread samples averaged 141 parts per billion of glyphosate, compared to 14 parts per billion for conventional white breads (and 6.5 parts per billion for gluten-free breads).[27]

There you have it. Not only does wheat mess with your brain and your appetite, it also messes with the trillions of body-weight regulators in your gut!

The Side Effects of a Wheat-Free Diet

Like Lucy, who stopped eating bread in order to lose weight but wound up losing her headaches, you may find that some other health conditions you've been worried about improve substantially if you cut out wheat. In fact, the elimination of wheat is a perfect example of the "side effects" of low-carb diets. You remove a food everyone has told you is healthy and necessary (wheat) because of its demonstrated connection to high blood sugar and fat storage, and you end up not only losing weight but improving health in literally dozens of ways across dozens of conditions.

Are you beginning to see why, in the beginning, I said you are "lucky"?

Fructose Makes You Fat—And It's Metabolic Poison

The other "food" that should get the pink slip on your low-carb diet is fructose. More specifically, (1) *high-fructose corn syrup*, which consists of 55%

fructose and 45% glucose, and its kissing cousin, (2) *sucrose*, which is ordinary table sugar, composed of 50% fructose and 50% glucose.

Because high-fructose corn syrup (HFCS) has gotten so much heat in the press, some food manufacturers now proudly advertise that their products contain none of it, and are instead sweetened with "natural" sugar (meaning ordinary sucrose). Meanwhile, the National Corn Growers Association, essentially a lobbying arm of the sugar industry dedicated to whitewashing HFCS, has claimed that high-fructose corn syrup is being unjustly targeted and is no worse than "regular" sugar.

Sadly, they're right. But that's a little like saying that diarrhea is "better" than Montezuma's revenge.

Fructose is the damaging part of sugar, and whether you get that fructose from regular sugar or from HFCS doesn't make a whit of difference. That doesn't absolve HFCS; it just means that "regular" sugar is *just as bad* as HFCS. It's the fructose in each of them that's causing the damage, and here's why.

Fructose and glucose are metabolized in the body in completely different ways. As "sugars," they are *not* identical. Glucose goes right into the bloodstream and then into the cells. It raises your blood sugar, causing a surge of insulin—the "fat-storage hormone"—leading to weight gain as well as the many other problems discussed in this book. Fructose *doesn't* raise blood sugar, but it damages the body nonetheless, albeit via different mechanisms. The end result is it still makes you fat, and it does some other significant damage as well.

Fructose is metabolized by the body like fat, and it turns into fat (triglycerides) almost immediately. "When you consume fructose, you're not consuming carbs," says Robert Lustig, MD, professor of pediatrics at the University of California, San Francisco. "You're consuming fat." Once fructose enters the body, it goes right to the liver. A substantial amount of research has now implicated fructose in non-alcoholic fatty liver disease.[28] "Fructose is 'alcohol without the buzz,'" says Lustig. "[It's] a dose-dependent chronic hepatotoxin."[29] Research has shown that fructose is many times more likely than glucose to form artery-damaging, free radical–generating factories called AGEs (advanced glycation end-products). AGEs are dangerous compounds that play a major role in heart disease.[30] Research by Kimber Stanhope at the University of California Davis has shown that when people consume 25% of their calories from fructose or high-fructose corn syrup, several factors associated with an increased risk for heart disease—including triglycerides and a nasty little substance called apolipoprotein B—go up significantly.[31]

The perfect example of how sugar is related to fat *and* to heart disease is *insulin resistance.* Insulin resistance is discussed throughout this book and is included in many of the diets we will review later, but here's the short definition so you don't have to go look it up: Insulin resistance is the condition in which the cells stop "listening" to insulin. That means insulin is *less* effective at getting sugar out of your bloodstream, even though the pancreas continues to pump out more and more of it in a futile attempt to make blood sugar go down. Eventually you have both high blood sugar *and* high insulin and you're basically—excuse my French—screwed. High blood sugar and high insulin are two of the features of metabolic syndrome, and when you have it, you're well on the road to diabetes, heart disease, or both. And you'll almost definitely find it impossible to lose weight.

The way in which sugar—especially fructose—damages the heart can be directly traced to insulin resistance. Varman Samuel of the Yale School of Medicine, a top researcher in the field of insulin resistance, told the *New York Times* that the correlation between fat in the liver (fatty liver) and insulin resistance is remarkably strong. "When you deposit fat in the liver, that's when you become insulin resistant," he says.[32]

And all together now, class: What causes fat to accumulate in the liver? Fructose.

If you want to watch a bunch of lab animals become insulin-resistant, all you have to do is feed them fructose. Feed them enough fructose and sure enough, the liver converts it to fat which then accumulates in the liver—with insulin resistance right behind it. This can take place in as little as a week if the animals are fed enough fructose, whereas it might take a few months at the levels we humans normally consume. In studies done by Luc Tappy in Switzerland, feeding human subjects a daily dose of fructose equal to the amount found in 8 to 10 cans of soda produced insulin resistance and elevated triglycerides within a few days.[33]

Fructose found in whole foods like fruits, however, is a different story. There's not all that much fructose in, for example, an apple, and the apple comes with a hefty dose of fiber, which slows the rate of carbohydrate absorption and reduces insulin response. But fructose extracted from fruit, concentrated into a syrup, and then inserted into practically every food we buy at the supermarket, from bread to hamburger buns to pretzels to cereals—well, that's a whole different animal.

High-fructose corn syrup was first invented in Japan in the 1960s and made it into the American food supply around the mid-1970s. It had two advantages over regular sugar, from the point of view of food manufacturers.

Number one: because it's sweeter, theoretically you could use less of it. (Theoretically.) Number two: it is significantly cheaper than sugar. Manufacturers found that low-fat products could be made "palatable" through the addition of HFCS, so before long they were adding the stuff to everything. (Doubt this? Take a field trip to your local supermarket and start reading labels. See if you can find any processed foods that don't contain it.)

The result is that our fructose consumption has skyrocketed. Twenty-five percent of adolescents today consume 15% of their calories from fructose alone! As professor Robert Lustig, MD, points out in his brilliant lecture "Sugar: The Bitter Truth" (available on YouTube), the percentage of calories from fat in the American diet has gone down at the same time that fructose consumption has skyrocketed, along with heart disease, diabetes, obesity, and hypertension. Coincidence? Lustig doesn't think so, and neither do I.

Remember metabolic syndrome? It's that collection of symptoms—high triglycerides, abdominal fat, hypertension, and insulin resistance—all of which seriously increase the risk for heart disease. Well, rodents consuming large amounts of fructose rapidly develop it.[34] In humans, a high-fructose diet raises triglycerides almost instantly; the rest of the symptoms of metabolic syndrome take a little longer to develop in humans than they do in the rat experiments, but develop they do.[35] Fructose also raises uric acid levels in the bloodstream. Excess uric acid is well known as the defining feature of gout, but it also predicts future obesity and high blood pressure.

Fructose and glucose behave very differently in the brain as well, as research from Johns Hopkins has suggested. Glucose decreases food intake while fructose increases it. If your appetite increases, you eat more, thus priming you for obesity, and likely an increased risk for heart disease. "Take a kid to McDonald's and give him a Coke," says Professor Lustig. "Does he eat less? Or does he eat more?"

M. Daniel Lane, PhD, of the Johns Hopkins University School of Medicine says "We feel that [the findings on fructose and appetite] may have particular relevance to the massive increase in the use of high-fructose sweeteners (both high-fructose corn syrup and table sugar) in virtually all sweetened foods, most notably soft drinks. The per capita consumption of these sweeteners in the USA is about 145 lbs/year and is probably much higher in teenagers/youth that have a high level of consumption of soft drinks."[36]

AGAVE NECTAR SYRUP: HOPE OR HYPE?

Agave nectar is an amber-colored liquid that pours more easily than honey and is considerably sweeter than sugar. The health-food crowd loves it because it is gluten-free and suitable for vegan diets—*and*, most especially, because it's low-glycemic (we'll get to that in a moment). Largely because of its very low glycemic impact, agave nectar is marketed as "diabetic friendly." What's not to like?

As it turns out, quite a lot.

Agave nectar has a low-glycemic index for one reason only: it's largely made of *fructose*, which, although it has a low-glycemic index, is now known to be a very damaging form of sugar when used as a sweetener. *Agave nectar has the highest fructose content of any commercial sweetener (with the exception of pure liquid fructose).*

All sugar—from table sugar to HFCS (high-fructose corn syrup) to honey—contains *some* mixture of fructose and glucose. The proportion in table sugar is 50/50; HFCS is 55/45. Agave nectar is anywhere from 57% to a whopping 90% fructose, almost—but not quite—twice as high as HFCS.

In the agave *plant*, most of the sweetness comes from a particular kind of fructose called *inulin* that actually has some health benefits: it's considered a fiber. But there's not much inulin left in the actual syrup. In the manufacturing process, enzymes are added to the inulin to break it down into digestible sugar (fructose), resulting in a syrup that has a fructose content that is *at best* 57% and—much more commonly—as high as 90%.

"It's almost all fructose, highly processed sugar with great marketing," said Dr. Ingrid Kohlstadt, a fellow of the American College of Nutrition and an associate faculty member at the Johns Hopkins School of Public Health. "Fructose interferes with healthy metabolism when (consumed) at higher doses," she told me. "Many people have fructose intolerance like lactose intolerance. They get acne or worse diabetes symptoms even though their blood (sugar) is OK."

Agave nectar syrup is a triumph of marketing over science. True, it has a low-glycemic index, but so does gasoline—that doesn't mean it's good for you.

If you've read my book *The Great Cholesterol Myth*, you already know that I think cholesterol is a very minor player in heart disease, and it doesn't predict heart disease very well at all. But hypertension, high triglycerides, and a high ratio of triglycerides to HDL cholesterol all *do*. Sugar, or more specifically *fructose*, raises *every single one* of those measures.

On top of that, high levels of sugar and insulin *damage* cholesterol particles, making them far more likely to start the process of inflammation. And even if you *don't* accept the theory that inflammation is at the "heart" of heart disease, it's worth pointing out that the metabolic effects of sugar are highly inflammatory to your artery walls.

And, by the way, to the brain. Elevated levels of glucose (sugar) in the brain actually impair the ability of nerve cells to repair themselves and regenerate, something greatly needed for cognitive health. It may be no coincidence that diabetics have almost twice the risk for Alzheimer's and cognitive impairment than non-diabetics do.[37]

The fact that sugar is far more damaging to the heart—and to the brain—than either fat *or* cholesterol has never stopped the diet establishment from continuing to stick to their story that fat and cholesterol are what we ought to be worried about.

THE CASE AGAINST SODA

One clever study by Kimber Stanhope and her colleagues at Stanford investigated the effects of "moderate" soda drinking on health.

They took 29 healthy, normal-weight male subjects and ran each one of them through six different three-week experiments. In the first condition, the men drank what was called a "medium fructose" beverage; in the second condition they drank a "high fructose" beverage. In the third and fourth conditions they drank a "medium glucose" beverage and a "high glucose" beverage, and in the final two conditions they drank "medium sucrose" and "high sucrose" beverages.

So, again, we had two conditions where they drank beverages sweetened with plain sugar (sucrose), two conditions where they drank beverages sweetened just with glucose, and two conditions where they drank beverages sweetened with just fructose.

The results were not good news for soda drinkers.

First of all, in all conditions, fasting blood sugar and high-sensitivity C-reactive protein increased significantly. (C-reactive protein, by the way, is a measure of inflammation, so this study clearly shows that sugar in all forms is very inflammatory.) Second, particle size of their LDL—the so-called "bad cholesterol"—was reduced in both the high-fructose group and in the high-sucrose group. This is a really bad thing because we now know that the small pellet-sized LDL molecules are the ones that cause the most damage, so shrinking the particle size of LDLs is a really bad outcome!

In addition, all the interventions containing fructose resulted in a significantly higher waist-to-hip ratio and there was a significantly higher percentage of body fat in the high-fructose intervention.

In another study, overweight and obese adults were instructed to eat their usual diet along with sugar-sweetened beverages. One group was asked to consume 25% of the day's calorie requirement as a specially made beverage sweetened with glucose. The other group was given an identical beverage sweetened with fructose. Both groups were allowed to eat as little or as much of their usual diet as they wanted, but were required to drink the sugar beverages.

"The subjects did not eat 25% fewer calories from their usual foods to make room for the sugar beverage calories. Instead, most of them ate more than their calorie requirement," Kimber Stanhope told me. Not surprisingly, all subjects gained weight. "But what was interesting and novel—and is a finding that needs to be confirmed—is that the fructose subjects gained intra-abdominal fat, whereas the glucose subjects did not," Ms. Stanhope said.

Why does this matter? Because intra-abdominal fat—the kind that makes you more of an apple than a pear—is the most dangerous kind of fat to carry around. It puts you at greater risk for diabetes, heart disease, and the constellation of symptoms called metabolic syndrome, an almost certain path to either heart disease or diabetes. "There was a definite increase in fasting insulin and in fasting glucose with the fructose consuming subjects," Stanhope explained. Elevated levels of fasting insulin and glucose (blood sugar) are both associated with a greater risk of metabolic syndrome and diabetes.

While the research is preliminary and needs to be borne out by future studies, high-fructose consumption could well be setting consumers up for atherosclerosis. "The overweight men and women assigned to drink the fructose-sweetened beverages developed a more athrogenic lipid profile in just two weeks," said Stanhope. "In 2006, five different publications came out showing that adolescents, college students, and adults under

50 were consuming as much as 15–20 percent of calories just from sugar-sweetened beverages—and that doesn't include the sugar calories from cakes and desserts."*

* Stanhope, et al., "Consumption of Fructose and High Fructose Corn Syrup Increase Postprandial Triglycerides, LDL-Cholesterol, and Apolipoprotein-B in Young Men and Women" *The Journal of Clinical Endocrinology & Metabolism* 96, no. 10 (October 2011): E1596–1605.

So let's review the "side effects" of a low-carb diet. Less likelihood of fatty liver disease, lowered markers of inflammation, and a lower risk for heart disease, metabolic syndrome, and diabetes just for good measure.

Not exactly a shabby list of accomplishments, lowered markers of inflammation, and a heck of a lot better than the side effects of many medicines.

CHAPTER 5

The Cholesterol Connection: Have We All Been Misled?

I t's been about 15 years since the first edition of *Living Low Carb* (then called *Living the Low-Carb Life*) was published. During that time I've witnessed a much greater appreciation for the value of low-carbohydrate eating, and a greater acceptance of the principles of low-carb among many (but not all) segments of the health professions.

But the conversation I listened to in between doubles sets on the tennis court the other day tells a much different story.

"My doctor says I have high cholesterol, so he put me on a statin drug," said one guy. "I can't understand why. I eat really healthy! No red meat, hardly any fat, lots of whole grains. Makes no sense!"

"My doctor just told me to eat low-fat foods and cut out meat. My cholesterol is OK, so I guess I don't have to worry," chimed in a second guy.

"I lost a ton of weight on that Atkins diet," said a third, "but my doctor told me it's really unhealthy. He says I might have lost weight, but I was putting myself at risk for heart disease from eating all that fat and osteoporosis from eating all that protein."

OK everyone, calm down and take a deep breath. We've got a lot of work to do.

The innocent conversation that took place on the tennis court in southern California—a conversation, mind you, among four reasonably smart, educated middle-aged men all of whom are health conscious enough to engage in regular exercise and affluent enough to afford good medical care—is a perfect object lesson in everything that's wrong with our collective thinking on diet and health.

Let me explain.

Low-Carb and Heart Disease: The Big Lie

"The big lie" was an expression coined—sorry to say—by Adolf Hitler, who used it in a completely different context. It's shorthand for the idea that if enough people repeat an untruth often enough, it becomes "accepted knowledge." Hitler meant it to refer to propaganda techniques. Though he was delusional about *who* was lying and what they were lying *about*, he was entirely correct about the propaganda part. Get enough people—and enough respected, mainstream organizations that dispense advice—to say that the world is flat, and before you know it, anyone who says differently is either crazy or subversive. After a while, everyone "knows" the world is flat, and anyone who says otherwise must be nuts.

Welcome to the modern world of alternative facts.

Which brings us full-circle to low-carb diets and heart disease.

Those men who were worried about their cholesterol all bought into the "big lie" that cholesterol causes heart disease. (To disassemble this "big lie" would take a whole book. Cardiologist Stephen Sinatra, MD, and I wrote one: it's called *The Great Cholesterol Myth*. I hope you read it.)

What's important for our purposes here is the stuff that logically follows from that "big lie." The "big lie" that cholesterol causes heart disease—and the secondary fib that saturated fat always raises cholesterol—was the impetus for several decades' worth of dietary advice that has led us down a path of ever-expanding waistlines and a virtual epidemic of obesity and diabetes. The dietary guidelines that flowed quite logically from the "big lie" about heart disease were nonsense when they were first issued in the late '70s and '80s, and they continue to be nonsense today.

If you think about it for a moment, every single time you've been warned off saturated fat it's for one reason only: it raises cholesterol. But really, it's not cholesterol you care about—it's heart disease. And they are *not* the same thing, though if you read the mainstream media, you'd never know it. The mainstream media and many mainstream medical organizations have got you convinced that cholesterol and heart disease *are* the same thing. By conflating cholesterol and heart disease they convinced us to avoid eating fat (especially saturated fat) since it *may* increase cholesterol.

Since "everybody knows" that high cholesterol spells heart disease, anything that increases cholesterol *must* be bad, and that's precisely why your doctor tells you to avoid low-carb diets.

But if cholesterol isn't the demon mainstream medicine thinks it is, then the admonition to eschew saturated fat collapses like a house of cards. If the only "bad" thing saturated fat does is raise blood levels of an innocuous molecule that is turning out to have very little to do with heart disease anyway, then why are we avoiding saturated fat?

Fat and the Big Lie

Fat is the Rodney Dangerfield of the modern diet: "it don't get no respect."

For years we tried to eliminate it from what we eat, even though it's been a basic (and necessary) part of our diet since at least the first recorded Homo sapiens in Africa about 200,000 years ago, and likely from the beginning of the genus Homo roughly 2.4 million years ago. More recently, experts have begun—almost grudgingly, it seems—to admit that some fat is good, but a good number of them still continue to recommend that you reduce it as much as possible. (And—with the exception of the universally appreciated omega-3 fats—many experts are still for the most part woefully uninformed about which fats are actually "good" and why.) It's common for health-conscious people to collapse the terms "healthful" and "low-fat" as if they were synonyms (trust me, they're not). And the majority of fitness books continue to repeat low-fat nonsense that should have gone out of style a decade ago.

So it's probably safe to say that fat is the single most misunderstood component of the modern diet. And our thinking about fat deeply colors the way we think about low-carb diets.

Here's why: Suppose, for the moment, that you're eating a typical American diet of 2,500 calories (or more), of which about half (or more!) comes from carbohydrates. If you remove a big chunk of the carbohydrates from your diet (the definition of a low-carb program, right?), one of two things *has* to happen: One, you simply cut out the carbs but keep everything *else* the same, effectively eating half as much food as before (this never happens). The second much more common and realistic option is that you replace all or some of those carbohydrate calories with something else.

Since there are only three other calorie-containing substances on the planet that you can replace those carbs with (protein, fat, or alcohol) and since most people don't replace their carbohydrates with a fifth of vodka, chances are your controlled-carb diet is now higher in either protein or fat (or both) than it was before and someone will soon be screaming bloody murder about how dangerous your diet is because of "all that fat" and how you will quickly die of heart disease.

So, as you can see, it's all but impossible to speak about low-carb diets and evaluate them properly without treading on a lot of preconceived ideas about fat.

In case you've just joined us from another planet and haven't heard the argument that's been repeated ad infinitum for the last few decades, here it is in a nutshell: low-carb diets are bad *because* they have too much fat, and too much fat (especially saturated fat) is bad *because* fat raises cholesterol, and high cholesterol is bad *because* it increases the risk for heart disease.

Now, if your first thought on reading the above argument was "*Well, sure, that makes sense,*" it's only because you've heard this argument so many times that you no longer question whether any of it is true. The association of fat and heart disease has become what philosophers call a "meme"—a generally accepted cultural notion that is deeply embedded in the national consciousness. To question it almost puts you in the category of the crowd with the tinfoil hats.

Hence this chapter. Because we've been taught so much gibberish about fat, and because the *fear* of fat is intimately entwined with *both* the fear of cholesterol *and* the general prejudice against low-carb diets, arming yourself with some basic info on fat may help you understand why a higher fat diet is nothing to fear. Sure, the "conventional wisdom" says otherwise, but in this case the conventional wisdom is only conventional. It is anything *but* wise.

Bear with me if you know this stuff—and even if you think you do, it's probably worth reviewing. I'm going to question some widely held beliefs now, including some choice tidbits of information you may be sure are true, but remember—sacred cows make the best burgers!

And one more thing: I promise to make this short and sweet, and my mission is to write it in such a way that your eyes don't glaze over.

Interested? Read on.

Everything You Ever Wanted to Know About Fat (But Were Afraid to Ask)

"Fat" is actually the general, colloquial term for a collection of smaller units technically (and properly) called fatty acids. Each of these fatty acids has a team identity—it belongs to a *group* (saturated, unsaturated). When we call something like butter or olive oil a "fat," what we actually mean is that it's a *collection of individual fatty acids.* (When a food is "high in fat," that just means it's got a lot of fatty acids in it.)

Almost all fats in food are some combination of the three main types of fatty acids—saturated, monounsaturated, and polyunsaturated—although we tend to identify a fat in food by the type of fatty acid that's *predominant* in the mix. For example, many foods that we characterize as having "saturated fats" (like butter or steak) actually contain many "unsaturated" fatty acids, and most foods that we refer to as "unsaturated fats" (like olive oil) contain some "saturated" fatty acids as well. And sometimes the mixture is actually quite different than you might think. (Would it surprise you to know, for example, that a typical sirloin steak has more *monounsaturated* fat than it does *saturated?* Or that fish oil—the ultimate unsaturated fat, and an omega-3 source to boot—is about 25% saturated fatty acids? Both are true.)

In addition to belonging to one of the three major "groups" of saturated, monounsaturated, or polyunsaturated fats, each individual fatty acid *also* comes with a molecular description (don't ask) and a name (e.g., stearic acid, lauric acid). This is important because some individual fatty acids have important health benefits and have distinct effects on the body. Lauric acid, for example, is a saturated fatty acid found in coconut that has immune-system–boosting properties—it's both antimicrobial and antiviral. Stearic acid, another saturated fatty acid, has virtually no effect on cholesterol.

Every single fatty acid on the planet—regardless of whether it's saturated, monounsaturated, or polyunsaturated—is basically a *chain of carbon atoms* linked together by chemical bonds. Think of a row of circles (carbon atoms), holding hands. You can also imagine these chains of carbon atoms as a bunch of little school kids on a day outing, joined together with one of those ropes that kindergarten teachers use when they take their kids on a field trip.

Now just as each of those kids in the kindergarten class has two arms that can "hold" something (like a book bag), each carbon atom has two "places" to which something can attach. In the case of the carbon atom, the only "thing" that can attach to those places are hydrogen atoms.

When all the "places" to which hydrogen atoms can attach are "filled" (i.e., "no seats left on the train"), the fatty acid is said to be "saturated." It's literally *saturated* with hydrogen. There's no more room at the table, so to speak. The places on the individual carbon atoms in the fatty acid are basically all occupied, so the fatty acid can't hold any more hydrogen passengers. (Trans-fats are a kind of "hybrid" saturated fat that's basically created in a lab by taking an "unsaturated" vegetable oil and blasting it with hydrogen atoms from the chemical equivalent of a turkey baster, forcing some hydrogen into the empty seats and producing "partially hydrogenated vegetable oil,"—or, as I like to call it, poison.)

Are you with me so far?

Good. Now, when there is one seat or more that's "unoccupied" on that chain link of carbons, the fatty acid is called *un*saturated—there are still places that could be occupied by hydrogen atoms. In other words, it's not yet a "full house." (If there's only *one* spot "open," it's called a *mono*unsaturated fatty acid; and if there's *more* than one spot "open," it's called a *poly*unsaturated fatty acid. More on that in a moment.)

So what happens when there's still "seating" on the carbon chain? Well, instead of holding on to two hydrogen atoms, that carbon atom takes its two empty hands and creates what's called a "double bond" with the next carbon in the chain. (Think of each school kid in the line holding *both hands* of the kid facing him. And because both his hands are now occupied, he can't hold anything else.) When there's just *one* such *double bond* in the chain, the fatty acid is called a—can you guess?—*mono*unsaturated fatty acid.

Fat Architecture

Now let's clear up all this stuff about "omegas." In fatty acids, as in real estate, there's one rule—location, location, location. Recall that if there's only *one* double bond in our little carbon atom chain, we're dealing with a *mono*unsaturated fatty acid. And if the *location* of that single double bond is on the 9th carbon counting from the end of the line, it's known as an *omega-9* fatty acid. How simple is that? The most famous source of omega-9 (monounsaturated) fat is olive oil, believed by just about everyone to be a "healthful" fat.

*Poly*unsaturated fatty acids simply have *more than one* double bond (hence the name "poly," which means "many"). Those that have their *very first* double bond on the 3rd position (counting from the end of the line) are called *omega-3s*. Those that have their very first double bond on the 6th position (again counting from the end of the line) are *omega-6s*.

OK, just in case your eyes are glazing over, there really *is* a good reason to know this stuff, and it's this: omega-3s and omega-6s are *building blocks* out of which the body makes distinct compounds (called *prostaglandins* or *eicosanoids*) that have different—and opposite—effects. For example, omega-3s are the building blocks for *anti*-inflammatory prostaglandins. Omega-6s are building blocks for *inflammatory* ones.

You might think: Hey, if omega-6s make inflammatory compounds, what do I need them for? Good question, and here's the answer: you need them because inflammation is a natural part of the body's healing response.

Let's say you injure your foot by stepping on a nail. What happens? Your foot swells up, because the body mounts a defensive reaction to that injury. Fluid and white blood cells rush in to surround the area, hoping to destroy any pathogens or bacteria that might have gotten into the wound, in an attempt to prevent an infection. You *need* the building blocks for that inflammation response* in your body, or you wouldn't have great "defenses" against what the body perceives as an attack.

But those inflammatory and anti-inflammatory prostaglandins need to be *in balance* in order for you to have an optimally functioning body. If your "pro-inflammation" factory is working overtime and your "anti-inflammation" factory is understaffed, you're in deep doo-doo. And that's exactly what's happened to most people eating a Western diet, which now has a ratio of about 20:1 in favor of omega-6 to omega-3. (The ideal ratio is between 1:1 and 4:1.)

You can't swing a rope without hitting an omega-6 fat—they're everywhere in our diet. Corn oil, soybean oil, vegetable oil, safflower oil, canola oil—all high in omega-6s. Those of us who have been taught the mantra "saturated fat *bad*, vegetable oil *good*" might think for a minute about consuming huge amounts of "unsaturated" vegetable oils without an appropriate amount of anti-inflammatory omega-3s to balance that intake.

You might think inflammation is no big deal, but you'd be making a huge mistake. Most of us are walking around with low-grade inflammation in our bodies that flies below the radar. Inflammation damages our vascular and circulatory systems and contributes to virtually every degenerative disease known to humankind, from heart disease to Alzheimer's, from cancer to diabetes. Not for nothing did *Time* magazine do a cover story called "Inflammation: The Silent Killer." There's a good deal of emerging evidence, by the way, that controlled-carb diets—even those higher in saturated fat—actually *lower* inflammation in the body.[1]

Here's something else to think about: we've done such a good job of demonizing saturated fat that it's effectively been replaced in our kitchens (and in fast-food restaurants) with the supposedly more healthful "vegetable" fat, most of which is stunningly high in omega-6s. The problem is that omega-6s are "unstable" fats. When used (and reused) for frying as they are in most fast-food restaurants, they actually get badly damaged and create carcinogenic compounds. Researchers at the University of Minnesota have

---

* In fact, one particular omega-6 fat—linoleic acid—is actually an essential fatty acid, meaning that it's required for health but your body can't make it, so you must get it from your diet.

shown that when unsaturated (omega-6) vegetable oils are heated at frying temperature (365° F) for extended periods—or even, for goodness' sake, for a half hour—toxic compounds will form. One in particular—HNE—is associated with a number of very bad chronic diseases that you really don't want to have.[2]

Saturated fats—because they are highly *stable*—do *not* create these toxic compounds when heated to high temperatures. Many people who really understand fat chemistry will tell you that they would much prefer deep frying in real lard (not Crisco®!) to reused canola oil any day of the week. It's far less damaging to the body. (My favorite oil for cooking at high temperatures in a wok or frying pan is Barlean's organic coconut oil.)

In addition to creating toxic compounds when heated repeatedly, vegetable oils used by fast-food restaurants often contain *trans-fats*, probably the most damaging fat on the planet (and one whose dangers dwarf the supposed dangers of saturated fat). Up until very recently, foods like margarine were loaded with the stuff. Kind of ironic, isn't it, when you think that the whole reason for the popularity of high omega-6 vegetable oil products like margarine was the desire to eliminate the "dangerous" saturated fat from our diet—talk about the "law of unintended consequences"!

So we have nothing to fear from a higher percentage of fat in our diet, particularly when it's "good" fat—by which I mean fat that has *not* been damaged by repeated high heat, fat or oil that is *not* highly refined (like some cooking and vegetable oils and *all* man-made trans-fats). Some cold-pressed unrefined omega-6s in the diet are fine, omega-9s are fine, omega-3s are better than fine, and—yup—*saturated fat is fine too*, especially when it comes from whole natural foods such as eggs, coconut, organic butter, and the like.

Now, here's an interesting factoid about fats: the only fatty acid that the body actually *makes* is palmitic acid—a saturated fat! Your body takes that palmitic acid and gets to work on it with a system of enzymes. It adds carbons, thus *lengthening* the chain—these enzymes are called *elongases* (they elongate the chain). It also *removes* pairs of hydrogens from some of the carbons that are saturated, thus creating new double bonds. The enzymes that do this are called *desaturases* (by removing some of the hydrogen passengers, they turn that saturated fat into an unsaturated one). Through this system of elongases and desaturases, the body—starting with saturated fat—winds up with a whole menu of fatty acids to serve different purposes. (We also get a variety of different fatty acids directly from our diet—like, for example, omega-3s directly from fish or flaxseed.)

If saturated fat were inherently so bad for us, why would it be the very fat our body makes naturally from food?

Saturated Fat and Heart Disease: What's the Real Connection?

In the context of today's conventional wisdom, it almost sounds ludicrous to put that question out there, so deeply accepted is the idea that saturated fat and heart disease are married forever in some metabolic Universe of Bad Things. But more and more researchers are asking that identical question, and the ones who are looking honestly at the data are not so convinced that the conventional wisdom is right. Over a decade ago, in 2008, the American Society of Bariatric Physicians, in conjunction with the Metabolism Society, presented an entire two-day conference in Arizona named "Saturated Fat and Heart Disease: What's the Evidence?"

I attended that conference, in which some of the smartest researchers investigating this issue participated; and I can sum up the answer to the question "What's the Evidence?" for you in two words: Not much.

In the ten plus years since that conference, we've had at least two major meta-analyses that further absolved saturated fat of a causal role in heart disease.[3] A 2015 systematic review and meta-analysis of randomized controlled trials,[4] performed by the prestigious Cochrane Collaboration, included 15 randomized controlled trials with more than 59,000 participants. These studies all reduced saturated fat in the diet or replaced it with other types of fats. Each one lasted more than two years and investigated what are called "hard end-points," which are the things we *really* care about, like actual heart attacks and deaths, not just a slight bump in cholesterol. At the end of the 2 years, the Cochrane group found that people who lowered their saturated fat intake were *just as likely* to suffer from heart attacks and strokes, or to die, as the people who *didn't* lower their saturated fat intake. This study confirmed an earlier 2011 study by the same group.[5]

And then there was Zoë Harcombe, who, for her PhD thesis in public health nutrition, undertook a systematic reevaluation of the evidence on which all low-fat dietary recommendations were based. These are the same recommendations we've been hearing globally for the better part of 40 years, the ones that demonize saturated fat and that recommend some form of a low-fat, high-grain diet to prevent heart disease. The results of her stunning research, which electrified the nutrition world, were published in *Open Heart.*[6] The title says it all: "Evidence from randomised controlled trials did not support the introduction of dietary fat guidelines in 1977 and 1983: a systematic review and meta-analysis."

I'm sure you're thinking right about now, "*What about all those studies I've read about that 'link' saturated fat consumption with heart disease?*" Well, to unpack the problems with those studies is a bigger project than I can take on in this book. But let's consider just a few of the issues worth thinking about before you buy—hook, line, and sinker—the idea that saturated fat is always "bad."

First—and this is an incredibly important point—the "fate" of saturated fat in the body varies significantly, depending on what else is eaten. "Saturated fat is a completely neutral fat," says my friend Mike Eades, MD. "It burns like any other fat." If you're eating a high-carb diet, the effect of saturated fat may indeed be deleterious, but *if you're eating a low-carb diet, it's a whole other ballgame.* "If carbs are low, insulin is low and saturated fat is handled more efficiently," said Jeff Volek, PhD, RD, one of the major researchers in the area of diet comparisons. "When carbs are low, you're burning that saturated fat as fuel, and you're also making less of it."

One study tested what happens when you take obese patients and put them on a high-saturated-fat diet—but without starch. The researchers took 23 patients with atherosclerotic cardiovascular disease and put them on a high-saturated-fat diet, but one in which all the starch had been removed. Here's what happened: body weight decreased, body-fat percentage decreased, total triglycerides decreased. The researchers concluded that a high-saturated-fat/starch-avoidance diet resulted in weight loss after 6 weeks *without adverse effects on serum-lipid levels.*[7] I suspect the results would have been very different indeed if the participants had been eating a lot of carbs along with that saturated fat.

The Paradox

Remember, when you're dealing with a diet in "free-living" humans—as opposed to lab rats—you have four dietary variables (at least) to deal with: total calories, percent protein, percent carbs, and percent fat. *It is impossible to change one without changing the others.* So whenever you "test" a diet that's *high* in one of those elements, it's by definition also *lower* in another (and vice versa).

Let's say, for example, that you have a 1,500-calorie diet made up of 70% carbohydrates, 15% fat, and 15% protein. If you now raise the fat intake by 20% (from 15% to 35%), keeping overall calories and protein the same, you've automatically *lowered* the carb intake by the same 20% (from 70% of the diet to 50%). That decrease in carb intake may produce—in certain populations—a very beneficial effect, lowering both insulin levels and triglyceride levels (and possibly increasing HDL in the process). In such a scenario, it would be entirely possible to say that an *increase* in fat (even saturated fat!) was associated with a *lowered* risk for heart disease.

And that's exactly what one study showed. Research by epidemiologist Dariush Mozaffarian, MD, at Harvard found that a "higher saturated fat intake is associated with *less* progression of coronary artery disease." What? Saturated fat *good* for you? In research done at Harvard? How can this possibly be explained?

Well, some folks at the prestigious *American Journal of Clinical Nutrition* wondered the same thing. They wrote a fascinating editorial in the November 2004 issue titled "Saturated Fat Prevents Coronary Artery Disease? An American Paradox." The authors posed the not-unreasonable question, "*How can this paradox be explained?*"

How, indeed. Since, as the authors point out, it's an article of faith that saturated fat raises LDL cholesterol and *accelerates* coronary artery disease, how are we to account for a study that shows the exact opposite?

The answer that keeps emerging from the research is this: the metabolic fate of saturated fat—what it actually *does* or *does not do* in the body—depends largely on what *else* is eaten. Eat way fewer carbohydrates and way less sugar, and how much saturated fat you eat may not matter so much.[8]

This is the explanation most scientists who are now researching low-carb diets believe accounts for their findings that higher saturated fat aren't a problem, as *long as people are not eating high amounts of carbohydrate.* But once you're eating a ton of carbs, all bets are off. If you're eating the standard Western mixed diet, high in sugar, high in processed carbs, high in fast food, and hugely high in calories, then yup, adding more saturated fat is a really bad idea. Added to a high-calorie, high-carb diet, saturated fat won't be burned as "fuel" and will tend to get stored on your hips. In the context of that kind of diet, the "low-fat" folks are probably right.

But a much *better* approach would be to cut out the sugar and processed carbs! In that case, the amount of saturated fat you're consuming probably wouldn't matter so much. Remember that in the early part of the twentieth century, the percentage of the American diet was much higher in saturated fat, and we had much lower rates of heart disease. Of course, we also consumed less food in general, fast food hadn't been invented, we ate much less sugar, and we moved around more. The point is that it's not saturated fat that's the demon here.

A second reason that saturated fat has been demonized, in my opinion, is that much of the research on diet and disease has lumped saturated fat together with trans-fats. Trans-fats weren't even a health issue until relatively recently, and for decades researchers didn't distinguish between the two when doing studies of diet patterns. Why does this matter? Because man-made trans-fats really are the spawn of Satan. They clearly raise the risk for heart disease and stroke, and, according to Harvard professors Walt Willett and Alberto Ascherio, are responsible for 30,000 premature deaths a year,[9] so obviously a study that lumps trans-fats together with saturated fat is going to show some nasty associations. The question is: Are those nasty health effects caused by the trans-fats, or by the saturated fats?

I think it's pretty clear that it's the trans-fats; and if you separate the two and look at their effects on the body as two distinct entities, you're going to see some very big differences. If you lump them together—as many researchers did before we knew what we know now—saturated fats are likely to be tainted by the negative actions of trans-fats.

Even the cholesterol-raising effect of saturated fat may be influenced by the presence of trans-fats. One study showed that palmitic acid (a saturated fatty acid) had no effect on cholesterol when the intake of omega-6 is greater than 4.5% of calorie intake; but if the diet contained trans-fats, the effect was completely different—LDL went up and HDL went down.[10] (How much this even matters is a whole different question. Still, it's important to point out that the combination of saturated fat and trans-fats has a different effect than saturated fat alone.)

The third reason saturated fat has such a bad reputation is that much of the saturated fat people consume comes from really crummy sources. Fried foods are not a great way to get fat in your diet. Neither are processed deli meats nor hormone-treated beef. But the saturated fat from healthy animals (like grass-fed beef or lamb) or the saturated fat in organic butter or in egg yolks is a whole different story. In fact, studies of dairy fat and heart disease have failed to show any compelling relationship between the two,[11] and recent literature reviews have shown that dairy fat can actually *protect* against obesity![12]

I've never seen one convincing piece of evidence that saturated fat from *whole-food sources* like the ones I just mentioned has a single negative impact on heart disease, health, or mortality, especially when it's part of a diet high in plant foods, antioxidants, fiber, and the rest of the good stuff you can eat on a controlled-carbohydrate eating plan!

The Big Reason Saturated Fat Has Been Demonized: The Cholesterol Connection

And finally, the zinger—the *major* reason saturated fat has been demonized over the years is this: *cholesterol.* The perception that saturated fat *always raises cholesterol* is enough to scare anyone exposed to conventional health "wisdom," and is so embedded in the national (and international) consciousness that it would take more than a crowbar to pry it loose from our belief system.

The truth about saturated fat raising cholesterol is this: Sometimes it does. And sometimes it doesn't.

And the bigger truth—hold on to your hats—is this: *it may not even matter.*

The Cholesterol Controversy

When we focus on cholesterol, we're *not telling the whole story.* In fact, we're not even telling the most *important* part of the story, and—according to many—the part of the story we *are* telling may actually be virtually irrelevant.

Here's why.

You don't really *care* what your cholesterol level is; what you *care* about is your risk for *heart disease.* And you've come to believe they're essentially the same thing. The only reason you even *know* your cholesterol level is that it has become embedded in your consciousness (as it was in mine) as an *important marker for heart-disease risk.* In fact, for many people, it is *synonymous* with heart-disease risk. (Doubt that? Try this party trick: ask five friends to say the first thing that comes to mind when you say the term "risk for heart disease." Case closed.)

But here's the thing: Fully half of the people with heart disease have perfectly "normal" cholesterol levels. And half the people who have what's considered "elevated" cholesterol have perfectly normal hearts.

As long ago as 1994, a study published in the conservative and august *Journal of the American Medical Association* demonstrated a complete lack of association between cholesterol levels and coronary-heart-disease mortality in persons over 70 years old. It also demonstrated a complete lack of association between cholesterol levels and mortality from any cause in that same population.[13] Since we already know that the rate of heart disease in 65-year-old men is many times that of 45-year-old men, does it make sense that cholesterol suddenly "stops" becoming a risk factor when you get older? It makes *more* sense that it wasn't that big of a risk factor in the first place! This is akin to suggesting that smoking causes lung cancer in young men, but somehow stops doing it in older men!

Consider also a classic study conducted in France over a four-year period from March 1988 to March 1992 and published in the journal *Circulation* in 1999.[14] The study—called the Lyon Diet Heart Study—looked at 605 patients who had already had a first heart attack. These folks were *not* in great shape—they had classic risk factors, high cholesterol, many were smokers, the whole ball game. Half of the 600 or so subjects were given the standard advice about eating a "prudent" diet (lower fat, lower cholesterol) and the other half were given instructions on following what we call the "Mediterranean diet"—high in olive oil, vegetables, fruits, and so on. (Neither group was given the standard treatment for high cholesterol, a statin drug.)

Are you ready for the results?

Those following the Mediterranean diet had a 72% decrease in coronary events and a 56% decrease in overall mortality.

The results were so stunning that the study had to be stopped in the middle so that everyone could go on the diet program that had produced such outstanding results.

But that's not even the best part. Get ready for the kicker:

Though people were dying at less than half the rate expected, and were having coronary events at about one-quarter the rate expected, *their cholesterol levels hardly budged.*

Did you get that? An almost 75% decrease in heart disease *without a budge in cholesterol levels!*

Now let's fast-forward to a drug study completed in 2006, the widely publicized ENHANCE trial. If you were following the news in 2008, you couldn't have missed this one, because it made the front pages of the newspapers and all the television news shows. Here's what happened.

A combination cholesterol-lowering medication called Vytorin® had been the subject of a huge research project, the results of which were finally coming to light and being given enormous negative attention. One of the many reasons for this negative attention—besides the actual results, which I'm going to share with you in a moment—was the fact that the companies jointly making the drug (Merck and Schering-Plough) waited almost 2 years before releasing the results of the study.

No wonder. The results stunk. Which was the *other* reason this drug test made the front pages. The new "wonder" drug *lowered cholesterol just fine.* In fact, it lowered it *better* than a standard statin drug. So you'd think everyone would be jumping for joy, right? Lower cholesterol, lower heart disease— let's have a party for the shareholders!

Not quite. Although the people taking Vytorin saw their cholesterol plummet just fine, they actually had *more* plaque growth than the people taking the standard cholesterol drug. The patients on Vytorin—low cholesterol and all—actually had almost twice as great an increase in the thickness of their arterial walls, a result you definitely don't want to see if you're trying to prevent heart disease.

So their cholesterol was wonderfully lowered and their risk for heart disease went up: shades of "the operation was a success, but the patient died."

Taken together—and there are countless other examples—I think we might be able to at least *question* the widely accepted dogma that *cholesterol is what we need to be focused on when it comes to heart disease.*

But wait! If cholesterol is not the huge deal everyone thinks it is, then it's reasonable to ask the question: Why are we so afraid of saturated fat? After all, isn't the big "rap" against saturated fat that it raises cholesterol? If that's not as big a deal as we thought, why are we so afraid of saturated fat?

Now you're beginning to get it.

Fact is, according to a ton of research by Jeff Volek, PhD, RD, and others, saturated fat *sometimes* raises cholesterol and sometimes doesn't. And then there's the question of exactly what "kind" of cholesterol it does raise.

Size Matters

As we touched on in chapter 3, there are several different subtypes of HDL (so-called "good" cholesterol) and several different subtypes of LDL (so-called "bad" cholesterol). In short, the large fluffy subtype of LDL is associated with much lower heart-disease risk than small, dense LDL. These subtypes of LDL—combined with the total number of LDL particles hanging out in our blood—are far more interesting to us than the total cholesterol content measured by standard cholesterol tests (even though that's the number that most people focus on).

In recent years, studies have begun to look at the factors that affect these particle sizes.[15] We are finding out that while the traditional high-carb, low-fat diet may in fact lower *overall* LDL, it *raises* the dangerous pattern B molecules and *lowers* protective HDL cholesterol. So while your overall cholesterol number may go down, your overall risk may go *up*. What often happens on a high saturated-fat diet is that LDL goes up—*but this is not the whole story*. When scientists look at the *actual particle sizes* of that LDL cholesterol, they find that higher saturated-fat intake (in the context of a low-carb diet) usually results in a significant shift to *more* of the harmless big fluffy particles and *fewer* of the much more dangerous little ones. Quite often, this happens without an increase (and sometimes even a decrease) in the total number of LDL particles we have—which is turning out to be a consistently important risk factor for heart disease.

And we haven't even begun to talk about triglycerides.

Triglycerides, which don't get nearly as much attention as cholesterol, are a far greater risk factor for heart disease than cholesterol is.[16] (They're also a significant risk for strokes.)[17] And triglyceride levels always come down on a low-carb diet. Always. Not sometimes; all the time. (Which makes sense—the body takes all that excess sugar and packages it into triglycerides, so the less sugar in the diet, the less triglycerides in the blood.)

Furthermore, according to a Harvard study published in *Circulation*,[18] the ratio of triglycerides to HDL cholesterol is a much better predictor of heart disease than cholesterol is. Also, according to many experts (including the Metabolic Syndrome Institute), that ratio can serve as a good "surrogate" marker for insulin resistance. Personally, if you show me a person with a ratio of 2 (triglycerides to HDL) who doesn't smoke, works out, isn't overweight, and has low markers of inflammation (CRP and homocysteine, for example), I'll bet you my life savings he's not going to have a heart attack, and I don't care what his cholesterol numbers are.

But that's just me.

Now let's reexamine the effects of this mythical low-carb diet on our mythical patient whose doctor is furiously prescribing statins.

PRE–LOW-CARB DIET	POST–LOW-CARB DIET
Triglycerides 175	Triglycerides 100
TOTAL CHOLESTEROL: 200	TOTAL CHOLESTEROL: 240
HDL: 50	HDL: 60
Triglyceride-to-HDL ratio: 3.5	Triglyceride-to-HDL ratio: 1.66
LDL cholesterol: 130	LDL cholesterol:150
LDL "fluffy" particles: 65	LDL "fluffy" particles: 110
LDL "small" particles: 65	LDL "small" particles: 40

Post–low-carb diet, this guy should be taking that blood test home and jumping for joy. His lipid profile is vastly improved. By every measure, he's doing way better than he was before the diet.

But his cholesterol went up.

To which I say: So what?

There are currently tens of millions of Americans on cholesterol-lowering medications. As of 2006, two of the five top-selling drugs in America were cholesterol-lowering medications, and they collectively rang up sales of over 18 billion dollars. Even without throwing in the annual budget of the National Cholesterol Education Program, it's safe to say that well over 20 billion dollars a year rides on the effort to get Americans to lower their cholesterol and fat. Current guidelines are to reduce saturated fat to 7% of the diet,[19] and there's a movement afoot to recommend lowering it even more. The American Academy of Pediatrics now recommends cholesterol screening for some children as young as 2, and treatment with statin drugs to lower cholesterol for some children as young as 8.[20]

Statin drugs probably do save some lives (though the number is probably way less than you've been led to believe, and the cost remains to be seen). However, whether they do so by reducing cholesterol is an open question. What the statins do *in addition* to lowering cholesterol is to reduce *inflammation*, which *is* a cause of heart disease. They also slightly reduce platelet aggregation (blood clotting) by thinning the blood. What they do to cholesterol, in my opinion, is their least important function in the body. You can reduce inflammation by consuming omega-3 fatty acids and reducing consumption of grains without the possible side effects of statin, including liver toxicity and mitochondrial damage, and without the increased risk of death from other causes associated with excessively low cholesterol numbers. (And you can thin the blood with a baby aspirin!)

Are we likely to see a moratorium on the demonization of fat and cholesterol and a move toward eliminating the real health-robbers in our diet, like sugar and processed carbs? Not bloody likely, and probably not anytime soon. As the author Upton Sinclair put it: *"It is difficult to get a man to understand something when his salary depends upon his not understanding it."*

The bottom line is that if you're eating a very-low-carb diet, I don't think you have much to worry about if it contains a relatively high amount of saturated fat, and you certainly don't have anything to worry about if it contains a nice mix of fats from omega-3s, 6s, 9s, and saturated fat. If you're downing six or seven meals of fast food a day with an average daily intake of 3,500 calories (or more!), adding more saturated fat *is* going to have a negative effect—you can count on it. Added to a high-calorie, high-carb diet, saturated fat is *not* a great thing. It won't be burned as "fuel" and will tend to get stored on your hips. If that's the kind of diet you're eating, the "low-fat" folks are probably right.

But a much better approach would be to cut out the sugar and processed carbs (and lower your calories to boot), in which case the amount of saturated fat you're consuming probably wouldn't matter half as much.

Now, before we wrap this up, let's be clear about one thing: I'm *not* saying you should go out and start drinking oodles of saturated fat. (I *am* saying you shouldn't be terrified of it, but that's a different statement.) The important thing to remember is this: *the metabolic effect saturated fat has on your body—its "fate," if you will—depends entirely on what else it's consumed with.*

In 2000, Walter Willett, MD, PhD, arguably the world's most respected nutritional epidemiologist, chairman of the Department of Nutrition at the Harvard School of Public Health, and the lead researcher on the Nurses' Health Study and the Health Professional Follow-Up Study, was interviewed by Harvard's *World Health News*. This is what he said:

"We have found virtually no relationship between the percentage of calories from fat and any important health outcome."[21]

Amen to that.

CHAPTER 6

The Biggest Myths About Low-Carb Diets

Over the years, there have been many criticisms leveled at low-carbohydrate diets. Some of these have been repeated so often that they are now taken as gospel, even though some have never been closely examined; while others have long ago been proven false, although they continue to be repeated as if the research debunking them had never happened. Some of these beliefs are based on complete misunderstandings of biochemistry and physiology, and some on an astonishing distortion of the program being criticized. (For example, one supposedly reputable health information website criticized the Zone on the basis of the "fact" that "the Zone diet contains less than 1,000 calories," which is patently false.)

Some of these beliefs are nothing less than cultural memes. They're rarely examined—they just "are." Examples of memes are tunes, catchphrases, or basic foundational beliefs—i.e., things "everybody knows" (like "the world is round," "birds fly," "you need eight glasses of water a day," and "saturated fat causes heart disease"). Some memes are useful and true, but some are in dire need of reexamination and should ultimately be dumped in the cultural wastebasket.

You'd think "science," with its reliance on experiment and validation and objective measurement, would be immune to the vagaries of beliefs and prejudices. However, you'd be sadly wrong. Scientists are first and foremost people, and they can be just as shockingly petty, proprietary, and stubborn as the rest of us. And entrenched beliefs and theories don't die easily. The history of science is littered with theories that lasted 50 or 100 years or more before people finally came to accept that they weren't valid.* Decades' worth of the prevailing medical and dietetic beliefs can be summed up in six words: low-carb diets will hurt you.

Luckily, the tides have—slowly and reluctantly—started to turn. Although most mainstream nutrition authorities still clutch tightly to the anti–low-carb dogma, the public is wising up. In May 2018, a survey conducted by the International Food Information Council Foundation found that a growing number of Americans believe carbohydrates—particularly sugar—is responsible for weight gain (33% of respondents cited sugar as driving weight gain and 25% cited carbohydrates, compared to only 16% blaming fat).[1] Even more exciting, dieters are hopping en masse on the low-carb bandwagon: according to this same survey, 24% of dieting respondents were following a reduced-carbohydrate eating pattern (including paleo, low-carb, Whole30®, high-protein, and ketogenic).

Nonetheless, some myths just refuse to die—even among folks who've been convinced, whether by science or by experience, that low-carb diets really *are* all they're cracked up to be. Let's take on a few of the most commonly held assumptions here and see where it takes us. At the very least, perhaps some of what I'm about to say will give you pause next time you hear one of these myths repeated with great authority as if it was gospel truth.

MYTH #1: You "Need" Carbs

When I do live workshops and talks, I often do the following demonstration: I tell everyone in the audience to pretend they are on the show *Survivor*

---

* Two famous examples come to mind. One, when Kilmer McCully, MD, of Harvard first hypothesized that homocysteine was at least as great a risk factor for heart disease as cholesterol, he was literally ridiculed out of his lab at Harvard. Twenty-five years later, homocysteine tests are routinely performed; homocysteine is widely recognized as a risk factor for heart disease, stroke, and Alzheimer's; and McCully is back at Harvard. Second example: when Jonas Folkman, MD, proposed angiogenesis as a mechanism by which cancer cells were able to thrive, he too was ridiculed, laughed at, and ostracized from the scientific community. (Establishment medicine, contrary to popular belief, does not like mavericks.) Angiogenesis is now widely accepted, and Folkman—now dead—is recognized and acclaimed as the brilliant and innovative pioneer that he was. Doctors, unfortunately, do not always take kindly to those who question their most cherished assumptions (see, for example, how the brilliant scientists who populate the International Network of Cholesterol Skeptics are treated by the conventional medical establishment, most of it documented on their website, http://www.thincs.org—it's not pretty).

and we're going to divide the room into two teams. Everyone in the room is going to be on a desert island for one year. Then I draw an imaginary line in the middle of the room and make everyone to the left of the line "Group One" and everyone on the right of the line "Group Two."

Then I say the following:

"Everyone in Group One will be fed absolutely nothing but protein and fat for one year. You will get zero carbohydrates in your diet. Everyone in Group Two will be fed nothing but carbohydrates for one year. You will get zero protein and zero fat."

Then I pause for the punch line, which is this:

"Everyone in Group Two will be dead within the year. Everyone in Group One will be doing just fine."

The fact is—hold on to your seats now—there is no physiological need for carbohydrates in the human diet.[2]

None.

Now, before you throw this book down and decide that I'm completely crazy for making such an outrageous statement, take a look at what the august and esteemed Institute of Medicine (renamed the National Academy of Medicine in 2015) had has to say about this in its reference manual, *Dietary Reference Intakes: Energy, Carbohydrate, Fiber, Fat, Fatty Acids, Cholesterol, Protein, and Amino Acids.* In case you don't want to bother looking it up, here's what it says on page 275:

"The lower limit of dietary carbohydrate compatible with life apparently is zero, provided that adequate amounts of protein and fat are consumed."[3]

In other words, just consume enough protein and fat and you'll be fine, even without carbs—much like Group One in my example above.

The Institute of Medicine went on to say: "There are traditional populations that ingested a high fat, high protein diet containing only a minimal amount of carbohydrate for extended periods of time (Masai), and in some cases for a lifetime after infancy (Alaska and Greenland Natives, Inuits, and Pampas indigenous people) (Du Bois, 1928; Heinbecker, 1928). There was no apparent effect on health or longevity. Caucasians eating an essentially carbohydrate-free diet, resembling that of Greenland natives, for a year tolerated the diet quite well (Du Bois, 1928)."

You've probably heard that the brain requires a minimum 120 grams of carbs a day in order to function. Actually, that's technically inaccurate—it does indeed need 120 grams of glucose (sugar) to function, but it can make that glucose perfectly well from certain amino acids (found in protein) and from the glycerol backbone of triglycerides. Let's not confuse dietary carbs with glucose. They're not the same thing.

OK, now that we've got that out of the way, let me back up a minute.

The fact that there is no dietary need for carbohydrates simply means we can survive without them. It does not mean—and I am not saying—that we shouldn't eat them (see myth #2).* I'm simply pointing out a basic fact in biology. Our bodies will and can run on ketones[4]—quite nicely, thank you very much—and whereas we will die without protein and fat, we will not die without carbohydrates. However, we would not die without hot and cold running water, nor without indoor plumbing. Nor without someone to cuddle with every night. That doesn't mean we shouldn't have them.

I do think it's curious that groups like the American Academy of Nutrition and Dietetics continue to recommend that the lion's share of our calories come from the one macronutrient we could actually survive without! But don't get me started.

Of course, we can also play devil's advocate here and make the case that while we do need dietary fat to survive, that "need" is only for small amounts of the aptly named *essential fatty acids* (linoleic acid, an omega-6 fat, and alpha-linolenic acid, an omega-3 fat). According to the World Health Organization, getting 2.5% of our daily calories from linoleic acid and 0.5% of our daily calories from alpha-linolenic acid covers our entire dietary fat needs.[5] Thus, there's no such thing as an essential saturated fat or essential monounsaturated fat, as delicious as they may be—those can be manufactured inside the body from other nutrients.

Not surprisingly, some challengers of low-carbohydrate eating have thrown this back as a retort to the "no biological need for carbohydrates" argument. And it's fine to admit they have a point. If our bodies only require tiny amounts of two specific omega fats, why promote a higher intake of all these other "non-essential" fats?

Here's where that logic falls apart.

While we can technically survive on low levels of fat (keeping in mind, there's a *big* difference between surviving and thriving), fat keeps us healthy by playing a number of secondary roles that carbs simply can't fulfill. In addition to providing some *essential fatty acids*, dietary fat often comes with important fat-soluble vitamins (and, not to mention, assists with their absorption), satiates appetite, and helps produce hormones. Meanwhile, carbohydrates bring exactly zero of these benefits to the table.

---

*And I don't mean to imply that the august researchers at the Institute of Medicine believed we shouldn't eat them either. They were simply saying that we appear to be able to survive quite well without them, pointing out: "The amount of dietary carbohydrate that provides for optimal health in humans is unknown."

BOTTOM LINE

Although carbohydrates like fruits, vegetables, and beans provide an array of important nutrients, dietary carbohydrates are not physiologically necessary in the human diet.

MYTH #2: In a Low-Carb Diet, You'll Be Missing All the Vitally Important Nutrients that You Get from Carbs

Well, this myth would have some validity *if* low-carb advocates actually suggested cutting out all carbs.

But most don't. (For the first three editions of this book, that sentence read "But no one does." That's no longer true, as there is a small but persuasive group of low-carbers on basically all-meat diets, also known as the Carnivore Diet (see page 264), AKA the zero-carb diet.

But as of this writing, the zero-carbers are a *very* small minority and are likely to remain so if only because an all-meat diet is not practical for a lot of people. The majority of low-carbers believe that carbs—from vegetables and fruits and legumes—provide fiber, phytochemicals, and a wealth of nutrients, vitamins, and minerals. Controlled-carb does *not* have to mean no-carb. Controlled-carb eating does usually mean a no-*junk* diet, and one with a lot less sugar and starch.

What's more, you can eat a ton—and I mean a *ton*—of vegetables and even fruits, and still be on the "low" end of the carbohydrate spectrum.

Consider this: you could eat—*on a daily basis*—the following carbohydrate foods and still be consuming *under* 140 grams of carbohydrate, which is *less than half* of what most Americans now consume:

- 5 cups of spinach = 5.45 grams carbs (3.5 fiber)
- 2 cups cooked broccoli = 22.4 grams carbs (10.1 fiber)
- 1 cup of raspberries = 14.69 grams carbs (8 fiber)
- 1 medium apple = 25.13 grams carbs (4.4 fiber)
- 20 grapes = 17.74 grams carbs (0.8 fiber)
- ½ sweet potato = 11.8 grams carbs (1.9 fiber)
- ½ bowl of oatmeal = 13.5 grams carbs (2 fiber)
- ½ cup of Brussels sprouts = 5.54 grams carbs (2 fiber)
- ½ cup of blueberries = 10.72 grams carbs (1.8 fiber)
- 2 medium carrots =11.68 grams carbs (3.4 fiber)

Considering that most people in America aren't even getting 5 (let alone 7 or 9) servings of fruits and vegetables, and considering that the above list represents roughly *16 servings*, you can see that I picked a pretty extreme menu. But even so—16 servings of carb foods and you're still *under* 140 grams (138.63 to be exact, but who's counting?).

But wait: it gets better.

Most people in the low-carb world don't count fiber as part of their "carbohydrate" intake, since it has absolutely no effect on blood sugar. They subtract fiber from total carb count, and call what's left either "net carbs" or "effective carbs," which is pretty much the way it should be. The above 16 servings give you a whopping 37.9 grams of fiber, one of the most important nutrients for health on the planet. (The average American gets between 4 and 11 grams, and every major health organization recommends between 25 and 38 grams.)

If you subtract those 37.9 grams of fiber from the overall carb total of 138.63, you are left with about 100 grams of carbs a day. That might be enough to make the American Academy of Nutrition and Dietetics apoplectic, but who cares? I defy anyone on the planet to show me how a diet that includes the above 16 servings of fruits and vegetables, *plus* plenty of protein (grass-fed meat, wild salmon) and fat like olive and coconut oil, nuts, avocados, and even a glass of red wine and a bite of dark chocolate, is "unhealthful." Show me. Please. I'll be right here waiting.

And I'll be waiting a hell of a long time.

Now, some people in the low-carb world would not consider 140 grams of carbs a "low-carb" diet. It's almost certainly not a ketogenic diet. And for some people—particularly the very insulin-insensitive, or those with metabolic conditions in which every single gram of carbohydrate must be counted—140 grams might be too high. But let's talk for a minute about the general reader: you, perhaps. A diet that reduces carbs to that very reasonable amount, and at the same time front-loads it on vegetables and fruits, is going to represent an improvement that's literally light-years ahead of what most folks are currently eating. It's going to extend your life, increase your energy, stabilize your weight, and improve your health.

MYTH #3: Low-Carbohydrate Diets Cause Calcium Loss, Bone Loss, and/or Osteoporosis

This criticism of low-carb (or high-protein) diets is based on the fact that higher levels of protein result in higher levels of calcium in the urine, leading some people to the erroneous conclusion that protein causes bone loss.

KILLER CARBS

Ever wonder why you're hungry for more after you eat a high-carb snack or meal?

Research by Zane Andrews, MD, and his team at Monash University in Australia identified key appetite-control cells in the human brain.* These appetite-control cells are attacked by free radicals after eating, but the attack is bigger and stronger following a meal rich in sugar and carbohydrates.

"The more carbs and sugars you eat, the more your appetite-control cells are damaged," said Andrews, the lead researcher on the study. The result? You eat more.

The forces that compel you to eat and the forces that tell the brain "Hey, this dude is full!" are constantly at war. When your stomach is empty, it triggers the release of a hunger hormone called ghrelin. When you're full, a set of neurons known as POMC's (proopiomelanocortins) kicks in.

Free radicals normally created in the body attack both the "hunger" neurons and the "antihunger" neurons, but the "hunger" neurons are naturally protected. This tips the scale in the direction of hunger and cravings.

And carbs create the most damage of all.

According to Andrews, people in the age group 25 to 50 are most at risk. "The neurons that tell people in that crucial age range not to overeat are being killed off."

Yet another reason to limit your sugar and processed carbs if you don't want to be the victim of constant cravings.

* Monash University, "Killer Carbs: Scientist Finds Key to Overeating as We Age," *Science Daily* (August 21, 2008). http://www.sciencedaily.com/releases/2008/08/080821110113.htm.

But a tremendous number of recent studies are showing something quite the opposite.

Want Strong Bones? Eat More Protein!

The Framingham Osteoporosis Study investigated protein consumption over a 4-year period among 615 elderly men and women with an average age of 75. The amount of protein eaten daily ranged from a low of 14 grams a day to a high of 175 grams. And guess what? The people who consumed *more* protein had less bone loss! Those who ate less protein had more bone loss, both at the femoral bone and at the spine. The study also found that "higher intake of animal protein *does not appear to affect the skeleton adversely.*"[6] [Emphasis mine.]

Calcium is better absorbed on a higher-protein diet, even if there is somewhat more *urinary* calcium excretion. High-protein diets in two recent studies resulted in *significantly more* calcium absorption than the low-protein diets, which were associated with *decreased* absorption.[7] Interestingly, the actual "low-protein" diet that caused decreased calcium absorption in these studies had about the same amount of protein that the government recommends for adults! The authors concluded that this fact "raises new questions about the optimal amount of dietary protein required for normal calcium metabolism and bone health in young women." And a 2002 study in *Obesity Research* looked at a high-protein versus low-protein diet to determine whether the protein content of the diet impacted bone mineral density. It did. *Bone mineral loss was greater in the low-protein group.*[8]

In other words, without enough protein, you just ain't gonna build (and preserve) strong bones, and the definition of "enough protein" may turn out to be a lot more than we previously thought.

The Verdict on Protein: Not Guilty

So, how did protein get this bad reputation for causing calcium loss and osteoporosis? It partly stems from something in the body called the acid–base balance. All foods eventually digest and present themselves to the kidneys as either acid or alkaline (base). When there is too much acid, the body needs to buffer it, and calcium is one of the best buffering agents—including the calcium deposited in your bones. Meats—along with many other foods, especially grains—are known to be acid-producing (meaning they produce more acidic ammonium than alkaline bicarbonate after reaching your kidneys); hence the deduction that high-protein diets would cause a leeching of calcium from the bone in order to alkalize the acid content.

But here's the thing: we now know that if you take in enough alkalinizing nutrients, this doesn't happen. If you balance your high-protein foods with calcium (and potassium), you will not lose calcium from your bones! An interesting side note: you can take all the supplemental calcium you want; if you don't get enough protein, it's not going to make much difference to your bone health. The studies are very clear on this: *extra calcium is not enough to affect the skeleton when protein intake is low.*[9]

In short, it doesn't matter if there is a little more calcium in the urine as long as the body is holding on to more calcium than it's losing (i.e., is in "positive" calcium balance). And it will do that when there's plenty of protein plus calcium (and other minerals) in the diet.

BOTTOM LINE

Higher protein intakes do not cause bone loss or osteoporosis, especially in the presence of adequate mineral intakes. In fact, lower protein intakes are associated with more bone loss.

MYTH #4: High-Protein Diets Cause Damage to the Kidneys

You will often hear that a high-protein diet damages the kidneys. Not so. Consider the example of step classes, which everyone knows are great calorie burners. They get the blood and oxygen flowing, are good conditioners of the cardiovascular system, and, with certain variations, can even be good for muscle toning. So step classes are a good thing, right?

Yup.

Unless you have a broken leg.

If you have a broken leg, or a sprained ankle, or shin splints, I'm going to suggest that you stay away from step classes until the injury heals. Under these special circumstances, the very weight-bearing that does so much good for the normal person is going to be more stress than you need during the healing phase. I'm going to tell you to stay off the leg, let it heal, and avoid putting additional stress on it at this time.

Does the fact that step class is not good for a person with a broken leg mean that the step class *led* to the broken leg?

No. And ketogenic diets do not—I repeat, *do not*—cause kidney disease. If your doctor says they do, politely ask him or her to show you the studies. (They don't exist.) Ketogenic diets may *not* be a good thing if you have an *existing kidney disease*, much the way a step class is not a good thing if your leg is already broken. Check with a keto-friendly doctor.

High Protein Causes Kidney Disease? Not.

The oft-repeated medical legend that high-protein diets cause kidney disease came from reversing a medical fact. The medical fact is that reducing protein (up to a point) lessens the decline of renal (kidney) function in people who already have kidney disease. Because restricting protein seems to be a good strategy for those with *existing* kidney failure (or even some kidney weakness), some people drew the illogical conclusion that the reverse must also be true—that large amounts of protein *lead* to kidney failure.

In any case, it is not proteins per se that cause problems, even for those who already have renal disease: it is the *glycolated* proteins. These sticky proteins, you may remember, are the result of excess sugar in the blood bumping into protein molecules. These sugar-coated proteins are called AGEs, advanced glycolated end-products. The AGEs themselves then stick together, forming even bigger collections of molecules, which are too large to pass through the filtering mechanisms of the *glomerulus*, the network of blood capillaries in the kidneys that acts as a filter for waste products from the blood. This reduces GFR (glomerular filtration rate), a measure of kidney function.

High-protein intake *does not* cause this to happen in normally functioning kidneys. In 2003, a study of 1,624 women enrolled in the Nurses' Health Study concluded that "high protein intake was *not* associated with renal function decline in women with normal renal function."[10] Another study in the *American Journal of Kidney Diseases* showed that protein intake had *no effect* on GFR in healthy male subjects.[11] And a third study in the *International Journal of Obesity* compared a high-protein with a low-protein weight-loss diet and concluded that healthy kidneys adapted to protein intake and that the high-protein diet caused no adverse effects.[12]

If you don't currently have kidney disease, a low-carbohydrate diet is actually an ideal way to help control the blood-sugar levels that can eventually lead to kidney disease. Of course, just to be safe, you should check with your doctor to make sure you don't have any undiagnosed kidney impairment; but if you don't, you're sure not going to develop it from being on a low-carb diet.

BOTTOM LINE

Higher protein intakes do not cause any damage whatsoever to healthy kidneys.

MYTH #5: The Only Reason You Lose Weight on a Low-Carb Diet Is Because It's Low in Calories

The short response to this myth is simple: That's probably not true, but even if it were, *so what?*

This accusation—that low-carb diets work only because they are low in calories—is particularly amusing because it is never made against high-carb weight-loss diets that are *equally* low in calories. In fact, there is only a

121-calorie difference between the most stringent induction phase of the Atkins diet and the Dean Ornish ultra-low-fat diet. And after the first couple of weeks, when you get into the ongoing weight-loss phase of Atkins, you're actually consuming 354 calories more than you would be on the Dean Ornish diet and 165 calories *more* than you would be on Weight Watchers![13] Yet you never hear the establishment say that the Ornish low-fat diet works only because it's low-calorie!

Look, on virtually every weight-loss diet in the world, you ultimately wind up consuming fewer calories than you did while you were putting on weight. I don't care if the diet is low-fat, high-fat, low-carb, high-carb, vegetarian, Food Guide Pyramid, raw food, you name it: ultimately, they are *all* — compared to your previous "weight-gaining" diet— reduced-calorie diets. One of the primary reasons most of them fail is hunger. By now, we know that insulin is called the hunger hormone for a very good reason, and insulin is elevated *most* by high-carbohydrate diets. So if you have a choice of gritting your teeth and staying on a 1,200-calorie, low-fat, high-carbohydrate diet that leaves you hungry and craving sweets all the time—or of going on a diet with the *same number of calories* that allows you to eat rich, satisfying, natural foods and doesn't leave you hungry all the time, which would *you* pick?

Exactly. That's why the short answer to this myth is: "Who cares?" Even if it were true that low-carb diets work only because they are low-calorie, who gives a rat's ass? If two "diets" with an equal number of calories produce equal weight loss but one is easier to stay on, why in the world wouldn't you go with it?

More Food on a Low-Carb Diet?

Because a low-carbohydrate diet is able to reduce insulin levels and is far more likely to induce hormonally balanced states than conventional high-carb diets, it is possible—though we're not 100% sure—that you may be able to consume somewhat more calories on a low-carb diet than you would on a high-carb diet and still lose weight. One dramatic study compared a low-fat diet to an Atkins-type diet in two groups of overweight adolescent boys. After three months, the low-carb group lost more than twice as much weight as the low-fat group (19 pounds for the low-carb group and 8.5 pounds for the low-fat group); the low-fat group averaged 1,100 calories a day, while the Atkins group averaged 1,803![14]

Recently, a number of studies have come out showing that weight loss is actually greater on a low-carb diet than on a conventional low-fat diet that has the same number of calories.[15] To be fair, there are plenty of studies showing that both diets produce identical weight loss. (Interestingly, there are virtually no studies that show that low-carb diets produce less weight loss!) But even in the studies that show identical weight loss, triglycerides and HDL levels almost always improve on the higher-protein diets. For example, Alain Golay, a respected researcher who is no particular advocate of low-carb diets, once tested a low-carb (25%) diet against a typical higher-carb (45%) diet for weight loss and found that, while there was not much difference in weight loss, the low-carb group had significantly greater improvements in fasting insulin and triglycerides.[16] In another study, he pitted a low-carb (15%) diet against a higher-carb (45%) diet and again found similar weight loss but marked improvements in glucose, insulin, cholesterol, and triglycerides on the low-carb diet only; no such benefits were seen on the high-carb diet.[17] If two "diets"—high-protein/low-carb and high-carb/low-fat—are equal in calories and produce equal weight loss but the first produces significantly improved blood chemistry and lowers the risk for heart disease and diabetes, why in the world wouldn't you choose that one?

Many studies have been done comparing all kinds of different diets for weight loss; but the truth is that very few studies have lasted more than a year or two, leading many experts to conclude that while you can basically lose weight on any diet, we really have no idea whether any particular regimen is easier to stay on over the long haul. The action is clearly in *maintaining* weight loss; and since the lower-carb diets seem to be much more satiating, we can speculate that they may turn out to be a lot easier to maintain as a lifestyle than a diet that simply reduces fat, which is turning out to be a lot less important than previously thought. In fact, in 2002, Dr. Walter Willett, chairman of the Department of Nutrition at Harvard University's School of Public Health and one of the most respected researchers in the field, declared in two articles—one in *Obesity Reviews*[18] and one in the *American Journal of Medicine*[19]—that dietary fat is *not* a major determinant of body fat and plays virtually no role in obesity. What about calories?

Since most low-carb-diet authors do not advocate counting calories (at least at first) and because most low-carb diets are based on the premise that it is critical to control the hormonal responses to food, many people have gotten the idea that low-carb theorists think calories don't matter at all. This isn't so. As I wrote in a previous book, calories are still on the marquee; it's just that they are not starring players anymore. Of *course* calories still count—there isn't a responsible low-carb diet writer out there who would argue the point. But controlling hormones counts *at least as much*, if not more, especially when it comes to slaying hunger and losing weight without fighting your body every step of the way.

On the other hand, to play devil's advocate, if I take in 15,000 calories, all from fat with a little protein, producing the absolute minimum amount of insulin, I'm *still* going to gain weight. Why? Because there is simply no reason for my body to *release* any of the fat inside my cells for fuel, because I'm already consuming way more fuel than I could possibly need.

Yes, calories count. But so do hormones, and way more than the dietary establishment believes. When it comes to losing weight (and actually *maintaining* that loss), keeping hunger at bay is key—and this is where low-carbohydrate diets blow the competition out of the water.

BOTTOM LINE

Calories count, but so do hormones. Many studies find that reducing energy (calorie) intake comes more easily and more spontaneously on high-carb diets, and there's some evidence that more of the weight you lose comes from fat. Even those studies that show equal weight loss invariably show better blood chemistry on the low-carb diets. Lowering fat in the diet is not the answer to obesity.

MYTH #6: Low-Carb Diets Increase the Risk for Heart Disease

In Denmark, the number of storks is positively correlated with the number of babies born.

This interesting fact was taught to me in graduate school by a wonderful psychology professor named Dr. Scott Fraser, who used it to teach a lesson about scientific studies that has allowed me to understand a great many things about research. I will pass it on to you, and you may never look at research studies in quite the same way.

So let's repeat: in Denmark, the more storks, the more babies. This positive correlation holds up year in and year out.

OK, class, what shall we conclude from this?

I know you're curious about what's *actually* going on here (how could you not be?) so here's the answer.

In the particular part of Denmark where the study was done, single people live mainly in the cities. When they get married and decide to raise a family, they move to the suburbs. The architectural design of the suburbs in Denmark favors angled roofs made of tar. Storks nest in angled roofs made of tar. Both storks and young married couples wanting to have children gravitate to the same area, albeit for somewhat different reasons.

But they are *found together*, consistently, year after year. They are *positively correlated*.

The lesson: *correlation* does not equal *causation*. When two variables are found together, it does not mean that one caused the other. Diabetes went way up during the Clinton presidency, so an increase in diabetes is positively correlated with the Clintons. Statistical studies have also noted that the number of new radio and television sets purchased correlates with an increased number of deaths from coronary disease.[20] In Stockholm, Sweden, there was a correlation between the municipal tax rate and coronary mortality, leading to the interesting proposition that if tax rates were lowered, there would be less heart disease![21]

One scholar described this as the "yellow finger" phenomenon. Men with yellow fingertips are more likely to die of lung cancer. The reason: they are smokers. That's why they *have* yellow fingers. The yellowed tips of their fingers are the result of holding 20 cigarettes a day for 20 years. Washing off the yellow will not reduce their risk for lung cancer.

This brings us to cholesterol, heart disease, and the low-carb diet.

The Birth of the Diet-Heart Hypothesis and the Demonization of Saturated Fat

When the diet-heart hypothesis—the idea that saturated fat causes heart disease—was first proposed in the 1950s by Ancel Keys (see chapter 2), very little was known about either fat or cholesterol. Cholesterol, which is actually not a fat at all but a waxy molecule classified as a sterol, is the parent molecule for all the sex hormones in the body. Without it, you would not have testosterone, the estrogens, progesterone, or DHEA, not to mention cortisol and aldosterone. Most of the cholesterol in your body is *produced* by your body. *Dietary* cholesterol has virtually *no effect* on the amount of cholesterol in your blood. Two major long-term studies, Framingham and Tecumseh, confirm this (see the tables on the following page);[22] they showed that those who ate the most cholesterol had exactly the same level of cholesterol in their blood as those who ate the least. Even Keys, the author of the diet-heart hypothesis, knew this and said, in 1991: "*There's no connection whatsoever between cholesterol in food and cholesterol in blood and we've known that all along. Cholesterol in the diet doesn't matter at all unless you happen to be a chicken or a rabbit.*"[23]

What we do know is that dietary fat has an effect on serum cholesterol. What is a lot less clear is whether it matters much. (Michael and Mary Dan Eades call "Cholesterol Madness" the most important chapter in their book, "not because we believe cholesterol is such an important

CHOLESTEROL INTAKE—THE FRAMINGHAM HEART STUDY		
Average Cholesterol From Food	Below Average Cholesterol From Food	Above Average Cholesterol From Food
	Blood Cholesterol	
mg/day	mmol/L	mmol/L
Men 704 ± 220.9	6.16	6.16
Women 492 ± 170.0	6.37	6.26

CHOLESTEROL INTAKE AND BLOOD LIPIDS—THE TECUMSEH STUDY			
Blood Cholesterol in Thirds	Lower	Middle	Upper
Daily Intake of Cholesterol (mg)	554	566	533

problem but because *everybody else does.*" I'm with the Eadeses, as I discussed in more detail in chapter 5.) Fully 50% of heart attacks happen to people with completely normal cholesterol numbers.[24] The Tokelauan Islanders get 63% of their diet from the healthy saturated fat in coconuts, and, though their cholesterol levels are a bit high, they have virtually no heart disease.[25]

Fats: The Good, the Bad, and the Ugly

We know a lot more about fat than we did back in the '50s and even in the '80s, when the message was "All fat is bad." Most people are now aware that there are "good" fats and "bad" fats, and most people believe that the bad fats are saturated. Not so fast. It's turning out to be even more complicated than that. We now know that there is a type of fat far more dangerous and insidious than saturated fat: *trans-fat;* and virtually all of the historical data we have that "links" saturated fat with heart disease did not distinguish between *saturated* fats and *trans-fats.* Therefore, it is almost impossible to know whether or not saturated fats got the blame for something that was really being done by trans-fats.[26] Saturated fats, for example, *lower* lipoprotein(a), a risk factor for heart disease, and *raise* protective HDL cholesterol; trans-fats not only do the exact opposite but also raise LDL cholesterol![27] Many of us now believe that saturated fats have gotten the blame for damage that is actually caused by trans-fats. Virtually every low-carbohydrate diet, by definition, contains incredibly low amounts of trans-fats.

A LITTLE INTERNET HUMOR

1. *The Japanese eat very little fat and suffer fewer heart attacks than the British or Americans.*

2. *The Mexicans eat a lot of fat and suffer fewer heart attacks than the British or Americans.*

3. *The Japanese drink very little red wine and suffer fewer heart attacks than the British or Americans.*

4. *The Italians drink excessive amounts of red wine and suffer fewer heart attacks than the British or Americans.*

5. *The Germans drink a lot of beer and eat lots of sausages and fats and suffer fewer heart attacks than the British or Americans.*

Conclusion: Eat and drink what you like. Speaking English is apparently what kills you.

Furthermore, we also know that "saturated fat" is not a homogeneous entity. It consists of many different types of fatty acids, and some of them are downright beneficial for health. For example, lauric acid has antimicrobial and antiviral properties and is able to fight bacteria. Caprylic acid is used to fight yeast. Short- and medium-chain saturated fatty acids like those found in coconuts and MCT (medium chain triglyceride) oil are actually much more likely to be burned for fuel than stored as fat, and can be a great adjunct to a weight-loss program.[28] And others, like stearic acid, have no effect whatsoever on cholesterol, except to possibly *raise* protective HDL.

Consider this, as the brilliant investigative reporter and three-time National Association of Science Writers' Science in Society Award–winner Gary Taubes did in an article in *Science.* A porterhouse steak cooks down to about half fat and half protein. Of that fat, 51% is monounsaturated, mostly all from oleic acid, the same monounsaturated fat found in heart-healthy olive oil. Forty-five percent is saturated, but a third of that is stearic acid, which at worst is harmless and at best raises HDL cholesterol. The remaining 4% is polyunsaturated. Thus, a porterhouse steak may actually be better for your heart—especially if eaten with a generous helping of vegetables— than a no-fat meal of high-glycemic, triglyceride-raising pasta.[29]

Do Low-Fat Diets Prevent Heart Disease?

So, then, what about that famous Dean Ornish study that showed that low-fat diets reverse heart disease?

Actually, it showed no such thing. The Ornish study took forty-eight middle-aged white men with existing moderate to severe coronary heart disease. The researchers then did five—count 'em, *five*—simultaneous interventions with these men. They put them on a stress-reduction program. They got them to stop smoking. They gave them group therapy and support. They had them do daily aerobic exercise. *And* they put them on a very high-fiber diet, which also happened to be low in fat. Why anyone would conclude that it was the low-fat part of this multiple intervention that caused their improvement is a mystery. If we put those same men on a program of exercise, stress reduction, smoking cessation, group support, and meditation and included a pack of M&M's in their diet every day, would we conclude that M&M's reduce heart disease? I would argue that Ornish would have gotten the same results—perhaps even *better* ones—using all those good interventions plus a diet loaded with fiber, absent of trans-fats, absent of sugar, containing very low amounts of vegetable fats, *and* containing plenty of good-quality protein from grass-fed animals plus saturated, monounsaturated, and omega-3 fats. We'll never know, because when five factors are involved, it is impossible to say which of them—or what combination of them—is responsible for the results.[30]

On a personal note: in researching this book, I read through literally hundreds of studies on cholesterol, fat, and heart disease. I could have rented a cot in the National Library of Medicine. I read the papers that appeared in the medical journals, I read the reanalysis of the data by scholars who questioned the cholesterol/saturated-fat hypothesis of heart disease, I studied their arguments, I read the rebuttals to their arguments, and I read the rebuttals to the *rebuttals*.

I have, I confess, come to believe—along with a growing number of health professionals—that saturated fat and cholesterol are, for the most part, innocent bystanders. They were in the wrong place at the wrong time, Your Honor, and they hung out with the wrong crowd. As I mentioned earlier, virtually every epidemiological study that linked saturated-fat consumption with increased risk of cardiovascular diseases failed to separate saturated fat from its extremely dangerous cohort, trans-fatty acids.[31] Nor did the studies implicating saturated fat distinguish the *source* of the saturated fat consumed: saturated fat from natural foods like butter, eggs, and grass-fed cattle is *not* the same as saturated fat from fries and burgers; most people in industrial nations consume their saturated fat from hot dogs, fast-food hamburgers, and processed deli meats like salami and bologna. The people consuming the most saturated fat in those studies ate few fruits and vegetables and little fiber. And for the most part, people in those studies did not exercise. (Add to all that the 152 pounds of sugar per year that the USDA estimates to be the average American's yearly intake,[32] and a pattern begins to emerge.) And while it's extremely convenient to blame a single factor (like saturated fat) for heart disease, the fact is that a matrix of lifestyle and dietary characteristics such as the ones just mentioned are found *together*. In my opinion, saturated fat and cholesterol are not the bad guys here.

New research is beginning to support this. When a recent study in the *British Medical Journal* factored in fiber intake, the usual association between saturated fat and coronary-disease risk practically vanished. The study concluded that the adverse effects of saturated fat and cholesterol are "at least in part explained by their low-fiber content and their associations with other risk factors." The researchers further stated that "benefits of reducing intakes of saturated fat and cholesterol are likely to be modest *unless accompanied by an increased consumption of foods rich in fiber*." The study also commented on how the inclusion of omega-3 fats in the diet had a protective effect on the heart.[33]

However . . .

I realize that this is a radical position and a hard sell to a population that has been raised on the premise that saturated fat and cholesterol are basically the children of Satan. So let me put you at ease: to do a low-carb diet, you do not have to accept the position that cholesterol and saturated fat are relatively harmless. In fact, there are low-carb advocates that don't accept that position either, so you won't be alone.

Just keep in mind that on virtually all low-carb diets, blood-lipid chemistries improve. That's what is important, and that is the take-home point here. Even those studies that showed identical weight loss with low-carb versus high-carb diets demonstrated this: low-carb diets beat the pants off high-carb diets every time when it comes to lowering triglycerides and raising HDL, even in those few cases where weight loss was identical.[34]

And here's the pièce de résistance. If you and/or your doctor are still concerned about the amount of fat in low-carb diets, consider the following (see the table below): if you are a male who is 40 to 50 pounds overweight, you have probably been consuming a diet of *at least* 3,500 calories a day (probably more: one fast-food order of fries alone is 700). Let's say you've been adhering to the dietary guidelines of no more than 30% of your calories from fat, with no more than 10% of the total diet from saturated fat.

That means you have been consuming about 1,050 calories a day from fat, of which 350 are from saturated fat.

Now look at what happens if you go on a typical low-carb weight reduction diet. You would consume in the ballpark of 1,700 satisfying,

		% Total Fat	Fat Calories	% Saturated Fat	Saturated-Fat Calories
	Calories				
Current diet (follows dietary guidelines for fat)	3,500–4,000	30%	1,050–1,200	10%	350–400
Low-carb, high-fat diet	1,700	50%	850	20%	340

MALE, 40 TO 50 POUNDS OVERWEIGHT: FAT INTAKE ON CURRENT DIET COMPARED WITH LOW-CARB DIET

filling calories. Let's give the worst-case scenario, from your doctor's point of view, and say that a full 50% of those 1,700 calories come from fat— that's 850 fat calories, definitely a high-fat diet in anyone's book. Say that 20% (twice the dietary guidelines) of your total calories comes from saturated fat (340). Even with these numbers, you would actually consume 20% *less* overall fat on a low-carb diet than you were before, when you were following the dietary guidelines. This should put both you and your doctor at ease.

BOTTOM LINE

Low-carbohydrate diets do not increase the risk for heart disease. If anything, they improve blood-lipid profiles.

CHAPTER 7

But What About the China Study?

With fair regularity, I get an e-mail or blog comment that takes me to task for recommending low-carb diets, for suggesting that humans usually do better with some animal products in their diet, for questioning the significance of cholesterol as a risk factor for heart disease, and for completely dismissing the obsolete notion that cholesterol in the diet makes a whit of difference to anything. These letters are often snarky, mean-spirited, and condescending, and more than a few of them end with the same rhetorical question: "*Didn't you ever hear of the China Study?*" The sarcastic tone is always the same, as if they were asking a heathen, "*Didn't you ever hear of a little thing called the Bible?*"

Well, yes, actually, I have heard of the China Study. Not only have I heard of it, but I've read the book *and* seen the movie *Forks over Knives*. I've also heard of the work of Joel Fuhrman, Caldwell B. Esselstyn, John McDougall, Neil Barnard, and all the rest of the good folks who believe, deeply in their DNA, that animal products are bad, bad, bad, and that fat should be mostly avoided (especially saturated fat!) and that a whole-foods, plant-based diet is the best answer to obesity, diabetes, cancer, and heart disease.

So yes, I'm quite familiar with the China Study. But unlike my vegan friends who treat it as some kind of final authority, I'm not at all convinced that T. Colin Campbell's book *The China Study*—or even the *real* China project on which it's based—is the be-all and end-all of nutritional research. Nor am I convinced by the pro-vegan arguments of Campbell, Fuhrman, or any of their rabidly fanatic followers.

Oh, heck, let me be real: I think the argument advanced in *The China Study* is basically bunk.

First, some background. Campbell's book is not the *actual* "China Study"; it's an *interpretation of* an 894-page behemoth of a book called *Diet, Life-style, and Mortality in China: A Study of the Characteristics of 65 Chinese Counties,* authored by four researchers, of which Campbell was one. (The other three are Chen Junshi, Li Junyao, and Richard Peto.)

Diet, Life-style, and Mortality in China is an enormous book consisting of data on 367 variables measured in 65 different counties and involving no less than 6,500 adults. The book is physically imposing—about the size of the *Physicians' Desk Reference,* and weighing nearly as much. Only the first 80 pages are text. After that, you get 800 pages of pure numeric data, densely packed on the page and looking like ticker-tape printout from the New York Stock Exchange. Understand, now, that they took 367 variables and correlated each one with the other 366, generating over 100,000 data points (or associations), of which 92,000 were statistically meaningless. (The other 8,000 were statistically significant.) Any way you slice it, that's a whole lotta numbers.

The first thing to know about *Diet, Life-Style, and Mortality in China* is that it's an *observational* study, not a clinical one. The original data from *Diet, Life-style, and Mortality in China* represent thousands and thousands of *associations* between variables. An association simply means that *two things are found together.* Statisticians call such associations *correlations.*

The great danger in observational studies is to believe that *correlation* is the same as *causation.* It's not. Cases in point: Whenever it rains, lots of umbrellas suddenly seem to appear. An observer from another planet might notice this pattern—umbrellas everywhere, every time it rains. And they might well conclude that umbrellas cause rain. A disturbingly high percentage of the nutrition "wisdom" that's been passed down through the ages is based on these kinds of observational, correlation studies that prove exactly nothing about causality, despite the fact that everybody acts as if they do. We'll come back to this later on.

The China Study is Campbell's popular book in which he basically presents his own theory that animal protein causes cancer as well as all sorts of other unpleasantries. He bolsters his antiprotein argument by using a very select group of those 8,000 associations from the original China Study that, taken out of context, could be used to promote his case. (These numbers sound all the more impressive if you haven't been trained in statistics and interpretation.) Interestingly, only 39 of its 350 pages are devoted to the *actual* China Study. *The China Study* is Campbell's *interpreta-*

tion of the findings from that enormous study as well as a few other studies he worked on, woven together with his own personal philosophy about how we should all eat. (A more appropriate title for his book would have been *A Manifesto for Veganism.*)

As anyone who watched the political debates in the early 2010s knows, it is entirely possible to have two experts examine a hugely complex set of figures and facts and draw entirely different conclusions about what they mean. (Debt reduction and health care costs, anyone?) Campbell looked at the massive raw data accumulated in the China Study, chose certain things to highlight (it's called "cherry-picking the evidence"), and connected the dots in a particular way to make a particular case. It is entirely possible to connect them in a completely *different* way and reach completely different conclusions (more on that in a moment).

Campbell—a lovely, sincere man who has made some important contributions to the field of nutrition—is proselytizing for a cause he truly believes in. Since I share his love for animals, I'm sympathetic. (Campbell is on the advisory board of the Physicians Committee for Responsible Medicine, which describes itself on its Facebook page as "a nonprofit organization that promotes preventive medicine, conducts clinical research, and encourages higher standards for ethics and effectiveness in research,"[1] while featuring a profile picture with the legend "Bacon is a Killer," reflecting the PCRM's close allegiance with People for the Ethical Treatment of Animals [PETA] and other animal rights groups.)

The problem is there's more than a little fuzzy math in *The China Study,* and his arguments are full of holes.

Full disclosure: Campbell's book and arguments have been brilliantly, methodically deconstructed elsewhere, point by point and statistical fallacy by statistical fallacy, by others, and I'm particularly indebted to four of them. Denise Minger has written several lengthy and cogent pieces, widely available on the Internet, that rebut Campbell point by point (see *Resources,* page 325). Her critique—a cogent, well-argued, and heavily referenced work noticeably absent of malice—went viral the moment it appeared and garnished so much attention that Campbell himself was compelled to offer a reply. The brilliant, irascible Anthony Colpo has written some damning critiques of the China Study as well, as has the always-dependable Chris Masterjohn. My friend Mike Eades, MD—whose blog at proteinpower.com never disappoints—has decimated it as well. Rather than reinventing the wheel, I'll summarize a few important points made by these four analysts, but I urge you to read their original pieces on the China Study if you want to delve into all the microscopic details. I'm deeply indebted to all four, particularly Minger, for the material that follows.

So, ladies and gentlemen, without further ado . . . here are a few selected points to consider about *The China Study*.

Cherry-Picking the Evidence: How to Lie With Statistics

To really understand the holes in Campbell's arguments, you have to know just a little about statistics and research design, and that's been one of the greatest challenges in getting people to understand the problems with *The China Study*.

Let's say you're interested in studying multivitamins and in finding out whether people who take them actually live longer. So you take a large sample of people, track them for 30 years, and see whether the vitamin users live longer than those who *don't* take vitamins. At the end of the 30 years, you have some good data to show that people who take vitamins live longer than people who don't. You would have shown a *positive correlation* between vitamin use and a longer life.

If you're trying to make the case for multivitamin use, you can just stop there. You've made your point, and it can sound pretty impressive, especially if you're only talking to the public and not to other scientists. But what you actually have on your hands is a massively worthless study.

To make the study useful, you have to ask (and answer) a few more questions: Are vitamin takers more likely to exercise? To go to the doctor? To pay attention to the nutritional labels? To avoid trans-fats? These are all things that could easily affect the outcome of your study.

The finding—that vitamin use is associated with longer life—is called an *unadjusted correlation*. It's just raw data. It doesn't answer any of the above questions, and researchers know this. That's why, in most studies, they use sophisticated statistical techniques to "adjust" for the possible influence of these extraneous variables. Most commonly, researchers make "adjustments" for age, sex, history of disease, medications, body mass index, and other factors that are known to influence outcomes in these kinds of studies. By "leveling" the playing field statistically, they hope to eliminate the contribution of these factors to their data.

So back to the vitamin study. If our researchers now "adjust" for such variables as exercise, age, sickness, medications, and so on, they have a much more accurate picture of whether vitamins extend life. If, after all these adjustments, vitamin use still correlates strongly with longer life, we can be much more confident that it's the vitamins—and not, say, the regular exercise vitamin users tend to engage in—that's responsible for the results.

Back to Campbell and his unadjusted data.

When Campbell's raw data showed a positive relationship between plant food consumption and health, he quoted these *unadjusted correlations* with no problem. (They supported his beliefs that animal foods are the spawn of Satan and that we'd all be better off eating carrots.) But when making the case *against* animal foods, he suddenly switched to *adjusted* correlations. That's fine—but shouldn't the same statistical standard be used for both?

As Minger points out, had he used the same (*un*adjusted) correlations for animal food variables, he would have found only neutral or inverse correlations between cardiovascular disease and animal products. If you want to make the argument that only adjusted correlations count, fine, count me in. But then why not use them on the plant food data? Perhaps Campbell felt that if he applied the same loose standard to the plant food data as he did to the animal food data, all those glowing positive correlations between plant food and health might collapse, and his pro-vegan case might dissolve.

Then there's the problem of "cherry-picking the evidence"—quoting associations that bolster your case while conveniently ignoring those that don't.

Here's an example: One of the counties studied in the original China Study was Tuoli. Look at the diet of the Tuoli residents and you'd think the whole darn county was on the Atkins diet. Forty-five percent of their diet was fat (!), and they consumed roughly 135 grams of animal protein a day. (For comparison, the FDA recommends 50 grams a day as the "Daily Value"* for most Americans.) So according to Campbell's theory, these folks must be dead men walking. Yet the raw data tells a different story. According to the data in the China Study, they had low rates of cancer, low rates of heart disease, and were generally extremely healthy, more so than some of the counties that were nearly vegan.

Here's another example: Campbell makes much of associations between *animal products* and various diseases, yet fails to explore a much

---

* I put "Daily Value" in quotes because no one—including some highly educated health professionals I informally surveyed—can give a cogent explanation of what the heck "Daily Value" means. And if we health professionals are confused by that ridiculous nomenclature, how confusing is it to ordinary Americans?

stronger correlation (r=0.67) between wheat and heart disease. Yet he's been aware of the possibility of a wheat–heart disease connection since at least 1998, when he wrote in another paper, ". . . *enhancement of coronary artery disease risk by wheat consumption may be a possibility.*"[2] Further, by Campbell's own admission, wheat flour intake correlates significantly with *greater* body weight, *and* with *lower* blood levels of the omega-3 DHA and monounsaturated fats, both of which are very heart-protective.[3]

Speaking of wheat, even a cursory glance at the data discussed in cardiologist William Davis's excellent book *Wheat Belly* would lead any thinking person to suspect that wheat is *at least* as likely a culprit in heart disease as animal foods. Yet this avenue of investigation is ignored or dismissed by Campbell.

It's an interesting omission. Campbell makes much of his correlations between animal protein and cardiovascular disease yet conveniently forgets that the data from the China Study clearly show that wheat flour has a correlation of .67 with heart attacks and coronary heart disease. Similarly, Campbell talks about the possible role cow's milk plays in causing type 1 diabetes, but he leaves out the fact that wheat gluten does the same thing.[4] (How do you manage to forget that? Simple. You don't. You just ignore it, since it doesn't bolster your case.)

Wheat flour also has a correlation of .46 with cervical cancer, .54 with hypertensive heart disease, .47 with stroke, and .41 with diseases of the blood and blood-forming organs. You could be forgiven for suspecting that this stuff wasn't discussed very much since it doesn't support Campbell's vendetta against animal foods as the main driver of Western diseases.

So Campbell looks at these 8,000 associations and, incredibly, sums them up thusly: "People who ate the most animal-based foods got the most chronic disease."[5]

But—as Minger, Masterjohn, and others have pointed out—when you compare Campbell's "summary" with the actual data, the result paints a very different picture. Sugar, certain carbs, and even fiber all have associations with cancer mortality that's about seven times the magnitude of the association with animal protein. Didn't know that from reading *The China Study*, did you? I'll bet you also didn't know that the only statistically significant association between a macronutrient and cancer mortality was—get this—a slightly *negative* association between cancer mortality and total fat intake, meaning those eating the *most* fats and oils had slightly *fewer* deaths from cancer. Oh, did Campbell omit that fact? Imagine that!

The Protein and Cancer Argument

Campbell never really said protein *causes* cancer, though you could certainly be left with that impression from a cursory reading of his book. What he *did* say was that carcinogens *initiate* cancer, but diet can *promote* it. I have absolutely no problem with this idea, which I like to call the "Miracle-Gro" theory. Fertilizer won't magically grow plants where there are no seeds, but it *will* promote growth once the seeds are firmly planted in the ground.

So how did Campbell come to focus on protein (and animal products in general) as the big promoter of cancer?

Glad you asked.

It all started with Campbell's early studies on rats (and ended with him becoming the poster child for veganism). You see, cancer is often induced in rats by feeding them *aflatoxin,* a nasty chemical found in peanuts. Researchers found that once cancer was induced, a diet of 20% casein (a protein in milk) *promoted* the cancer, while a diet of only 5% casein did not. What's more, when the same rats were fed plant protein (instead of casein), it didn't seem to matter how much they ate—plant protein, in any quantity studied, did not promote cancer in the same way that casein did. From this, Campbell concluded that animal protein was a likely suspect in the development of cancer.

So how exactly does protein promote cancer, you ask? Certain liver enzymes convert aflatoxin into a really nasty substance that Campbell believes initiates the formation of cancer. Feed a rat lower amounts of protein, he says, and you lower the activity of this enzyme; feed it a lot more protein and you up the activity of this enzyme. Hence the conclusion that protein is associated with cancer.

Sounds plausible (almost) until you realize that in this experiment, sugar (sucrose) was eaten along with the protein. But in experiments when *starch* was used (instead of sugar), the impact of the protein was far less. So protein and sugar *together* may produce an effect, but protein with *starch* produces much less of one. "Who knows whether or not it's even the protein that has the effect and not the sugar?" asks Mike Eades. "It can't be shown from this study."

Campbell generalizes from casein to all animal-food protein. But this conclusion is hardly warranted by the data. Another component of milk protein—whey—actually has a *protective* effect against colon cancer.[6] Was that mentioned? Nope. Why would it be? It doesn't support Campbell's anti–animal products agenda.

And as far as plant protein *not* contributing to the promotion of cancer, that may have more to do with adaptation than it does with anything else.

Rats on farms like to hang out in hay and grain, which are two of their favorite foods. Both hay and grain are common places for the growth of the fungus that produces aflatoxin. Eades suggests that over multiple genera-tions, rodents have clearly adapted to this combo of plant protein and aflatoxin. "In my opinion," writes Eades, "making a huge issue of the fact that rats didn't get cancer after dosing with aflatoxin irrespective of how much plant protein they ate is pretty disingenuous."

Campbell even ignores his own previous findings in his quest to demonize all animal products. In an earlier experiment, he studied three groups of carcinogen-exposed rats.[7] All three groups were fed about 20% protein and 20% fat, but the protein and the fat came from different sources. One group was fed casein (a protein from milk) plus corn oil (which is high in omega-6 fat). The second group was fed fish protein and corn oil, while the third group was fed fish protein plus fish oil (which is high in omega-3 fats).

So what happened? There were significant increases in precancerous growths (known as *preneoplastic lesions*) in the casein/corn oil group and the fish protein/corn oil group. (Was it the protein? Or was it the corn oil? I'm betting on the corn oil, but we'll never know.) Point is, the *third* group—fish protein plus fish oil—had a completely different result. The fish oil, in Campbell's own words, "had a dramatic effect both on the development in the number and size of preneoplastic lesions." What's more, "no carcinomas . . . were observed in the F/F (fish protein/fish oil) group, whereas the F/C (fish protein/corn oil) group had an incidence of 3 per 16 with 6 total carcinomas."

Here's the conclusion, in Campbell's own words:

"[A] 20% menhaden oil diet, *rich in omega-3 fatty acids*, produced a *significant decrease* in the development of both the size and number of preneoplastic lesions when compared to a 20% corn oil diet rich in omega-6 fatty acids. *This study provides evidence that fish oils*, rich in omega-3 fatty acids, *may have potential as inhibitory agents in cancer development*."[8] [Emphasis mine.]

Let's remember that Campbell's whole theory is that nutrients from animal-based foods *increase* tumor development while nutrients from plant-based foods *decrease* tumor development.

As Minger wryly notes, "Last time I checked, fish oil ain't no plant food.

"Why does Campbell avoid mentioning anything potentially positive about animal products in *The China Study, including evidence unearthed by his own research*? For someone who has openly censured the nutritional bias rampant in the scientific community, this seems a tad hypocritical."

The Protein and Heart Disease Problem

Campbell loves to quote Dean Ornish and Caldwell Esselstyn, two doctors who have gotten some impressive results in reversing heart disease with plant-based diets. Yet he conveniently omits the equally impressive research of George Mann on the heart-healthy Masai who practically live on milk, meat, and blood, or the extensive research of Weston Price, who studied fourteen different primitive cultures, many of which were absolutely thriving on high intakes of animal foods.

What's even more interesting is that the China Study itself contains data that—at the very least—questions the central thesis of Campbell's book *The China Study*.

Let me explain.

You see, different regions of China have vastly different rates of heart disease mortality. Out of every 100,000 deaths, Fusui—one of the counties studied—has a measly 1.5 deaths due to heart disease while Dunhuang—another county studied—has 184. (For reference, out of every 100,000 deaths in the United States, 165 are attributed to heart disease.) When you compare the five counties with the highest heart disease rates (Dunhuang, Longxian, Tulufan, Yongning, and Jiangxiang) with the five counties with the lowest heart disease rates (Fusui, Qiyang, Cangwu, Mayang, and Linwu)—some very interesting contrasts show up.

But they're not exactly what you'd expect if you buy Campbell's theory.

Compared to the high heart disease regions, the heart-healthy regions had *higher* intakes of animal protein, animal fat, saturated fat, and dietary cholesterol.

The healthier regions also consumed less fiber, less plant protein, less vegetable oil, and less wheat flour.

Again, correlation doesn't prove causation, but still it's impossible to ignore the fact that some regions in China consume an awful lot more animal foods than the average Chinese while having extremely low rates of heart disease. Nor the fact that out of all the counties studied, Longxian—the county that consumed the absolute *lowest* amount of animal foods—had the *next-to-highest* rate of heart disease mortality. Did I say "impossible to ignore"? Sorry. It's not impossible at all—Campbell ignored it just fine.

A side note: Denise Minger created a series of visually compelling and instructive graphs comparing the five counties that had the healthiest hearts with the five counties with the highest rates of heart disease. Taking data from the actual China Study,[9] she compared the two groups on such metrics as total animal fat intake, total animal food intake, total saturated fat intake, percent of calories from animal protein, percent of protein from animal foods, and so on.[10] If Campbell's interpretation of the raw data were correct, we'd expect to see a clear relationship between animal protein consumption and heart disease. Instead, we see nothing of the sort.

The Mortality/Overall Health Problem

Another thing Minger did was to look at the mortality differences between the five counties that ate the most animal foods and the five counties that ate the least. Counties were all over the place in terms of protein consumed, with animal protein consumption ranging from almost zero to nearly 135 grams a day. So, if Campbell's theory is true, you'd expect to see some huge differences in health risks between the counties that were practically vegan and the counties that were practically Atkinsian. Especially since, according to Campbell, "*even relatively small amounts of animal-based food*" increase the risk of disease.

Minger painstakingly graphed the mortality rates (deaths per 1,000 inhabitants) from cervical cancer, breast cancer, stomach cancer, leukemia, lymphoma, brain and neurological diseases, diabetes, stroke, heart attacks and coronary artery disease, and deaths from all cancers for each of the five "near-vegan" counties and each of the five "near-Atkins" counties.[11] It's a set of graphs worth looking at, but I'll summarize them in three words: *not much difference*. Overall mortality rates for both sets of counties are quite similar, with the high-animal-food counties coming out more favorably in death from all cancers, heart attacks, brain and neurological diseases, lymphoma, and cervical cancer. Though, as Minger correctly points out, this little 10-county sample doesn't carry a ton of scientific clout because of its small sample size, it sure blows some serious holes in Campbell's "summary" of the important points:

"*People who ate the most animal-based foods got the most chronic disease . . . People who ate the most plant-based foods were the healthiest and tended to avoid chronic disease.*"

As Jon Stewart might say, "Hmm . . . not so much."

OK, you say, you don't trust Minger, who by her own (incredibly modest) self-description is just "some girl with a blog." How about Harvard researchers? Here's what the two lead researchers on the Nurses' Health Study had to say about the original China Study. As you can see, they interpreted the data quite differently than Campbell did in his book *The China Study*:

"A survey of 65 counties in rural China, however, did not find a clear association between animal product consumption and risk of heart disease or major cancers."[12]

The Protein/Calcium Problem

In an article in the Cornell *Chronicle,* Campbell claimed that animal protein *"almost certainly contributes to a significant loss of bone calcium while vegetable-based diets clearly protect against bone loss."*[13]

But the actual study on which he based this comment—"Dietary Calcium and Bone Density among Middle-aged and Elderly Women in China"—a paper on which *Campbell himself was one of the authors*—tells quite a different story.[14] Here's what Campbell and his coauthors wrote in that very paper:

> The results strongly indicated that dietary calcium, especially from dairy sources, increased bone mass in middle-aged and elderly women by facilitating optimal peak bone mass earlier in life . . .
>
> Nondairy calcium . . . showed no association with bone variables after age and/or body weight were adjusted for. . .
>
> . . . calcium from dairy sources was correlated with bone variables to a higher degree than was calcium from nondairy sources, probably resulting from the higher bioavailablity of dairy calcium"[15]

Protein and calcium have an interesting symbiotic relationship when it comes to bones. Protein works great for strong bones when you're taking in enough calcium. But high-protein intakes can work against you when calcium intake is low. So it wouldn't be entirely surprising if a higher protein/weaker bone connection showed up in areas of China like Changle, which, on average, took in the highest amount of nondairy animal food but *also* took in the least amount of calcium. Was it the protein? Or the combination of protein *with* a low-calcium intake?

What's more, a number of studies have shown the exact opposite of what Campbell claims is a universal truth regarding protein and bones. One study investigated the diet of a cohort of women from the Iowa Women's Health Study and followed them for 1–3 years. In this study, a clear association was found between increased dietary protein intake—*especially from animal sources*—and a reduced risk of hip fracture.[16]

The Framingham Osteoporosis Study also looked at protein intake and bone loss in elderly people. "Lower protein intake was significantly related to bone loss," wrote the researchers, with "persons in the lowest quartile of protein intake [showing] the greatest bone loss." The researchers' conclusion was pretty clear: "Even after controlling for known confounders including weight loss, *women and men with relatively lower protein intake had increased bone loss*, suggesting that *protein intake is important in maintaining bone or minimizing bone loss in elderly persons.*"[17] [Emphasis mine.]

Then there was the Rancho Bernardo Study, which studied a cohort of 970 men and women between the ages of 55 and 92. They found a "positive association between animal protein consumption . . . and bone mineral density," which was statistically significant in women. But for both sexes, a *negative* association between vegetable protein and bone mineral density was observed.[18]

And finally, if there were any more doubt, the results of a study from the Agricultural Research Service of the USDA should put the issue to bed. The title says it all: "Controlled High Meat Diets Do Not Affect Calcium Retention or Indices of Bone Status in Healthy Postmenopausal Women." The researchers' conclusion: "Calcium retention is not reduced when subjects consume a high protein diet from common dietary sources such as meat."[19] So, not only do Campbell's *own* findings and studies directly contradict his conclusions, but so do several other independent studies that show absolutely no negative effect on bones or bone-mineral density from a diet that is high in animal protein. Quite the contrary.

It's instructive at this point to mention an absolutely stunning paper in the *American Journal of Clinical Nutrition*,[20] but first, a word of background. Nearly 80 years ago, it was shown that ingestion of protein increases the amount of calcium excreted in the urine. But most of this work was done with isolated protein feedings, and it wasn't at all clear whether the same thing would happen using real protein-containing foods. Robert P. Heaney, MD, the author of the paper I'm about to discuss, tried to test this notion using real people consuming real food. He did some early research showing that in free-living middle-aged women, the more protein they ate, the more calcium they excreted in their urine. "This study," he writes, "cited extensively since its publication, contributed to the widespread impression that protein is harmful to bone."

However, as Heaney points out in his paper "Protein Intake and Bone Health: The Influence of Belief Systems on the Conduct of Nutritional Science," that impression is absolutely incorrect.

The first thing he mentions in his paper is that taking a little extra calcium offsets the slight loss of calcium in the urine from higher protein intakes. So, at very *low* levels of calcium intake, protein may indeed have a negative effect on calcium balance. But this effect disappears as soon as calcium intake is adequate. "In brief," he writes, "if protein exerts a negative effect, it is only under conditions of low calcium intake."

Further debunking the idea that protein has a negative effect on bone strength, he states: "Since our study was reported, an impressive body of literature has proven that protein tends to have a positive effect on bone overall." Two randomized controlled trials showed that increased protein intake dramatically improved outcomes after hip fracture,[21] and subsequent work showed that protein supplements reduce bone loss at the contralateral hip in patients with upper-femoral fracture.[22]

Heaney—who, let's remember, did some of the original research upon which most of the "protein is death to bones" propaganda was based—essentially repudiates this interpretation of his work. "A ferment in the larger society has arisen out of opposition to the use of animal products," he writes. "Although only a tiny proportion of the general public or the nutritional science community holds this view, *the zeal of these groups and their eagerness to exploit any evidence that suggests harmful effects of animal products have had a disproportionate effect both on public consciousness and on the agenda of nutritional science itself.*"[23] [Emphasis mine.]

Think he might've been talking about the Campbell-Barnard-Fuhrman contingent?

Finally, he concludes by pointing out that there is exactly zero evidence that primitive humans had low intakes of either total protein or of animal protein. "That, coupled with the generally very robust skeletons of our hominid forbears, makes it difficult to sustain a case, either evidential or deductive, for overall skeletal harm related either to protein intake or to animal protein. Indeed the balance of the evidence seems to indicate the opposite."[24]

The Attribution Problem

Pitchers often throw sand over their left shoulders, thinking it brings them good luck. Rain men think their dances bring on the rain. Medicine men in primitive cultures often believe that disease is caused by demonic possession. This judgment about what causes what is called *attribution*, and it refers to the way humans construct the world and assign meaning to events they observe. There's even a whole theory in psychology (the Attribution Theory) that seeks to explain how we attribute *cause* to the events around us.

We humans are remarkably bad at attribution, which is to say that we are often clueless about causes. The point of science is to remove this natural human defect by applying all the tools—statistical and otherwise—of objective assessment, independent of our private beliefs or values. Unfortunately, it rarely works that way, even in science. Particularly when there is a massive amount of data—such as in the China Study—it is very easy to fall victim to what's called "confirmation bias," the tendency to interpret data according to something you already believe is true. Example: If you firmly believe your house is inhabited by ghosts, you will tend to hear every creak in the attic as "proof" of what you already "know."

Campbell—and his like-minded colleagues—are not people of ill intent. Far from it. They genuinely believe we'd all be healthier if we eschewed all animal products from our diet. But like all humans, they're not exempt from confirmation bias, letting those strong beliefs color the way they interpret the world.

Campbell isn't alone in reading masses of data and connecting just the dots that form the picture he wants to paint while leaving the rest of them alone. Neal Barnard (head of the radically vegan Physicians Committee for Responsible Medicine), John McDougall, Dean Ornish, Caldwell Esselstyn, and Joel Fuhrman have all advocated programs that eschew meat and animal products. Ask any one of them what makes their programs "successful," and they will undoubtedly focus on the elimination of those terrible animal foods that "everyone knows" cause heart disease. But a closer look at their programs tells a more nuanced story.

Ornish's original "reversing heart disease" study put men on a very-low-fat vegetarian diet, but it *also* employed anger management, stress reduction, low-sugar diets, smoking cessation, and exercise. Ornish may *attribute* his results to his low-fat diet, but it's impossible to know for sure. Esselstyn may believe that his (almost) zero-fat program at the Cleveland Clinic gets good results because of the elimination of saturated fat, but let's remember that his program *also* eliminates pro-inflammatory vegetable oils and refined grains, both of which are way more of a problem than saturated fat. Even the rabidly vegan Barnard advises readers to keep vegetable oils to a minimum and to favor low-glycemic foods. And McDougall's vegetarian program strongly recommends cutting back on four demons in the American diet: refined flour, refined cereals, soft drinks, and vegetable oils.

Though these fine gentlemen may well believe that animal foods are the real villains in our diet, we'll never know if the elimination of all that other crap (including refined, pro-inflammatory vegetable oils and sugar) was the real driver behind whatever positive results they've achieved with clients. Personally, I think that if you eliminate sugar, wheat, dairy, and high-glycemic processed carbs, it wouldn't much matter whether you ate a pound of grass-fed meat a day. But since all these guys are *already convinced* it's the animal foods, fat, and cholesterol that are causing all the damage, they simply assume that the "rest of the stuff" is just the icing on the cake.

The truth is "that other stuff" may be the cake itself.

Miscellaneous Untruths

In his quest to demonize animal foods while portraying plant foods as the savior of the human race, Campbell makes incredible and fully disprovable statements like "Folic acid is a compound derived exclusively from plant-based foods such as green and leafy vegetables,"[25] or "Eating foods that contain any cholesterol above 0 mg is unhealthy."

Point of information, Your Honor: chicken liver contains nearly four times the folate of spinach. A look through the USDA database[26] or a search for folic acid on Nutridata clearly shows that the foods highest in folate are meats like duck, goose, and turkey. (Pan-fried beef liver, for example, has 260 mcg of folate per 100-gram serving; spinach has 194.) And the idea that *eating* cholesterol raises *blood levels* of cholesterol is so far past its expiration date that it's hard to find even conservative nutritionists who still believe this. Even Ancel Keys, the man most associated with the "diet-heart hypothesis"—the idea that fat in the diet causes heart disease—didn't believe this nonsense. In 1997, he wrote: "*There's no connection whatsoever between the cholesterol in food and cholesterol in the blood. And we've known that all along. Cholesterol in the diet doesn't matter at all unless you happen to be a chicken or a rabbit.*"

Campbell makes the same mistake everyone else does in equating a blood marker (cholesterol) with a disease (heart disease). They're hardly the same. Even a study Campbell himself worked on concluded, "Within China, neither plasma total cholesterol nor LDL cholesterol was associated with CVD [cardiovascular disease]. The results indicate that geographical differences in CVD mortality within China are caused primarily by factors other than dietary or plasma cholesterol."[27]

That same study uncovered some associations that Campbell would probably like to forget, since they hardly support his thesis. Wheat flour and salt were *positively* correlated with cardiovascular disease, *positively* correlated with HHD (hypertensive heart disease) and *positively* correlated with stroke. And the total amount of polyunsaturated fatty acids in red blood cells—especially the pro-inflammatory omega-6 fats so prevalent in vegetable oils—was *also* positively correlated with coronary heart disease and hypertensive heart disease.[28]

THE BOTTOM LINE

The bottom line is that The China Study represents a point of view, not incontrovertible fact. It's a collection of carefully selected associations threaded together to support a particular point of view. As Minger and others have shown with painstaking detail, you could easily use a different collection of carefully selected associations from the very same database and arrive at an entirely different set of conclusions. Campbell ignores the substantial amount of data—both in the China Study and elsewhere—showing benefits for animal-based foods, and conveniently excludes all of the data that indicts plant foods as causative of disease (wheat flour for one).

Campbell has responded to the critical blogosphere on a couple of occasions. Quick summary of his rebuttals: "These people aren't professional researchers and besides, they have an 'agenda.' I'm a trained scientist. You should trust me, not your lying eyes."

It's a profoundly lame rebuttal. As Minger points out, "It doesn't require a PhD to be a critical thinker, nor does a laundry list of credentials prevent a person from falling victim to biased thinking."

CHAPTER 8

My Big Fat Diet: The Town That Lost 1,200 Pounds

I f you're interested in weight loss—or even if you're not—the headline is virtually guaranteed to grab your attention: "The Town That Lost 1,200 Pounds!"

That's exactly what readers first saw when they picked up the March 16, 2008 Sunday edition of the Canadian newspaper *The Province*. Here's how reporter Lena Sin started the story:

> His town was shrinking, and Greg Wadhams was determined
> to shrink with it. So on a cold December night in 2006, the
> 55-year-old commercial fisherman sat down to say goodbye to the
> past. He devoured a spread of chicken chow mein, fried rice and
> deep-fried prawns to triumphant delight. Then, with the final
> bite, he bade farewell to his favorite foods.
>
> Intrigued? Read on.

Greg Wadhams lives in the small fishing village of Alert Bay, off the northern tip of Vancouver Island in British Columbia. Most of the inhabitants of this sleepy town (population 1,500) are members of the 'Namgis First Nations people—the Canadian counterpart to what we would call American Indians. Obesity and diabetes are rampant here, about 3 to 5 times greater than the national average. Understanding why this is so can teach us a lot about diabetes and obesity—and about the value of low-carb diets.

The 'Namgis have always been fishermen. But the local fishing industry was collapsing. Wild salmon supplies were diminished, largely because sea lice from the increasing number of salmon farms were making their way into the oceans and killing thousands of the wild fish. Fuel prices had made it difficult, if not impossible, for local fishermen to regularly travel out and back to their usual fishing sites. Meanwhile, supermarkets had sprung up, and convenience foods were everywhere. Paralleling the experience of the formerly lean Pima Indians on the Arizona reservations—now among the most obese and diabetic people in the world—the 'Namgis had begun to consume vast amounts of packaged convenience foods, sugar, and other supermarket "staples."

The disastrous effects of this Canadian version of the "Standard American Diet" were even more pronounced with these First Nations people. Genetically, they are perfectly well adapted to a world in which food is hunted, fished, gathered, and plucked. They are supremely *ill*-equipped—as are most of us—to deal with a food supply that comes mostly from the 7-Eleven.

Jay Wortman, MD, a researcher from the University of British Columbia, had more than a passing interest in what was happening on Cormorant Island, which consists primarily of the village of Alert Bay. Several years ago, he had noticed that he was gaining weight. His blood pressure was rising, and he was constantly tired and thirsty. A vigorous guy who exudes good health from every pore, he slowly realized that he was exhibiting all the classic symptoms of type 2 diabetes.

"I stopped eating sugar and starch just to get my blood sugar down," Wortman said when I interviewed him. While he did not intend this dietary change to be a treatment for diabetes, a curious thing happened. "Cutting out sugar and starch literally reversed all my signs and symptoms of diabetes," he told me. His blood pressure normalized and his energy came back.

He began to wonder if similar dietary changes could make a difference to the First Nations people of Alert Bay.

With funding from Health Canada and the University of British Columbia, he decided to find out.

Wortman—along with colleagues Mary Vernon, MD, Eric Westman, MD, and nutritional biochemist Stephen Phinney, PhD—designed a 1-year study to see what would happen if the First Nations people returned to their "native" aboriginal diet. "People here traditionally got their calories mostly from protein and fat," Wortman told me. "If you 'reverse-engineered' their traditional diet, you would come up with something that looks—in modern parlance—like the Atkins diet." Wortman enrolled about 100 people in his study and got to work.

One of the first things he did was to go into people's homes and perform an exorcism on their kitchen. Gently but firmly, he removed all starch, cereals, rice, popcorn, flour, pasta, sugar, and breads. Gradually the participants got the idea. Burgers were served, but without the buns. Fries were banished. Salads came without croutons. Butter and cream were back on the menu.

The First Nations people traditionally got a large percentage of their calories from eulachon grease—a rich monounsaturated fat extracted from a little smelt-like fish (the eulachon) that was a staple of the native diet. In the "old" days, they ate tons of the stuff; but they had effectively banished it from their diet, believing all fat was bad. Eulachon grease—back on the table! Ditto with any kind of fish and traditional inland aboriginal foods like deer and roast elk. Salmon was cooked on an open fire and generously dipped in eulachon oil. Potatoes, bye-bye. "We supplemented the traditional diet with 'market foods' like bacon, cheese, and all the vegetables you could buy," said Wortman, "but the main thing was the avoidance of starch and sugar, because these were not components of the traditional diet."

And then a funny thing happened.

People who had struggled with weight for years started to shed pounds—lots of them. Jill Cook, a school principal who had struggled with weight all her life and who had previously managed to drop all of 7 pounds on a strict 4-month Jenny Craig routine, lost 58 pounds (not to mention 9 inches off her waist and 7 off her chest). Art Dick, a tribal chief who had been on a ton of medications for diabetes, was able to get off 75% of his meds within 4 days of starting the program. Andrea Cranmer lost 22 pounds and went from a size 16 to a size 12. The aforementioned Greg Wadhams lost 40 pounds and no longer requires drugs to treat his diabetes. "Our forefathers sure must've known something we didn't know, because when you eat [this] way you just feel good!" he told *The Province*.

While this might sound like the stuff of which infomercials are made, it all went into the database of the rigorously designed study. "The average weight loss was 7.5 kg (16.5 pounds) over 3 months, 11 kg (24.2 pounds) over 6 months," Wortman reports. "We saw a change in diabetes symptoms in as little as 3 days. Triglycerides went down about 30%—better than any drug we have. People lost weight, their lipid profile improved, their blood-sugar control got better, their A1c [a long-term measure of blood sugar and a risk factor for diabetes] went down," he told me. "All the things we hoped would happen seem to be happening."

As well as some things that were unexpected.

"There was a real change in attitude," Wortman told me. People started feeling good. "All my mental, emotional, spiritual, and physical aspects are finally feeling like they're in some kind of unity together, and that's so cool," said Andrea Cranmer. "What we didn't anticipate was the tremendous impact on the mental health of the community," Wortman told me. "People were happier. They spontaneously started forming support groups. It became a community affair."

So here's the question: how can a diet so filled with fat and protein— foods that the traditional health establishment tells you are "bad" for you—and lacking the cornerstone of mainstream dietary recommendations (grains, carbohydrates, cereals)—produce such impressive results in so many people?

A couple of reasons suggest themselves—besides the obvious one (that the mainstream dietary recommendations are for the most part bone-headed).

First, there's more and more evidence that saturated fat has a profoundly different fate in the body when it's consumed in the context of a very-low-carb diet. This is a critically important point, and one that has been made by a number of researchers, notably Jeff Volek, PhD, RD, of the University of Connecticut, who has done some of the most extensive and comprehensive research on low-carb diets. "Saturated fat is relatively passive," Volek told me. "[The thing that] controls what happens with saturated fat in the diet is the carb content of the diet. If carbs are low, insulin is low and saturated fat is handled more efficiently. It's burned as a fuel.

"In contrast," he continued, "when carbs are high, insulin is high. Then you're *inhibiting* the burning of saturated fat and potentially making a lot more of it, so you tend to see harmful atherogenic effects."

According to Volek—and many others—you can't really talk about saturated fat without considering the background levels of carbohydrate. "What happens with saturated fat is completely dependent on whether you're on a low-carb or a high-carb diet," says Colette Heimowitz, MSc, a nutritional scientist and coauthor of *The Atkins Advantage*. "Despite ingesting more saturated fat on low carb, the amount in the plasma (blood) is significantly less. Fat oxidation ('fat burning') is increased and fat synthesis (making new fat) is decreased."

So why do so many studies seem to show negative health effects of saturated fat intake? "All those studies are in the context of mixed diets," Heimowitz explained. "When you're on a high-carb diet, your saturated fat should probably be exactly what's recommended—no more than 10% of total calories, ⅓ of your fat. But when you're on a very low-carb diet, it's a whole different story."

Whenever I'm asked to explain this seeming paradox, the example I use is house paint. Pick your favorite color—mine is red—and then consider how it looks when you put it on a nice clean white surface. Now imagine that same color mixed with another one—say purple, or blue or green. Some of those combinations produce really hideous results. How the color "behaves" depends completely on what it's mixed with (if anything). By itself it's gorgeous, but mixed with a noncomplementary color . . . not so much.

"Although people on a high-fat, low-carb diet eat more saturated fat, their blood levels (of saturated fats) actually go down," explains Stephen Phinney, PhD, the nutritional biochemist who worked with Wortman on the Alert Bay study.[1] While the exact reason for that paradox is still being investigated, "the interim answer appears to be that when you take carbohydrates out of the diet, it causes less interference with the body's natural ability to handle fats and that the saturated fats are burned and not retained."

And what about the "side effect" of the dietary experiment, the fact that well-being improved and people seemed—well, happier?

One hypothesis has to do with inflammation. "When you have insulin resistance and metabolic syndrome, you have high inflammatory levels," Wortman reflected. "You have poor energy and you just feel crappy and you're irritable." Not so coincidentally, when you go on a low-carbohydrate diet, many of the pro-inflammatory foods in your diet are eliminated.

Research comparing the metabolic effects of low-fat and low-carb diets on inflammatory markers (such as TNF-alpha and interleukin-6) confirms this inflammation connection. A study by Jeff Volek and his associates published in the January 2008 issue of the scientific journal *Lipids* concluded that "a very low carbohydrate diet resulted in profound alterations in fatty acid composition and reduced inflammation compared to a low fat diet."[2] Richard Feinman, PhD, professor of biochemistry at SUNY Downstate Medical Center and one of the researchers involved in the study, comments: "The inflammation results open a new aspect of the problem. From a practical standpoint, continued demonstrations that carbohydrate restriction is more beneficial than low fat could be good news to those wishing to forestall or manage the diseases associated with metabolic syndrome."[3]

Another hypothesis has to do with oxidative stress, the technical name for what happens when nasty rogue molecules called "free radicals" attack and damage cells and DNA. Oxidative stress is known to be a significant component of aging, and it figures prominently in a host of diseases including atherosclerosis. "Inflammation might be one way the body has of responding to oxidative stress," Wortman suggests. Research has shown that a ketogenic (very-low-carbohydrate diet) "up regulates" (or turns on the production factory) for glutathione (GSH), a powerful antioxidant in the body, helping to protect DNA from damage.[4]

Could all these metabolic mechanisms help account for why the people of Alert Bay seemed so energized and felt so darn good? Who knows? Weight loss has so many overlapping dimensions—social, interpersonal, metabolic, hormonal—that it's hard to sort out what's responsible for what. One thing that's clear is that people lost a ton of weight, felt better about themselves, and—as a "side" benefit—seemed more connected and supportive as a community.

The "town that lost 1,200 pounds" also wound up gaining back an awful lot of wonderful things—things that had been lost for a very long time.

CHAPTER 9

Low-Carb Diets: From Paleo to Keto (and Everything in Between)

Living *Low Carb* first came out in the early 2000s.

The Atkins Diet had just been rereleased in its third edition, research on low-carb diets was starting to accumulate, and public interest in low-carb eating plans was at an all-time high. For a couple of years, right before low-carb became mainstream, specialized supermarkets started springing up to accommodate the explosion of low-carb food "products" (which, by the way, were no better than the low-fat products of the SnackWell generation). More importantly, there was an explosion of low-carb diet programs, and the public was massively confused about how they differed. People didn't know how to tell the Atkins and South Beach diets apart and which programs were "healthy" and which might not be, nor did they have any kind of GPS for what seemed like an endless number of low-carb programs, each promising love, life, happiness, and weight loss.

In the previous editions of this book, I reviewed the diets of the day— 14 in the original, which expanded to 38 in the next edition and dropped down to a mere 23 in the most recent book. (For the record, many of these diet programs never caught on or no longer exist.)

But that was then.

Low-carb is no longer considered a "fad" diet, even by the mainstream. (Truth is, it was never a fad diet—it was the way humans ate for most of our time on this planet!) And while there are still dozens of new diet plans cropping up every year, I feel that—at least on the low-carb end of things—

the plethora of diet plans can now essentially be lumped into two big "category trends:" paleo and keto.

If you understand the basic principles of these two "movements," you'll understand most of what you need to know about low-carb dieting.

For this edition, I'll be discussing different diets with a special focus on paleo and keto. For those interested in the evolution of low-carb thinking, I've included the original reviews of five of the most important of the earliest low-carb diets—in a section called The Founding Fathers—as well as reviews of other, more recent versions of low-carb that don't fit neatly into the paleo or keto templates (I've called this section The Rest of The Gang.)

So the chapter is now divided into four sections: The Founders (in which I discuss the Atkins Diet, Protein Power, The Rosedale Diet, the Zone, and the Fat Flush Plan®, all of which are still very much with us); The Paleo Diet(and its variations); The Keto Diet (and its variations); and The Rest of the Gang (in which I cover some of the terrific hybrid programs, such as Whole30®, that are worth knowing about). And just for comparison, I've included a brief discussion of the Mediterranean Diet, which has near-universal support among nutritionists. (Spoiler alert: It's actually quite possible to do a relatively low-carb version of Mediterranean eating!)

I've organized the diet chapter like this because I want to *eliminate* confusion, not add to it. A dozen "new" diet programs could appear just between the time I submit this manuscript and the time it gets published. My thought is that if you understand the basics—which you most definitely will once you understand paleo and keto—you'll be able to evaluate any program that comes down the pike much more effectively. Even more important, you'll have a tool kit that will let you mix and match ideas, using concepts or ideas from a variety of sources to come up with an eating plan that ultimately supports, nourishes, and sustains *you*.

I. THE FOUNDERS

Let's get started with the founders of the modern low-carb movement in America as we know it today. While the authors of two of these programs would probably reject the "low-carb" label, these programs still shared a healthy skepticism (to put it mildly) about the high-carb low-fat diets that were being prescribed and recommended pretty much universally for the second half of the twentieth century. All the programs discussed in this section offered terrific alternatives to the existing food-pyramid–based dietary advice. And all were courageous departures from what the diet dictators were telling us to do. For that, they each deserve to be included in the Low-Carb–Diet Hall of Fame.

1. THE ATKINS DIET
ROBERT ATKINS, MD

You can't really talk about low-carb diets without talking about Robert Atkins. Greatly misunderstood and misquoted, Dr. Atkins was an icon in the low-carb movement and with good reason: For all intents and purposes, it was Atkins who put low-carb on the cultural radar. He had far more knowledge of nutrition than the average doctor, and wasn't shy about telling the establishment where they'd gone wrong. Universally disliked by the medical establishment when he was alive, he nonetheless leaves an impressive legacy, all the more so because—on so many important things like the role of insulin in weight gain—he turned out to be right.

WHAT IT IS IN A NUTSHELL

An easy-to-follow, specific dietary plan in four distinct stages. Stage one is "induction": a very low-carb (20 grams or less) approach to jump-starting weight loss. You move through the four stages, adding more carbs in specific increments until you find the level of carbohydrate consumption at which you can continue to lose weight gradually and consistently. You stay at that level of carb consumption until you are within a few pounds of your goal, and then you transition into a lifetime maintenance plan.

About the Atkins Diet

The Atkins diet was introduced in 1972 with the first edition of *Dr. Atkins' New Diet Revolution* and immediately became an object of scorn and disdain by the conventional medical establishment. Why? Because it went completely against the accepted dietary truths of the time. In many ways it still does, though cracks in the cement are beginning to show, and the dietary establishment is finally becoming less certain that its nutritional commandments are actually true. As you may remember from chapter 6, the conventional wisdom that Atkins opposed included the following:

- To lose weight, you must eat a low-fat, high-carbohydrate diet.
- High-fat diets cause heart disease.
- Low-fat, high-carbohydrate diets prevent heart disease.
- All calories are the same.

Dr. Robert Atkins, a cardiologist and something of a visionary, was the first to bring to popular attention the influence of the hormone insulin on weight loss and to introduce the notion that *controlling insulin effectively is the key to losing weight.* By now, if you've read chapters 3 and 4, you are familiar with the central role that insulin control plays in virtually every carbohydrate-restricted diet and the reasons it occupies center stage. But in 1972, virtually no one in America who wasn't either a diabetic or a doctor had heard of insulin, let alone understood its role in weight gain and obesity. And it was not until much later that the public began to get a glimmer of insulin's role in heart disease, hypertension, and aging.

Atkins explained that insulin causes the body to store fat, that some people are metabolically primed to put out more insulin than others in response to the same foods, that sugar and carbohydrates were the prime offenders when it came to raising insulin, and that elevated levels of this hormone invariably resulted in increased body fat. He argued that it is not *fat* in the diet per se that makes you fat, but rather *sugar*—even more precisely, fat *in combination* with high sugar—and the resulting insulin that leads to weight gain. Atkins took serious issue with the idea that fat causes heart disease and claimed that his diet would actually *improve* blood-lipid profiles, measurements that show up in blood tests as risk factors for heart disease.

What is the actual diet that stirred such passionate controversy? Well, the Atkins diet is, and always has been, a four-stage affair, but most people think of it as synonymous with the first stage, "induction." During induction, you eat all the fat and protein you want, but you limit carbohydrates to 20 grams per day—an extremely low level of carbohydrate consumption equal to about 2 cups of loosely packed salad and 1 cup of a vegetable such as spinach, broccoli, Brussels sprouts, or zucchini. At stage one, you eat absolutely *no* rice, potatoes, cereal, starch, pasta, bread, fruit, or dairy products other than cheese, cream, and butter.

To anyone who has read a diet book in the last 10 years that wasn't written by low-fat guru Dean Ornish or his followers, this list of prohibited foods sounds pretty familiar. But you have to realize that in 1972, banning these foods for even 2 weeks was the nutritional equivalent of suggesting that every school and office in the country burn the American flag. These foods were the holy grail of the low-fat religion. Bagels were the breakfast of choice for health-conscious Americans. Oils, fats, butter, cheese, cream, steak, and the like were considered heart attacks on a plate, and here Atkins was making them the centerpiece of his eating plan.

The establishment thought him quite mad.

And if this weren't enough, Atkins spoke in downright loving terms of something called ketosis, which he termed "the metabolic advantage" and compared favorably to sunshine and sex. (For a much more detailed discussion of ketosis, see Keto, page 225.) For Atkins, being in ketosis was the secret to unlocking your fat stores and burning fat for fuel. Ketosis was the desired goal of the induction phase. Being in ketosis was a virtual guarantee that you were accessing your stubborn fat stores and throwing them on the metabolic flame, using your fat, instead of your sugar, for energy. A big part of the program involved checking your urine for ketones, which are the by-product of this kind of fat breakdown.

The problem was that mainstream medicine considered ketosis to be not only undesirable but dangerous, a metabolic state to be avoided at all costs. For the most part, they still do—see later in this chapter for a full explanation of why the common belief that ketosis is dangerous is wholly without merit. The emphasis on ketosis, coupled with the recommendation to eat unlimited amounts of fat, was enough to make Atkins a complete pariah in the medical establishment, and it is only now, more than 35 years after the publication of the original book and nearly a decade after his death, that we are beginning to see a turnaround in that evaluation.

Briefly, ketosis works this way: when there is not enough carbohydrate (sugar) coming into the body and when sugar stores (glycogen) have been essentially used up, the body is forced to go to its fat stores for fuel. Furthermore, because there isn't enough sugar to get fat into the usual slow-burning energy production cycles of the body (known as the Krebs cycle), the fat has to be broken down in another pathway, with the result that *ketones*—by-products of this incomplete fat-burning—are made and used freely for energy by most of the tissues, including the brain and the heart. Forced to run on a fuel of fat, the body drops weight as the fat is burned off.

The advantages of this plan are twofold. First, the severe restriction of carbohydrates and sugar in the diet immediately brings down your level of insulin, the hormone that is released in response to carbohydrates (and to some extent protein). By dialing down insulin production, you are forced to burn your own fat, a situation Atkins referred to as "biologic utopia." Since insulin is a "storage" hormone, less *insulin* means less *fat storage*. Dietary fat has no effect on insulin, so, Atkins reasoned, even if there *is* a lot of fat coming into the diet, there's not enough insulin to drive the "fat-storing" machinery.

Second, going into ketosis was a way of "tripping the metabolic switch" from a sugar-burning metabolism to a fat-burning one. Excess calories cause weight gain only when you're eating a lot of carbohydrates, said Atkins. Dump the carbohydrates, and the fat in your diet is not a problem. He also claimed, to the sputtering frustration of his detractors, that you could consume *more* calories on his program and *still* lose weight, precisely because the fat-storing hormone, insulin, remained at low levels.

Atkins argued that obesity exists when the metabolism is not functioning correctly, but that metabolic disturbances have little to do with the fat we eat; rather, they are caused by eating too many carbohydrates. According to Atkins, if you've been overweight for a long time, it's a virtual certainty that your body has problems processing sugar.

Atkins also believed that the biggest reason people gain back weight lost on a diet is hunger, and that hunger is just about inevitable when you go on a reduced-calorie, high-carbohydrate, low-fat diet. On his program, hunger was virtually eliminated, as were cravings and blood-sugar instabilities. There are good physiological reasons why the appetite is suppressed on a low-carbohydrate diet rich in protein and fat—for example, the release of the hormone CCK (which tells your brain you are full) and the possible suppression of a substance in the brain called neuropeptide Y, which stimulates appetite.

The rules of his induction phase are straightforward and simple. You do not count calories. You do not count protein. You do not count fat. You *do* count, however, grams of carbohydrate, and you can have up to 20 grams a day in the form of *either* 2 cups of loosely packed salad and 1 cup of uncooked vegetables chosen from a specific list, *or* 3 cups of salad. Period. As mentioned earlier, you can't have starches, grains, sugar, fruit, or alcohol. You cannot eat nuts, seeds, or "mixed" foods (combinations of protein and carbohydrate) like beans, chickpeas, or legumes. It is also suggested that you avoid the artificial sweetener aspartame and caffeine, the latter because it can lead to low blood sugar and stimulate cravings.

Weight loss in the induction phase is fairly quick and dramatic. Much, but not all, of the weight loss is water and bloat, largely because insulin's message to the kidneys is to stockpile salt (and therefore water) is no longer being sent. But the induction phase is only meant as a jump-start. Though Atkins felt it was perfectly safe to stay in the induction phase for a month or so, he encouraged dieters to progress to stage two, which he calls ongoing weight loss, or OWL.

The key to the success of OWL is finding what Atkins calls your *Critical Carbohydrate Level for Losing*, or CCLL. (Some version of this has been adapted by virtually every low-carbohydrate diet that uses the concept of "stages.") Here's how it works: After completing the initial induction phase, you slowly add back carbohydrates at a very specific rate of 5 grams *per week* (the amount of carbs in another cup of salad, half an avocado, or six to eight stalks of asparagus, for example). This would put you at 25 grams of carbs per week. If you continue losing, in the next week you go up to 30 grams. You continue this progression upward until your weight loss stalls, and then you cut back to the previous level. That level is what Atkins calls your CCLL.

The rules for OWL are simple: you still eat as much protein and fat as you want (stopping when you're satisfied, of course); you increase carbs by no more than 5 grams per week; you add one new food group at a time to see if it has any negative impact on cravings or symptoms (such as headaches, bloating, and so on); and you continue this way until you are close to your goal weight.

When you are 5 to 10 pounds from your goal, you move to stage three, "premaintenance." During premaintenance, you up your carbs by another 10 grams per week (for example, some typical 10-gram portions are ½ cup of almonds, filberts, or macadamia nuts; ¼ cup of yams or beans; and 1 cup of strawberries or watermelon). Again, you're looking for the level of carbohydrate consumption that will let you keep losing, albeit at a much slower rate. If you overshoot that level and stop losing completely or even start gaining, you drop back down a level. Simple.

Atkins stresses the importance of the premaintenance stage, but I imagine it's the one most people resist the most. Here's why: when you're within spitting distance of your goal, you are naturally tempted to keep doing what you're doing until you get there. Atkins wants you to actually *slow the weight loss down* during premaintenance to less than a pound a week for 2 to 3 months. Premaintenance is seen as a kind of driver's ed for lifetime maintenance. You're using this time to learn and master new habits of eating that will last the rest of your life. You need to do a great deal of experimenting and tweaking, as the difference between your Critical Carb Level for *Losing* and your Critical Carb Level for *Maintaining* is likely to be very small. Finally, when you do arrive at your goal, you increase the carbohydrate level—again in measured increments and very gradually and carefully—until you find the level that allows you to stay exactly at that weight. Now you're in stage four, "maintenance"; the number of grams of carbohydrate you're consuming is your Critical Carb Level for Maintaining, and that's what you continue eating to stay at your goal weight.

Atkins spends a lot of time discussing metabolic resistance to weight loss, which he defines as the inability to burn fat or lose weight. He identifies four major causes of metabolic resistance, which are discussed at length in chapter 20 of his *New Diet Revolution*. Obviously, excessive insulin and insulin resistance is one of the causes (see chapter 3 of this book for a full discussion on insulin resistance). Prescription drugs or hormones are another, and an underactive or malfunctioning thyroid is another. The last is yeast.

Atkins' discussion of yeast is useful reading for everyone who has had trouble losing weight. I believe yeast is a far more common factor in weight-loss problems than was previously thought. Atkins explains that yeast overgrowth is commonly found in conjunction with a sensitivity to mold, and that the combination may easily suppress metabolism. Dr. Alan Schwartz, medical director of the Holistic Resource Center in Agoura Hills, California, has said that yeast creates its own food source by literally demanding sugar to feed on (i.e., cravings), a theory that would dovetail nicely with Atkins's. Yeast, a living organism, also produces waste products and toxins, which can weaken the immune system and lead to food intolerances, another obstacle to weight loss. While the mechanisms are not completely understood, it's a good bet that Atkins was right about the yeast connection. Fortunately, the Atkins diet—at least the induction phase—virtually eliminates all of yeast's favorite foods, and the classic anti-yeast diet looks a lot like Atkins's induction.

Atkins identifies what he calls three levels of metabolic resistance: high, average, and low. How easily your body responds to carbohydrate restriction defines your level of metabolic resistance. He suspected that most people with a high level of metabolic resistance would wind up with a maintenance level of somewhere around 25 to 40 grams of carbs a day. Those with a low level of resistance would be in the 60-to-90–gram range, and regular exercisers would be at 90-plus grams of carbohydrate per day.

Atkins has been one of the most misunderstood diet authors and has been the target of more attacks than any other low-carb proponent, probably because his was the first and the most commercially successful of the plans and also, to the constant chagrin of the establishment, because he simply wouldn't go away. While some of the larger criticisms of the Atkins diet are applicable to all low-carb diets and have been dealt with in depth in chapter 6, some are specific to Atkins and are briefly addressed here.

One source of misinformation about Atkins came because many people confused the *induction* phase with the whole program. Atkins was very clear that induction was for a limited time only. A common criticism of Atkins is that he doesn't allow you to eat vegetables and fruits. Actually, he said no such thing. Atkins was a nutritionist, and a very good one at that—he did not want you to miss the incredible nutritional benefits of the phytochemicals found in vegetables and fruits, so he has you adding these back to the program in the subsequent stages of his plan. He never said you couldn't eat vegetables and fruits. He *did* say you couldn't eat junk carbohydrates.

Another problem with the public's (and the medical establishment's) perception of Atkins's program is that it was based solely on the first (1972) edition of his book. In that edition, where Atkins first put forth the radical proposition that cutting carbohydrates was the key to controlling insulin, he didn't pay as much attention to what you were *allowed* to eat, concentrating instead on the foods you had to cut out. Atkins in 1972 was like the doorman at an exclusive club who is given the order *"don't let in anyone wearing sneakers!"* and, as a result, is so focused on the ground that he doesn't realize he is letting in all kinds of other riffraff that just happen to be wearing leather shoes. Atkins revised the book twice (in 1992 and 2002), and with each edition he became more outspoken about the need to emphasize omega-3 fats, eliminate trans-fats, and include plenty of vegetables and fiber in the diet. But sadly, he could never shake the 1972 image as the diet doc who lets you eat pork rinds and lard, an unjustified characterization of his work if there ever was one.

Finally, it bears mentioning that the fully developed Atkins program is a three-pronged approach to health that involves not just carbohydrate management (he later called the diet a "controlled-carbohydrate approach to eating"), but also exercise and nutritional supplementation. In his New York clinic, only a small percentage of patients came in solely for weight loss. Atkins should be remembered for his marvelous work in the field of complementary and integrative medicine, as well as for his pioneering work on diet.

The Atkins Diet as a Lifestyle: Who It Works For, Who Should Look Elsewhere

While his last book, *Atkins for Life,* is a pretty good template for healthy living that almost anyone could benefit from (and is not wildly different from the Zone or the last stage of the Fat Flush Plan), the Atkins diet proper is likely to be most successful with, and most appreciated by, those who really have a fair amount of weight to lose and have had a great deal of difficulty getting it off. People with only 10 or 15 pounds to lose could certainly do the program, but the exacting and cautious approach to adding carbohydrates back 5 grams at a time is likely to be overkill for them.

In the next decade, I believe we will have an even better understanding of why different folks respond to different diets; but the fact is that some people do very well on higher-protein, higher-fat diets and some do not. Obviously, those with fat- and protein-friendly types of metabolisms are going to fare well on this diet and not find it nearly as difficult and restrictive as those with a different sort of metabolic blueprint.

JONNY'S LOWDOWN

Rereading the Atkins opus for the zillionth time in preparation for this book, I was once again struck by the disparity between what he actually said and what people think he said. The Atkins diet was never an "all-protein" diet; in fact, a recent statistical analysis put the induction phase at 35% protein and the maintenance phase at only 25%![1] He stressed vegetables, talked about fiber, went to great lengths to emphasize individual responses and the need for customizing, and thought that both exercise and nutritional supplements were absolutely vital for optimal health. The later version of his book—as well as the breezier Atkins for Life—is heavily referenced, with a superb bibliography of scientific studies.

Atkins's only real mistake was in portraying ketosis as identical to fat loss and making it seem as though calories didn't matter at all. He kind of boxed himself into a corner on this one. Ketosis doesn't cause fat loss; it is simply the by-product of fat-burning. Yes, ketosis occurs when you are burning fat for fuel, but you will dip into stored fat only if you are not getting enough fuel from the diet. If your diet is 10,000 calories made up of 90% fat, 9% protein, and 1% carbs, you will most certainly be in deep ketosis, but you will gain weight like crazy.

I don't think everyone who needs to lose weight must go on Atkins, but it is certainly a viable option and likely to be quite helpful for people with carb addictions, resistant metabolisms, significant insulin problems, and a fair amount of weight to lose.

2. PROTEIN POWER
MICHAEL EADES, MD AND MARY DAN EADES, MD

Michael and Mary Dan Eades are two of the true pioneers of the low-carb movement. Shortly after writing *Protein Power,* they published *The Protein Power Lifeplan.* It's their "this is how you live" book, and it's a darn good one. I've referenced both books in the section that follows.

Both Eadeses are still very active today. Michael Eades writes a very interesting and wide-ranging blog in which he talks about everything from nutrition and medicine to Freddy Mercury. (Search online for *The Blog of Michael Eades.*) *Highly recommended.*

WHAT IT IS IN A NUTSHELL

A three-phase plan in which you do the following:

- *Eat no less than a minimum calculated amount of protein per day (you are free to eat more, but not less)*
- *Eat no more than a maximum amount of carbohydrates per day (you are free to eat less, but not more)*

The maximum amount of carbohydrates depends on which phase of the diet you are in. Phase 1 is intervention and allows up to 30 grams of carbohydrates a day; phase 2 is transition and allows up to 55 grams; phase 3 is the maintenance phase, and the amount of carbs will vary according to the individual.

About Protein Power

In the Eadeses' plan, you first determine your protein needs through an easy-to-follow series of steps:

1. Measure your wrist, then your waist.

2. Refer to a chart to estimate your body fat from these measurements.

3. Now you calculate your total number of fat pounds. For example, if you're 200 pounds with 20% body fat, you would have 40 fat pounds.

4. Subtract the number of fat pounds from your total weight to get the number of lean body-weight pounds (muscle, bone, and the like). Using the above example, you would subtract 40 pounds from 200 and wind up with a lean body weight of 160 pounds.

5. Multiply your lean body weight by an "activity factor" to get your minimum daily protein needs (in grams). The activity factor ranges from 0.5 for someone who is completely sedentary to 0.9 for a competitive athlete. For example, if the 200-pound guy with 40 fat pounds and 160 lean pounds were sedentary, he'd multiply 160 by 0.5 for a total of 80 grams of protein per day, minimum.

Knowing your lean body weight also allows you to calculate a realistic weight goal, which is done using worksheets and very easy formulas.

Note: In *The Protein Power Lifeplan*, the authors have simplified the process even more. You don't even have to take your wrist or waist measurements, compute your lean body mass, or multiply by an activity factor. There's a simple table in which you look for your height and weight, and the table tells you immediately what your minimum protein requirement is. It couldn't be easier. It's not as refined and accurate as the method in the original *Protein Power*, but it will give you a decent estimate of your minimum requirement and is good for people who just don't want to do the calculations. (My personal opinion: the calculations are easy.)

Once you know your minimum daily protein needs, you simply decide what phase of the diet you're going to be on. Phase 1, intervention, is for those who have a lot of fat to lose and/or who want to correct a health problem. In phase 1, you take in 30 grams or less of carbohydrate a day (in *The Protein Power Lifeplan*, this number is amended to 40) plus, of course, *at least* your minimum protein requirement. Phase 2 is the one to go with if you want to lose a little fat, recompose your body (i.e., change the ratio of fat to muscle or, as people often say, "tone up"), or improve your general health. In phase 2, the maximum carb allowance is upped to 55 grams a day, in addition, of course, to the protein allowance determined above. You can eat *more* than your minimum protein requirement but not less, and you can eat *less* than your maximum carb allotment but not more. The rest of the diet comes from fat.

Nearly everyone will fall into one of four categories of minimum protein requirement—less than 60 grams a day, between 60 and 80 grams a day, between 80 and 100 grams a day, or between 100 and 120 grams a day. You find the category you belong to and then refer to the corresponding chart. The chart will tell you exactly what protein foods in what amounts you can have *per meal and snack*. For example, if you're in the 80-to-100–gram category, you should be getting about 34 grams of protein per meal. The chart shows you exactly how to make any combination you can think of from meat, fish, poultry, eggs, hard cheeses, soft cheeses, curd cheeses, or tofu to get the right amount of protein per meal.

Like nearly all the diet or lifestyle plans discussed in this book, Protein Power is all about controlling and balancing insulin. The Eadeses have a clever way of determining the actual insulin-raising (or active) carbohydrate content of foods. Even though fiber is not metabolically active, it's technically counted as a carbohydrate on food labels and the like. But it doesn't raise insulin at all, since it's not even digested. So the Eadeses have come up with a formula in which you subtract the fiber from the total carb content of a food to get what they call the "effective carbohydrate content," or ECC. That's the only number you have to pay attention to when counting your carbohydrate grams. For example, 1 cup of fresh raspberries has 14 grams of carbohydrate but 6 grams of fiber, so you'd subtract the 6 grams of fiber from the 14 grams of total carbohydrate to get a mere 8 grams of ECC, and only those 8 grams would count toward your carbohydrate allowance for the day. (This is now standard operating procedure for most low-carb diets, some of which call the number "effective carbs," some "net carbs.")

Protein Power has charts of the ECC for a huge number of foods, so you don't have to figure them out for yourself. You use these charts to put together your daily carbohydrate allowance (or, if a food is not listed in the chart, you can easily compute it yourself from the label's listing of total carbs and total fiber). Counting only effective carbs, you could easily have 1 cup of broccoli, 1 cup of cabbage, 3 celery ribs, 1 cup of green beans, 1 cup of lettuce, ½ cup of mushrooms, 1 cup of zucchini, 1 cup of spinach, and 1 cup of raspberries in one day on phase 1. Even though the total carb content of these foods is about 44 grams, 16 of them are fiber; subtracting the 16 from the 44 (all done for you in the charts) leaves you with only 28 grams of usable (effective) carbohydrate, well under the cutoff for phase 1 and not even close to the cutoff for phase 2.

Calories are barely mentioned in *Protein Power*. The idea is that calories are self-regulating if you are eating the foods that put you in correct metabolic balance (an idea that runs throughout many low-carb diet plans). The Eadeses do warn you that since you may not be as hungry on a low-carb plan as you were before, you can easily *under*-eat, so it's important to be sure that your calories don't fall below 850 to 1,000 a day. (The 850 figure seems really, *really* low—nearly every other weight-loss expert, including myself, uses 1,000 to 1,250 as the bare minimum, and some even suggest not dropping below 1,250. If the food eaten produces a hormonally balanced state and the calories are coming from good stuff, most women will drop weight on 1,250 calories and most men on 1,500.)

On the other hand, especially in *The Protein Power Lifeplan*, the authors explain that if you're doing everything right (i.e., eating the minimum protein requirement and not exceeding the maximum carb allotment) and you're *still* not losing weight, you might be consuming too many calories, especially calories from fat. Nuts seem to be a frequent culprit: since nuts are only fat and protein, many low-carbers munch on these with abandon because they have very little effect on insulin. But while a 1-ounce portion (which is pretty small!) may have only 160 calories and a few grams of carbs at most, three to four portions can add an awful lot of calories (and carb grams) to a diet plan and could effectively slow down or stop weight loss altogether. As with most low-carb plans, the message here is this: though calories are not the whole story by a long shot, they still matter, so don't ignore them.

Phase 3 is the maintenance phase, which is what you stay on once you've reached your goal. To get there, you add 10 grams of carbohydrate to your phase 2 daily allotment, and stay there and stabilize for about 5 to 7 days. Then you add another 10 grams. You continue in this way until you find the amount of carbs you can take in and still keep your weight stable. The Eadeses have found that *most* people will stabilize when they've reached the point at which the number of carb grams equals the number of protein grams, but they discuss the exceptions to this general rule and tell you what to do if you don't fit the template.

The maintenance phase is pretty cool. There is really no food you can't have "in some quantity at some time." The trick is knowing what you're doing. As the authors put it, there are foods that are "so rich in sugars and starches, such potent unbalancers of your metabolic hormones, that you cannot have unlimited amounts of them anytime you want unless you are willing to accept the consequences of that action." They even have recovery guidelines for those times when you throw caution to the wind and have a "nutritional vacation," such as on birthdays, holidays, and the like. You simply return to phase 1 for 3 days (or until you have lost any of the weight you might have gained), move to phase 2 for the rest of the week, and then return to your maintenance level of carb consumption.

The thing about *The Protein Power Lifeplan,* and to a lesser extent the original book, is that it is about so much more than just a diet. There is absolutely first-rate information about cholesterol and the "cholesterol hoax," plus wonderful explanations of how insulin works in the body and its relationship to heart disease, high blood pressure, diabetes, and obesity. There is a terrific exposition on the Paleolithic Diet. And in *Lifeplan,* the authors go into even more detail on all of these topics, plus they include discussions of antioxidants, leaky gut syndrome and autoimmune responses, sugar, iron overload, magnesium, brain health, and a further expansion of the nutritional plan.

Lifeplan also has a cool concept. It suggests three levels of "commit-ment" to health: the purist, the dilettante, and the hedonist. All of these approaches share the same requirements for protein, the same need for high-quality fat, the same prohibition of trans-fatty acids, and the same limitations of carbohydrate grams (depending on what phase you're in). (Even at the lowest level of commitment, the hedonist, you're still way better off than you would be following the standard American diet or, for that matter, the standard high-carb, low-fat diet.) All of the levels should theoretically give the same weight-loss results. The difference is in overall health benefits.

The purist regimen is really restrictive. Purists eat *no* cereal grains or products made from them. They eat *no* dairy or legumes (such as beans). (Spoiler alert: This has a lot in common with Paleo; see page 186.) They eat *only* organic fruits and vegetables and *only* natural meat and poultry—no processed foods, no sugars (except occasionally honey), no artificial sweeteners, no caffeine, and no alcohol. It's probably the most healthful diet in the world to follow, but can be difficult for most folks. However, for people with serious health issues, it may literally mean the difference between life and death.

Next up is the dilettante regimen. You aim for organic foods whenever possible but are not obsessive about it. You still avoid some grains (wheat, for example) but can eat others (like oats and rice). You eliminate high-fructose corn syrup but can have some other sweeteners, even table sugar (in very limited amounts), and the prohibition against alcohol and caffeine is lifted. This is the program the Eadeses themselves follow.

Finally, there is the hedonist, where anything goes, within the limits of your carbohydrate allowance. You still have to keep to the basic parameters of the program, but you can fulfill those requirements with just about any foods you wish. Obviously, the high-carb content of some foods, such as potatoes, may make it impossible to fit those foods into the phase 1 plan, when carbs are limited to 7 to 10 grams per meal and snack. But once you're on phase 2 or 3, you can eat anything you want as long as you don't exceed the maximum number of carbs for the day.

Protein Power as a Lifestyle: Who It Works For, Who Should Look Elsewhere

This is a great plan if you have a lot of weight to lose or if you have any of the health conditions discussed in the book. In its maintenance phase, it's a great plan to follow, period. But you've got to be willing to do a little figuring. You can't eyeball portions on the first two phases (like you can on the Zone or even on phase 3 of this plan). You've got to be exact about carb-gram content and about meeting your minimum protein needs. The calculations to figure out your protein needs could put some folks off (although it's a nonissue in *Lifeplan*). Having to check ECC for every food might be a pain and could be a real problem if you eat out often, unless you get really familiar with the carb content of a lot of foods. If you're willing to put in the effort, it's totally worth it. If you're not into counting, measuring, and keeping really clear records (in your mind, if not on paper), this is going to be a hard plan for you to follow, and you might be better off with a simpler formula.

JONNY'S LOWDOWN

It's hard to find anything wrong with this plan and the concepts and theories behind it. In some ways it's like the Zone with an induction phase, which may be why Barry Sears, whose Zone diet is way higher in carbs and lower in fat, is still able to endorse it (phase 3, the maintenance phase of Protein Power, is not far from Zone-like eating). Plus, The Protein Power Lifeplan *is a great general guide for anyone who just wants to live a healthy lifestyle and manage their weight.*

3. THE ROSEDALE DIET
RON ROSEDALE, MD

When I first started to study nutrition, Ron Rosedale was one of my heroes. He was doing "metabolic medicine" before they called it that. The Rosedale Diet had a brief period of popularity and then seemed to fade from view; but with the resurgence of interest in keto diets and the growing acceptance of high-fat diets in general, Dr. Rosedale is enjoying a much-deserved renaissance of popularity. He was one of the first popular diet-book authors to discuss *leptin*, the hunger-management hormone. He definitely deserves a place at the "Foundation Table."

WHAT IT IS IN A NUTSHELL

A novel higher-fat approach to low-carb that focuses on leptin, a hormone involved in the regulation of appetite.

About the Rosedale Diet

How can you fault any diet book that clearly states the following: "The high carbohydrate–low fat diet being prescribed to diabetic patients is precisely the wrong approach"? Answer: You can't.

The Rosedale Diet is a gem. It's is the creation of Ron Rosedale, MD, the doctor who, when Mike and Mary Dan Eades (of Protein Power fame) left Colorado to move on to other projects, took over the directorship of their clinic for metabolic medicine. Rosedale has long been one of the most sought-after educators in nutritional and metabolic medicine, and his book, which shares its name with his diet, is his first entry into the popular-diet world. It's a winner on every count.

While the Rosedale Diet is clearly a "low-carb" plan, it takes a somewhat different approach to weight loss, one that is focused on a hormone called *leptin*.

Here's the deal with leptin. Back in the '90s, researchers were excited to discover this protein hormone which seemed to regulate appetite. Leptin signals the brain that it's time to stop eating. Rats that were leptin-deficient ate a ton of food and, when injected with leptin, lost weight easily. The excitement in the research community was palpable. Researchers at the Rockefeller Institute believed they just might have found the holy grail of weight loss. They reasoned that obese people must be leptin-deficient, and that if leptin (or a drug that mimicked it) could be given to obese individuals, their appetite would be regulated automatically and the pounds would drop off.

No such luck. Turns out that what worked in rats didn't work at all in humans. Obese people, as it happens, have plenty of leptin.

The problem is, their bodies don't "listen" to it.

They are, to use the term Rosedale uses, *leptin-resistant*. "Leptin is produced by your fat cells," Rosedale explains. "It tells your brain when to eat, how much to eat and most important, when to *stop* eating." Just as type 2 diabetics have plenty of insulin (but their cells don't respond effectively to it), obese people have plenty of leptin, but all that leptin falls on deaf cellular ears. In obese or overweight people, leptin does not seem to be able to effectively communicate its message to "stop eating."

Rosedale explains it elegantly: "*When leptin levels can be properly 'heard,' it alerts your brain and other body tissues that you have eaten enough and stored away enough fat, and it's now time to burn off some excess fat. This feedback system is designed to prevent you from getting fat. In order for leptin to be heard clearly, however, leptin levels must remain stable and low. When leptin levels spike too high, too often, your cells stop listening to leptin. In medical terms, they become 'resistant' to leptin*." In other words, your brain continues to tell you "be hungry, eat, and store more fat!"

The Rosedale Diet is all about getting rid of "leptin resistance."

Interestingly, the same foods that aggravate *insulin* resistance—the central factor in obesity, diabetes, and metabolic syndrome—also promote *leptin* resistance: sugar and high-carb diets. The Rosedale Diet abandons the outdated classification of carbohydrates into "simple" and "complex" and instead classes them into "fiber" versus "non-fiber" (or what some people would call "slow-burning" versus "fast-burning"). Fiber, good; non-fiber, not so good. Not surprising, and totally accurate. On the Rosedale Diet, most grains are avoided (especially for the first 3 weeks), but non-starchy vegetables are plentiful.

Rosedale isn't of the opinion that protein should be unlimited, and I think he may be right on this. He recommends limiting protein to 50 to 75 grams a day. Remember, protein doesn't have a neutral effect on insulin (the way fat does). "Extra protein can be converted into glucose and burned as sugar, which causes spikes in leptin and insulin levels, which in turn cause sugar cravings," he points out.

Rosedale's variation on the low-carb theme is lower in protein than, for example, the Eadeses' program, and—perhaps counterintuitively—concentrates on fat. (Remember, fat is the one macronutrient that has virtually no effect on insulin!)

Rosedale's take on fat is some of the sharpest and most accurate writing I've yet seen, and should be read by everyone. For openers, he distinguishes between "good" and "bad" fat, but he actually knows what he's talking about. Don't expect the usual "saturated fat is bad, unsaturated fat is good" platitudes. "Some types of fat are bad for you all the time," he says, "and some types of fat are bad for you only some of the time. The health effects of fat often depend on what you eat with it."

Amen.

He warns against too much omega-6 (found in vegetable oils that the conventional establishment thinks are healthy all the time), completely forbids trans-fats, and even points out the fact that saturated fat sometimes has an *advantage* in the diet. But he doesn't recommend eating a huge amount of saturated fat since, in general, "it is the toughest fat to burn." "If you are looking to shed pounds, it is best to limit (not eliminate) your intake of saturated fat."

I have to give Rosedale credit also for being just about the only nutrition doctor I've ever read who actually questions the universal mandate that omega-9s (monounsaturated fat such as that found in olive oil) is great.

"I'm not convinced that monounsaturated or omega-9 fat has any special health properties, yet people who eat monounsaturated fats seem to be protected against certain common diseases." He suggests that the health benefits seen by people consuming the Mediterranean diet (which is famously high in olive oil) get those health benefits more because of the amazing beneficial phenols and antioxidants in olive oil and nuts rather than the omega-9 fat itself. "I believe that the major benefit of monounsaturated fat is what it is *not*," he says. "It is *not* bad for you and doesn't have any of the negative effects of other oils."

Clearly, Rosedale is a guy who thinks for himself.

The Rosedale Diet is divided into 2 levels: Level 1 and Level 2. "I consider Level 1 to be the healthiest possible diet," Rosedale says, "and one that will not only help you lose weight quickly, but will give you the best shot at longevity." On the diet program, you stay on Level 1 for at least 3 weeks, though you can opt to stay on it forever. "It is basically the diet that I follow most of the time," Rosedale says. Level 2 contains a wider variety of foods (a few more servings of fruits and starches) but is still a hugely healthful diet. On the first 3 weeks of the Rosedale Diet (Level 1), you'll eat nuts, nut butters, avocado, olives, all kinds of fish, poultry, game, veggie burgers, and even some selected dairy. Protein powders are OK, as is plain tofu, and there's the usual list of "free" vegetables, from asparagus to zucchini. A few high-fiber starches, limited legumes, tea, and just about any spice you can name round off the list. You don't count calories, but you eat until you're full, which winds up being less than "usual" because you don't crave sweets and your body is becoming less leptin-resistant.

After the first 3 weeks, you can opt to move to Level 2 and begin to add a wider variety of foods, including fruit and legumes, coffee and wine. Off the menu—pretty much permanently—are milk, most full-fat hard cheeses, processed meats, certain legumes (including peanut butter, which I'm not sure I agree with), very starchy vegetables, sugar, commercial fruit juices, soda, and all fried foods. (I have a few minor disagreements with some of the foods on the "banned" list, but for the most part I think he's nailed it!)

How long can you stay on the diet? The short answer is forever, if you want to. "I consider the Rosedale Diet the optimal diet for life and I urge patients to stay on it forever," he says. "If you keep your leptin levels down, you will not experience the constant hunger or food cravings that helped make you overweight and sick in the first place, and that make diets difficult or impossible to maintain."

The Rosedale Diet as a Lifestyle: Who It Works For, Who Should Look Elsewhere

For those who are metabolically suited to a hunter–gatherer diet of protein, vegetables, and fat (with a few judiciously chosen extras thrown in for good measure), this is a terrific weight-loss plan that you can actually stay on for life.

If you're OK bucking the conventional establishment "wisdom" on fat, this is a program definitely worth looking at. Your friends may think you're nuts for eating so much fat, but if you can ignore them, you'll be glad you did. The only danger here is the same danger that exists with Atkins—assuming that once you lose the weight, you can continue eating this way plus add back all the junky carbs you used to eat. This program works, but not when you add a bunch of useless carbs to it.

JONNY'S LOWDOWN

One thing you can say about the Rosedale Diet is that you will actually learn something from it. The information on leptin alone—and its relationship to insulin, stress, and aging—is worth the price of the book. The diet is designed to "turn off your hunger switch," which certainly makes sticking to a plan a lot easier than gritting your teeth and relying on willpower all the time. Well worth reading and well worth following.

The following two programs—written by two experts who have very similar visions about healthy eating and have been friends and colleagues for years—share a certain sensibility, if not a similar style. Both are "40/30/30" programs, meaning you get about 40% of your calories from carbs and 30% each from fat and protein. Technically, these are not low-carb programs, but because they came about at a time when all our dietary "experts" were advising that we eat 60–70% of our calories from carbs, they were *considered* "low-carb" (though not by their authors).

Both programs have a much more generous view of carbohydrates than the other ones we've been discussing, but both share a belief—novel for the time—that food has a hormonal effect. And both eschew "low-fat" diets, sugar, and empty calories.

4. THE FAT FLUSH PLAN
ANN LOUISE GITTLEMAN, PHD, CNS

WHAT IT IS IN A NUTSHELL

A 3-phase eating plan designed for both fat loss and detoxification. The idea is both to lose fat and to make your body more efficient at processing it effectively, largely by targeting a sluggish liver, the main organ for detoxification and fat metabolism in the body. The first phase is fairly (though not completely) carbohydrate-restrictive —you can still have two portions of fruit a day and a ton of vegetables—with each subsequent phase adding back more carbohydrates until you reach maintenance.

About the Fat Flush Plan

The Fat Flush Plan started life as a 2-week eating program that was originally chapter 16 in Ann Louise Gittleman's pioneering book *Beyond Pritikin*. Developed and expanded over the years, it eventually became the fully realized diet and lifestyle plan that is the cornerstone of Gittleman's book.

Fat Flush brings a different spin to low-carb dieting by concentrating on what Gittleman calls the "five hidden weight gain factors": an overworked liver, lack of fat-burning fats, too much insulin, stress, and something that Dr. Elson Haas has called "false fat."

The Liver

In addition to being the main organ for detoxification in the body, the liver is also responsible for fat metabolism. Bile, for example, is made in the liver (and stored in the gallbladder) and is responsible for helping the liver break down fats. But bile can't work efficiently if it doesn't have the proper nutrients that make up the bile salts, or if it is congested or thickened with toxins, pollutants, hormones, drugs, and other nasty stuff. Hence, inefficient bile production can slow weight loss.

Another example of how impaired liver function can slow weight loss is "fatty liver," a condition that many overweight people develop. It's not life-threatening, but it's also not something you want to put on your holiday wish list. A very early symptom of possible liver disease frequently seen in alcoholics, it basically means that fat is backed up in the liver like cars on a multi-lane freeway trying to get through a single toll booth.

Modern life puts a lot of stress on the poor overworked liver. The number of commonly used substances (including medications and even some herbs) that can harm the liver is enormous, and includes Tylenol, some cholesterol-lowering medications, some estrogens used in hormone-replacement therapy and in birth-control pills, alcohol, and a host of other stuff.

Getting the liver in tip-top shape is one goal of the Fat Flush Plan, and that's something that virtually no other diet program addresses. Fat Flush does it by including well-known bile thinners like eggs (high in an amazing liver-supportive substance known as phosphatidylcholine, which also has the ability to break up fats in the bargain) and hot water with lemon juice.

Fat-Burning Fats

Gittleman was a pioneer in debunking the popular '80s notion that a no-fat diet was a good thing (*Eat Fat, Lose Weight*), and she was especially credible because she had been chief nutritionist at the Pritikin Center, which was (and still is) Command Central for the low-fat contingent. She specifically recommends supplementation with GLA (gamma-linolenic acid, a fatty acid found in evening primrose oil, borage oil, and black-currant oil) because it stimulates a special kind of fat in the body called brown adipose tissue, or BAT. BAT is metabolically active fat that surrounds vital organs and can actually help *burn off* calories.

Excess Insulin

Virtually every low-carb diet plan exists precisely because of the theory that too much insulin is the culprit behind weight gain for a huge number of people. *The Fat Flush Plan* addresses this with the now-familiar prescription of healthful fats, lean proteins, and low-glycemic carbohydrates.

Stress

The connection between stress and fat gain is mediated by excess production of the stress hormone cortisol, and is firmly established by research. This connection made its way into the popular consciousness largely due to the pioneering work of Dr. Pamela Peeke. The connection is too lengthy to go into in detail here—those interested should check out Dr. Peeke's excellent book *Fight Fat After Forty*, or read the very good explanation of the stress–fat connection in *The Fat Flush Plan*. Here's the condensed version: *stress makes you fat*. The Fat Flush Plan addresses stress by offering suggestions for improving sleep, getting moderate exercise, and removing dietary cortisol boosters such as caffeine and sugar.

"False Fat"

People love this term. When I wrote about it for iVillage.com, my article got more hits than almost anything else I had ever written and was featured on the America Online home page. People are fascinated by the notion that they could actually be carrying around something that *feels* like fat, *looks* like fat, but maybe, just *maybe*, isn't *actually* fat at all! The term is the invention of the wonderful integrative physician and author Dr. Elson Haas, who wrote a book about it (*The False Fat Diet*), and Gittleman honorably credits him with the concept, which is central to her discussion of the five hidden weight-gain factors.

Here's the deal: Food sensitivities can trigger hormonal reactions in the body that lead to both water retention and cravings. Water retention happens because incompletely digested molecules or peptides from the food you're sensitive to enter the bloodstream and are perceived as invaders by the immune system, which then mounts a full-fledged Pac-Man–like attack, releasing histamine and flooding the area with extra fluid. (This extra fluid can be up to 10 or 15 pounds in some people—it's not really fat, but it sure feels like it, and it can easily make the difference between you being able to wear your "skinny clothes" and having to wear your "fat jeans.")

During this immune-system response, the body also overproduces the hormones cortisol and aldosterone, which in turn increase sodium retention, attracting even more water to the cells and tissues. This whole immune cascade will cause you to release endorphins (natural "feel-good" opiates), which can, over time, easily give rise to a feeling that you're addicted to the very foods you're sensitive to. (Think of sugar, wheat, flour, and the like. Ever notice how no one ever says they're addicted to Brussels sprouts?) Finally, your levels of serotonin—the feel-good neurotransmitter—drop when the immune system goes into full alert, because the same white blood cells that carry serotonin are now too busy fighting off the invaders to bother with serotonin. Lower levels of serotonin almost always lead to increased cravings for high-carbohydrate foods, which in turn spike your blood sugar, leading to a vicious circle of higher levels of insulin and more fat storage. Get it?

The Fat Flush Plan relies heavily on daily intakes of "cran-water," a mixture of unsweetened cranberry juice (not the "cocktail" stuff commonly found in supermarkets) and water. The juice contains arbutin, an active ingredient in cranberries that is a natural diuretic (as is the lemon in the hot-water-and-lemon-juice mix). The Fat Flush Plan also deals with the "false fat" issue by restricting the "usual suspect" foods that are likely to trigger food sensitivities: wheat, dairy, and sugar.

Phase 1 of the plan is about 1,100 to 1,200 calories (this is one of the few low-carb plans in which the author actually mentions caloric intake) and is designed to jump-start weight loss. It's also meant to be a good cleansing program that supports the liver. You stay on it for 2 weeks; if you've got more than 25 pounds to lose, you can stick with it for a month, though it might get pretty boring.

In phase 1, you avoid:

- hot spices (because of possible water retention)
- oils and fats (other than daily flaxseed oil and GLA supplementation)
- all grains
- all starchy vegetables (potatoes, corn, peas, carrots, beans, etc.)
- all dairy
- alcohol and coffee (you are allowed one cup of organic coffee in the morning)

Other than that, the diet is flexible. No counting carb grams, figuring out protein minimums, or counting calories. You eat:

- up to 8 ounces a day of almost any kind of protein
- *in addition*, up to two eggs a day
- one serving of whey protein powder (not in the book, but later added to the phase 1 food list on the website)
- unlimited amounts of almost any vegetable but the starchy ones (which get put back in during the next phase)
- up to two portions of fruit per day

You can sweeten with stevia (xylitol wasn't widely available when Fat Flush first came out, but I'm willing to bet that xylitol would be acceptable). Each day, you have a fiber supplement, a GLA supplement, flaxseed oil, and the cran-water mixture.

Phase 2 is for ongoing weight loss, and it ups the calories to between 1,200 and 1,500. You stay on phase 2 until you're at or near your goal weight. The main difference between phase 1 and phase 2 is that during phase 2, you slowly add back some carbohydrates from the "friendly carb" list—one serving per day for the first week and two servings per day for the second week and beyond. The cran-water drink gets replaced with pure water, and most everything else stays the same.

Phase 3 is 1,500 (or more) calories per day and is designed for ongoing maintenance. There are more liberal choices in the oil and fruit categories, and you can now add dairy products as well as choosing from a bigger list of "friendly carbs," working up to four servings a day. Most everything else remains the same—there are some minor changes in supplementation that are discussed.

The book also has sections on exercise (greatly expanded in *The Fat Flush Fitness Plan*), journaling, stress reduction, recipes, resources, and great FAQ.

The Fat Flush Plan as a Lifestyle: Who It Works For, Who Should Look Elsewhere

This is such an all-around sensible plan that it's hard to see how anyone wouldn't benefit from it. Within certain parameters (like the carb restriction and the prohibition on sugar), it's very flexible, and it's one of the few lower-carb plans where you can eat fruit right from the beginning. Gittleman seems to have a particular gift for writing for women, who appear to constitute the majority of her audience. Men do well on this plan, too, but need to make some adjustments. According to Gittleman, they should do phase 1 as is, but can usually jump to phase 3 so they can take in more carbohydrates right away. They also generally should increase the portion sizes of their protein and can double up on the whey protein powder.

People who need a lot of structure might find this plan too freewheeling for their tastes, and the maintenance plan allows more carbs than some people might feel comfortable with. In addition, if you suspect you have a carbohydrate addiction, the amount of carbs allowed on the maintenance phase could conceivably trigger binges.

JONNY'S LOWDOWN

When I first wrote Living Low Carb, *this was one of the half-dozen best low-carb approaches to health around, and it continues to have a loyal and devoted following. I have minor quibbles, with the emphasis on "minor": there is a lot of talk about cellulite and how the plan can reduce it, which I think is highly speculative, as is the section on food combining. I'd like to have seen alpha lipoic acid mentioned as an important supplement for liver health. In my opinion, there is disproportionate emphasis on flaxseed oil and not enough on fish oil, which provides equally important omega-3s that are harder for the body to make on its own. But with that said, the basic template—limited starch, some fruit, unlimited vegetables, lean protein, and high-quality fats—is a great program and would benefit anyone. The phenomenal success and public acceptance of this program is well deserved.*

5. THE ZONE
BARRY SEARS, PHD

WHAT IT IS IN A NUTSHELL

An eating plan consisting of 40% carbohydrates, 30% protein, and 30% fat. Zone orthodoxy calls for eating five times a day—three meals and two snacks, each of which should contain the 40/30/30 distribution.

About the Zone

Tell Barry Sears, creator of the Zone, that his eating plan is a high-protein diet, and you're likely to be met with either an icy stare or a frustrated sigh, depending on his mood. Most often, you'll get a resigned explanation that you sense (correctly) he's given a thousand times. "The Zone," he says patiently, "is *not* a high-protein diet: it is a protein-*adequate* diet. The amount of protein recommended on the Zone is very similar to what Americans are currently consuming. The amount of fruits and vegetables that are recommended on the Zone diet is nearly three times the amounts recommended by the U.S. government, even though the amount of total carbohydrates is lower."

He's got a point. This just might be the most misunderstood and falsely maligned popular dietary approach of all time, considering the fact that it has probably had the most influence on changing the dietary tenor of the times, especially in altering the prevailing attitude about fat as the demon behind obesity and disease. Let's go over just what the Zone is and what it isn't.

The Zone is not a high-protein diet, despite the fact that critics—who seem never to have read the book—continue to refer to it as such, especially in popular magazines. The amount of protein on the Zone diet could hardly be considered high. On a 1,500-calorie diet, 30% protein—the amount recommended by Sears—works out to 112 grams of protein (roughly 16 ounces) a day. That's about 4 ounces per meal and 2 ounces per snack for the average man, nowhere near an excessive amount. (In our book *Smart Fat*, Dr. Steven Masley and I recommend that 80–120 grams of protein daily should be adequate for the vast majority of people.)

The Zone is also not a low-carb diet. Do the math—you're always eating slightly more carbohydrates at every meal than you are eating protein or fat. In fact, 40% of your meal is carbohydrates, yielding, with the same 1,500-calorie intake, 150 grams of carbs a day. Just for comparison, Atkins allows 20 grams per day on the induction phase of his program. The Zone allows more than seven times that amount. The Zone diet gets most of its carbohydrates from fruits and vegetables and uses the starchy carbohydrates—breads, pastas, rice, cereal, and the like—sparingly: almost, says Sears, "as condiments."

The Zone was never meant solely as a weight-loss diet. It was designed to reduce heart disease through the control of inflammation, and its success and popularity surprised Sears as much as anyone. The fact that so many people lose weight and feel terrific on it—and that it has been adopted by a number of celebrities—put it in the public arena and made Sears either a hero or a monster, depending on what academic pundit you listen to.

The Theory Behind the Zone: A Short Lesson in Nutritional Endocrinology

Think of your body and its organs, glands, hormones, and other chemical compounds as one huge biological Internet, where messages (sometimes conflicting ones) are constantly being sent out, received, interpreted, misinterpreted, and acted upon. Hormones are particularly potent messengers; when you receive a message from a hormone in your biological e-mailbox, you pay attention. Insulin is a hormone—a major one. It's secreted by the pancreas in response to the increased blood sugar that you get after you ingest food (particularly carbohydrates). Insulin is intimately tied to levels of blood sugar. If you eat a candy bar, your blood sugar rises and the pancreas says "*Uh-oh, dude ate candy; let's get to work.*" It secretes some insulin. The job of that insulin is to bring the blood sugar back down into the normal range. It does this by "escorting" the sugar out of the bloodstream and into the cells. According to Sears, excess insulin is the culprit behind skyrocketing rates of obesity, a premise he shares with all low-carb diet writers.

There are two basic ways to raise insulin levels. One is to eat too many carbohydrates. The other is to eat too much food. Americans do both.

The word "zone" in the title actually refers to an *optimal range* of insulin levels. The diet claims to keep insulin levels from rising too high by replacing some of the carbs in the typical American diet with fat (which has no effect on insulin) and protein (which has some effect, but not as much as carbs). The balance among carbs, protein, and fat at each meal and snack is designed to prevent blood-sugar levels (or insulin levels) from going too high (or too low). This, combined with the fact that the diet is not too high in calories, is responsible for the weight-loss effects on the diet.

The *health* effects of the diet are caused by a different, though related, pathway. Remember that the Zone diet was birthed in the midst of a high-carb, low-fat diet mania. All of us in the field of nutrition were seeing clients who had virtually cut fat out of their diets (and almost always replaced it with carbohydrates). They thought they were eating healthfully. It was not unusual in those days (and even now, for that matter) to see a woman eating a bagel and orange juice for breakfast, a salad for lunch, a nonfat frozen yogurt for an afternoon snack, and pasta for dinner, then wondering why she wasn't losing weight. The Zone almost single-handedly put the argument for inclusion of good fats in the diet back "on the table." And it is through the inclusion of this fat that the Zone diet is thought to have one of its most significant health effects.

Here's how it works: The body makes an entire class of "superhormones" called eicosanoids out of the "raw materials" of essential fats. Eicosanoids are made by every one of the 60 trillion cells in your body. They don't circulate in the body—they're made in a cell, they do their action in the nearby vicinity, and then they self-destruct, all within a matter of seconds, like those little tapes they used to give Peter Graves on *Mission: Impossible*—so they are virtually undetectable in the bloodstream. But their importance on human health is incalculable. The 1982 Nobel Prize in Medicine was awarded for eicosanoid research. Your doctor may not know much about eicosanoids, but he or she has undoubtedly heard of prostaglandins. Prostaglandins are eicosanoids made by the prostate gland and were one of the first groups of eicosanoids to be studied.

The type of fat you eat influences the kinds of eicosanoids you make. Eicosanoids come in many "flavors" and types, but for our purposes we'll identify two major classes: the "good" and the "bad." The good are responsible for preventing blood clots, reducing pain, and causing dilation (opening) of the blood vessels, among other things. The bad are responsible for promoting blood clots, promoting pain, and causing constriction (closing) of the blood vessels. The point is not to get rid of *all* the bad ones, but to have a balance between the good and the bad. (For example, if you didn't have eicosanoids that promoted blood clots, you would bleed to death from a minor wound.) Aspirin works by knocking out *all* eicosanoid production for a while, which is a little like killing a fly with a sledgehammer. Corticosteroids do the same thing. The fat included in the Zone diet specifically fosters the creation of good eicosanoids and an optimum balance between the good and the bad.

The insulin connection is this: insulin stimulates the key enzyme involved in producing *arachidonic acid*, which is the "building material" of the bad eicosanoids. So by controlling insulin levels with the Zone diet, you not only lose weight, you also reduce many of the symptoms and health risks that come from an imbalance of good and bad eicosanoids. The promise of the Zone is that controlling insulin will result in increased fat loss, decreased likelihood of cardiovascular disease, and greater physical and mental performance. By controlling eicosanoids, you will have decreased inflammation and increased blood flow, which will help improve virtually every chronic disease condition and improve physical performance.

So, What Can You Eat?

A lot. The best protein choices on the plan are skinless chicken, turkey, all kinds of fish, very lean cuts of meat, low-fat dairy products, egg whites, tofu, and soy meat substitutes. For carbohydrates, Sears likes all vegetables except corn and carrots and all fruits except bananas and raisins. The heavy starches like pasta, bread, cereals, rice, and the like are used very, very sparingly. For fats, use olive oil, almonds, avocados, and fish oil.

It's really simple to make a Zone meal, actually, and doesn't require a lot of complicated calculations. All you have to do is divide your plate into thirds. On one third of the plate, put some low-fat protein—a typical portion would fit in the palm of your hand and be about the thickness of a deck of cards. Then fill the other two thirds of the plate with vegetables and fruits. Once in a great while, part of that two thirds can consist of pasta or rice, but again more as a condiment than a main dish. Add a dash of fat, and you have the basic Zone meal.

The Zone as a Lifestyle: Who It Works For, Who Should Look Elsewhere

The one criticism you hear about the Zone from the average person is that it is difficult to follow. Technically, if you're trying for the exact proportions of 40/30/30, that's correct. The fact is that you really *don't* have to achieve

Zone-perfect proportions to get the beneficial effects—an approximation works perfectly well—but the lack of precision may be a problem for people who like their diets very exact and specific. Some people find that thinking about food in terms of Zone "blocks" is cumbersome. If you happen to love doing the math, and the computations of grams, calories, and so on is something you eat for breakfast, this is the perfect diet for you.

This is a great program if you are not overweight but just want a healthful way of eating that will in all likelihood reduce your risk for a number of unpleasant diseases and conditions. If you are only moderately overweight and believe you are not insulin-resistant (i.e., do not have a particular problem with carbohydrates), it's a great way to eat, but you will have to watch calories. If you are very overweight or very sedentary—or both—this program is probably too high in carbohydrates for you, and you might be better off using one of the more carb-limited programs (such as Protein Power or Atkins), at least to begin with.

The other thing to consider in choosing this program as a lifestyle is whether you can tolerate this level of carbohydrate. If you are carb-addicted, getting 40% of your calories from carbs may seem outrageously high. The program *does* allow things that trigger carb cravings—like bread and even pasta, albeit in small amounts—but for some people, small amounts are too much. Remember, it *is* entirely possible to create Zone-perfect meals using only vegetables and fruits as carbohydrate sources, and if you're able to live with that, you will do fine.

JONNY'S LOWDOWN

It's hard to underestimate Dr. Sears's contribution to the current nutritional zeitgeist. He almost single-handedly forced the dietary establishment to reevaluate the prohibition of fats. I have a few minor disagreements—I don't believe saturated fats from natural sources like butter and eggs are a problem, and I also don't agree with his position that supplements aren't necessary if you are eating correctly (a position, to be fair, that he has modified considerably in recent years). That said, the Zone template of 40% carbs, 30% protein, and 30% fat is darn close to ideal as a starting point for a healthful diet. I'm a huge believer in biochemical individuality and not in the "one size fits all" diet mentality, but we still need a basic template from which to individualize our diets; the Zone is as good a basic template as exists anywhere. Some people may need fewer carbohydrates; some may even need more. But the 40/30/30 plan beats the USDA Food Guide Pyramid (or its updated version, My Plate) as a place from which to begin constructing an individual diet plan.

II. THE PALEO PHENOMENA

Saying that the Paleo Diet was "invented" in 1939 would be like saying America was invented in 1492. It might, however, be fair to say that the Paleo Diet became a "thing" in 1939. That's when the term made its way into the general lexicon, which ultimately led to some attempts to define it and test it in a number of different peer-reviewed studies, some of which we'll review briefly in a minute.

It all started with a mild-mannered, unassuming dentist named Weston Price who wanted an answer to a simple question: Why did all his patients have so many damn cavities?

He wound up undertaking one of the most profoundly important studies in the history of nutrition. Like many great pioneers, he accidentally discovered a lot more than he was looking for, and in the process has given us some of the most important data about human nutrition ever assembled. In 1939, he wrote a book about his studies—*Nutrition and Physical Degeneration*—that has influenced generations of nutritionists (it was one of the first books I was assigned when I began studying nutrition in the 1990s). It's arguably one of the foundational texts for what is now called the ancestral health movement.

Dr. Price investigated fourteen indigenous communities. He journeyed across the world to remote areas that were completely dependent on their own resources for food—they ate what they could hunt, fish, gather, or pluck. These areas were isolated from developing urban centers and, in many ways, untouched by the ways of a technology-centric industrial lifestyle. In most cases, Dr. Price was also able to compare "isolated" people who lived on their native diets with "modernized" members of the same community who had ventured into cities and whose lifestyle and diet had changed accordingly.

He investigated isolated and modernized individuals from the Lötschental Valley in Switzerland and the Outer Hebrides in Scotland, as well as Alaskan Natives, Native Americans, Melanesians, Polynesians, ethnic groups in central and eastern Africa, Aboriginal Australians, Torres Strait Islanders, New Zealand Maori, and indigenous peoples in Peru. Anyone who has ever seen his photographs comparing members of these groups will not soon forget them. The teeth of virtually every isolated individual looked as if they could appear in a toothpaste ad. They're strong, white, and even, and the faces that contain them radiate good health and cheer. The modernized tribespeople, on the other hand, have

THE ANCESTRAL HEALTH MOVEMENT VS. PALEO: WHAT'S THE DIFFERENCE?

The easiest way to explain the difference between the paleo movement and the ancestral health movement is that one says "eat like a caveman" and the other says "eat like your great-grandmother."
They're not exactly the same thing.
Remember, Weston Price conducted his field studies in the early part of the twentieth century. He studied hunter-gatherer societies, but they were hunter-gatherer societies living in modern times. (There were no scientists armed with measurement algorithms and notepads following around the cavemen while they hunted mammoths a few thousand years ago.) And many of these twentieth-century indigenous people consumed foods that were not on the caveman menu. For example, one group studied by Price lived in the Swiss Alps and practically lived on fresh cream, not exactly a paleo staple.
Consequently, there have been very public spats between the Weston A. Price Foundation and the paleo movement over things like dairy and legumes. Price's work definitely does *not* support a ban on dairy—the Foundation is all about raw, unpasteurized milk, for example. So let's refer to the Weston Price Foundation as ancestral-health friendly and the modern paleo movement as something that is related to Price's work, but differs from it on a number of issues.

uneven, missing, and decaying teeth, rot in their mouth and gums, facial and bone deformities, and an overall look that can't be mistaken for anything but general unhealthiness.

What can we conclude from these remarkable studies? Was there some magical, terrific food that all of these isolated societies ate that kept them relatively disease-free? Absolutely not. The diets of the healthy individuals studied by Dr. Price were extremely heterogeneous. Some were high in animal products, some were not; the diets of the people who lived near the water were high in seafood; the isolated inhabitants of Lötschental practically lived on fresh cream and raw milk; other diets contained no dairy whatsoever. Some diets included almost no plants, while others comprised a huge number of fruits, vegetables, and even grains.

But here's the kicker: None of these native diets—not a single one—contained *any* refined foods whatsoever.

There was no white sugar, no flour, no canned goods, no skimmed milk, no refined oils, no partially hydrogenated *anything*. The only preserving that went on was drying, salting, and fermenting, all of which, when done by hand, preserve the nutrients in the food and may even increase them.

These people were eating their factory-specified diet, a term coined by nutritionist Patrick Quillin to describe a diet with food from the natural environment. They were eating the foods that their bodies had adapted to eating, the ones that were found in their immediate environment, the ones they could catch, hunt for, gather, pluck, or dig up, and they were eating them in—for the most part—their natural state. Here's what they were *not* doing: going to the supermarket and choosing from a dazzling array of processed, refined, denatured food products that have long since lost any of their nutritional value and have been pulverized and processed into oblivion, then colored, sweetened, and preserved beyond recognition—all so they can sit on the shelf without spoiling. Meanwhile, their manufacturers devise brilliant ad campaigns to tell you how healthy and delicious they are and how living without them is a life of "deprivation."

Now obviously we can't all go back to Eden, but we can learn something about the factory-specified diet for humanity from these studies. The take-home point is this: *There is no one healthy diet.* But *all* healthy diets have certain things in common, and you can ultimately devise the best strategy by following these principles:

- The more you can mimic eating what you would have eaten in the wild, the better

- The closer your food looks to the way it is found in nature, the better

- The less stuff you eat that comes in packages, the better

- The better it is for shelf life, the worse it is for *your* life

- The less stuff you eat with ingredients you can't pronounce, the better

This leads us to the first—and maybe most important—lesson to be learned from studying the history of dieting. We learn it not from studying the dietary wisdom of the last twenty or thirty years, but from studying the dietary wisdom of the ages. Memorize it and remember it, for it will serve you well in devising your best eating strategy: the more food you eat that could have been grown, hunted, fished, caught, plucked, or gathered, the better off you'll be.

And that's the Paleo Diet in a nutshell. Now let's get into some details.

Why Paleo?

The thinking behind the Paleo Diet becomes very clear if you think, for a minute, about the giraffe.

Giraffes, with their majestically long necks, evolved to thrive in a particular environment. In their natural habitats in eastern or southwestern Africa, the tastiest and most nutritious food you can imagine—assuming you are a giraffe and you have an imagination—are the nourishing leaves that grow on the upper branches of acacia trees. These trees easily grow to 30 feet. Giraffes with shorter necks starve and pass on fewer "short neck" genes to the gene pool. Long-necked giraffes, on the other hand, thrive in this environment, reproducing and peppering the gene pool with more "long neck" genes. When this keeps happening over eons, you have the giraffe as we know and love it. The giraffe is a perfect—if wildly oversimplified—example of how genetics adapts to an environment in a way that ensures the continuation of its species.

The theory behind paleo—and it's pretty hard to argue with—is that we humans are also "genetically adapted" to a particular kind of food environment. But it's *not* the food environment we live in now.

Instead, we're genetically adapted to the natural food environment that existed for most of the 2.6 million years the human genus has been around. Food that you could hunt, fish, gather, or pluck has been the diet of *homo sapiens* for at least 100,000 years.

In contrast, the first supermarket opened in 1930—less than a 100 years ago—and the first McDonald's franchise opened in 1955. Which "fuel" should we base our diet on?

Exactly.

According to the paleo crowd, there's a punishingly cruel disconnect between the diet our genes are crying out for and the diet we actually *eat*. And therein lies the problem. "Ultimately, nearly every single major disease affecting modern human populations—whether bacterial, viral, parasitic or noncommunicable—has its roots in the mismatch between our biology and the world we have created since the advent of agriculture," writes geneticist and anthropologist Spencer Wells.

The technical name for this disconnect between the food environment we are genetically programmed for and the food environment we find ourselves in is the discordance hypothesis. It was first proposed by Stanley Boyd Eaton and Melvin Konner. Eaton and Konner are generally thought of as the founding fathers of paleo; they published what could be called the first major, peer-reviewed study on the subject in the *New England Journal of Medicine* in 1985, titled "Paleolithic Nutrition: A Consideration of Its Nature and Current Implications."

In its simplest form, the discordance hypothesis states that our genome evolved to adapt to conditions that no longer exist, a theme we'll be coming back to again and again. The discordance hypothesis also proposes that this mismatch between food environments can cause many common chronic diseases, from arthritis to heart disease. Eaton and Konner believe that some aspects of this discordance began around 10,000 years ago, right around the beginning of agriculture.

The discordance hypothesis is beautifully illustrated in the field studies of Dr. Weston Price, discussed earlier. Price, you'll remember, studied genetically similar people and compared those who lived in their native environment and ate foods from this environment with their relatives who had moved to the big industrial cities and had begun eating the typical Western diet. Research conducted since Price's original work has confirmed his observations: hunter–gatherers who had moved to the big cities and now suffered from type 2 diabetes "showed marked improvement . . . when they were experimentally returned to their former lifestyle."[2]

Twelve years after publishing their seminal 1985 paper, and joined by coauthor S. B. Eaton III, Eaton and Konner published an update called "Paleolithic Nutrition Revisited: A Twelve-year Retrospective on Its Nature and Implications";[3] and then in 2010, in conjunction with Professor Loren Cordain, they published "Paleolithic Nutrition: Twenty-Five Years Later,"[4] in which they wrote the following passage summarizing the benefits of a Paleo Diet:

> "Anthropological evidence continues to indicate that ancestral human diets prevalent during our evolution were characterized by much lower levels of refined carbohydrates and sodium, much higher levels of fiber and protein and comparable levels of fat (primarily unsaturated fat) and cholesterol. . . . Doubts have been raised about the necessity for very low levels of protein, fat, and cholesterol intake common in official recommendations."

The 25-year follow-up contained some modifications of their original findings. For example, in their earlier research they had estimated the fat content of paleo diets at around 20% of calories, but in the updated paper they had adjusted this up to a total fat intake of 20–35% of calories. Overall, the basic findings of the 1985 paper held up. The diet of our Stone Age forefathers was qualitatively and quantitatively different from our modern diet, and this discordance seemed to be at the root of much chronic modern disease.

What exactly did this diet of our Stone Age ancestors look like?

By estimating the food intake data from 58 technologically primitive societies, Eaton and Konner found that the average diet consisted of 35% meat and 65% vegetables. Of course, they point out, that paleo diet was not a fixed entity. Its individual components and the relative proportions of animal and vegetable components varied. It's also worth pointing out was that a paleo diet consisting of 35% meat would have had a lot less sodium than there is in the typical American diet. Much more important than the total amount of sodium, however, is the balance between sodium and potassium. Hunter-gatherers consumed significantly more potassium than we do, and they would have had a far more healthy sodium-potassium balance. Their vitamin intake would have substantially exceeded ours, "irrespective of the proportion of meat in the diet." They also got tons more fiber than we do—and little to none of it came from grains.

Though the mainstream press likes to parrot the standard trope that "there's no research on paleo diets," that's actually not true.[5] (I know—hard to imagine that the mainstream press would inaccurately report on nutrition!) In one study, 29 patients with heart disease plus either glucose intolerance or full-blown type 2 diabetes followed the Paleo Diet or the Mediterranean Diet for 12 weeks. The Paleo dieters showed a 26% reduction in glucose measurements, compared to a 7% reduction for the Mediterranean dieters. The Paleo dieters also saw a significantly greater decrease in waist circumference. For those who might think the improvement in glucose (blood sugar) was simply due to their losing inches around the waist, think again. In this study, glucose reduction was independent of inches lost on the waist.[6]

A randomized controlled trial that compared the Mediterranean Diet with a simulated hunter–gatherer diet found the latter to be more effective in improving insulin resistance and cardiovascular risk factors in type 2 diabetes.[7]

In the study referred to in the previous sentence, 13 patients with type 2 diabetes were placed either on a paleo diet of meat, fish, fruit, vegetables, root vegetables, eggs, and nuts or on a conventional diabetes diet prescribed by American Diabetes Association guidelines (evenly distributed meals, with whole-grain bread and other cereal products but less total fat). Participants went on each diet for 3 months. Subjects on the paleo diet had lower mean levels of hemoglobin A1c, lower triglycerides, lower diastolic blood pressure, and higher mean HDL cholesterol levels. The paleo folks also had lower weight, body mass index (BMI), and waist circumferences.

Hunter-gatherer carbs came from fruit, vegetables, and nuts—not from grains. Refined carbs such as sucrose contributed virtually nothing to the diet, and the plant foods available to hunter–gatherers were way higher in fiber than those we consume today.

Like many people who put forth a theory disliked by the establishment, Eaton and Konner were often misquoted and misrepresented. They never, for example, recommended that we follow a paleo diet. *"We did not then and we do not now propose that Americans adopt a particular diet and lifestyle on the basis of anthropological evidence alone; formal recommendations must rest on carefully executed laboratory, clinical and epidemiological studies."* What they *did* suggest—and what has turned out to be accurate—was that our standard dietary recommendations need more research "in light of the hunter–gatherer model."

Fast-forward to today. So, what are the principles of the *modern* Paleo Diet, anyway?

Glad you asked.

On Paleo, there are three things you won't be eating: dairy, grains, and beans—though, depending on the version of the diet you follow, there may be some wiggle room. (More on that later.) Virtually all processed foods are verboten, but just about everything else is cool. You'll be eating lots of meat, poultry, and fish plus berries, nuts, fruits, and vegetables. (The diet is very difficult for vegetarians and impossible for vegans.) You'll avoid cereal, bread, pasta, and rice. And you won't be drinking any milk, certainly not the homogenized, pasteurized kind that comes from factory-farmed cows. (Which, come to think of it, is not such a bad thing, since commercial dairy is one of the most common sources of food sensitivities.)

Did I mention that sugar isn't on the menu either?

Paleo proponents point out that crops like wheat, corn, and soy are all products of modern agriculture ("modern" meaning in the last 10,000 years, a mere blip on the 24-hour clock of human development). Not without some justification, paleo folks feel that our genetics have simply not had time to catch up with these newfangled foods.

What's worse, these same foods, particularly in their most processed and nutrient-poor form—have taken over the modern diet. They're not just used as occasional condiments and treats—they are our predominant source of calories. Not only are we eating foods that we have not *evolved* to eat, we're getting the majority of our daily calories from them.

People report far more energy on paleo than they had when eating their former (usually bad) diet. Weight loss is a frequent accompaniment. Some paleo gurus—like Robb Wolf, for example, author of *The Paleo Prescription*—originally turned to paleo to conquer serious gut problems (in Wolf's case, colitis). Many of these folks report vastly improved digestion and elimination, and a noticeable boost in well-being.

Although paleo and low-carb do not mean the same thing, the eating plans do overlap. However, you can eat far more carbohydrates on paleo than you'd ever get away with in the early phase of Atkins, where carbs can be limited to as little as 20 grams a day. All vegetables and all low-sugar fruits like berries and apples are virtually unlimited on paleo. This alone distinguishes it from most classic "low-carb" plans.

One area of controversy about paleo is the ban on beans. The reason given for the off-limits sign on beans and legumes is that these foods contain compounds called *lectins* (see Lectins: The Bad, the Ugly . . . and the Good?, page 194), which can frequently cause inflammation. But beans (and legumes) are among the best sources of fiber on the planet and pack a huge amount of antioxidant firepower. Some experts think the whole lectin thing has been exaggerated. "From my experience treating thousands of patients over the years, only about 10% of them react to lectins," says Steven Masley, MD, director of the Optimal Health Center in Florida and author of *The 30-Day Heart Tune-Up*.[8]

Luckily, Paleo programs can be fairly forgiving. Even Robb Wolf told me that he doesn't stick to the program 100 percent of the time, and orthodox paleo proponents like Cordain allow for about three "off-duty" meals a week where you can wander away from the basics. Some paleo gurus have even confessed to me—off the record—that they'll frequently experiment with beans for some of their clients. I haven't found any, however, who endorse dairy or sugar.

If by now you're thinking that I'm a big fan of the paleo style of eating, you're right. However, there are a couple of caveats.

Chris Kresser, LaC, author of *Your Personal Paleo Prescription*, points out that paleo is a starting place, not a destination. In a minority of cases, people making a quick switch to paleo may notice some digestive problems and sugar cravings. Kresser thinks—and I agree—that in the majority of cases, people who find themselves with digestive issues on paleo probably had them before they started paleo.

LECTINS: THE BAD, THE UGLY . . . AND THE GOOD?

Lectins are substances contained in legumes and grains that originally evolved to fight off insect predators. A portion of the lectin acts as a kind of metabolic super-glue that can bind with tissues in our body and create problems. (One of the founding principles of Dr. Peter D'Adamp's Blood Type Diet is that if you eat lectin-rich foods that are incompatible with your blood type, those lectins target an organ or bodily system and can begin to wreak havoc with the tissues in that area.[*])

Lectins figure prominently in papers about paleo. Loren Cordain, PhD, the aforementioned paleo guru and a highly respected researcher at the University of Colorado, published a paper in the *British Journal of Nutrition*[†] detailing a theory that dairy, legumes, grains, and yeast may be partly to blame for rheumatoid arthritis and other autoimmune diseases in genetically susceptible people, due in part to the lectin molecule.

According to Cordain, the lectins in food increase intestinal permeability (also known as "leaky gut"). They allow partially digested food proteins and remnants of gut bacteria to spill into the bloodstream and make the intestines easier to penetrate, impairing the immune system's ability to fight off food and bacterial fragments that leak into the bloodstream.

In 2017, a book by a former cardiac surgeon named Steven Gundry seemed to confirm Cordain's worst nightmares about lectins. This book, *The Plant Paradox*, received a ton of attention for claiming that the plant-based diet everyone seemed to be recommending contained what Cordain had referred to as "cellular Trojan horses." Gundry maintained that lectins were the root cause of both weight gain and many chronic illnesses. His book lists more than a dozen disorders that he believes come from lectin activity in the body, including diabetes, chronic fatigue, memory loss, and heart disease. His dietary recommendations are far more restrictive than Cordain's. Gundry counsels that we reduce grains of all kinds (especially whole wheat), beans and legumes (especially soy), nuts, fruits, vegetables, dairy, and eggs.

Meanwhile, back at the ranch, there are some studies that suggest that some lectins may have *positive* effects. They can bind to cancer cell membranes, which could conceivably inhibit tumor growth, or lead to cell death.[‡] One study discussed the clinical studies of plant lectins for their potential therapeutic effect in cancer treatment, and concluded: "These inspiring findings would open a new perspective for plant lectins as potential antineoplastic drugs from beach to clinic."[§] Lectins from mushrooms have been found to inhibit proliferation of cancer cells in the test tube.[**]

You also have a "leptin-skeptic" chorus of folks like Dr. David Katz of Yale University asking us to consider the question "*What happens overall to people who eat foods that are high in lectins?*"[††] He's referring, of course, to the countless epidemiological studies that show that populations that eat lots of beans (as well as many of the foods Gundry warns against) have significantly lower risk for a host of diseases like diabetes, cardiovascular diseases, cancer, and more.

To further complicate things, there are ways to prepare beans and legumes that may reduce lectin's negative effects. "Historically, most grains and legumes have gone through a system of soaking and sprouting which reduce the amounts and effects of various anti-nutrients (lectins)," Robb Wolf told me.[‡‡] "Modern processing tends to skip this step." Even Gundry himself agrees that cooking and soaking do help reduce lectins, but he is concerned that not all are inactivated.[§§]

Bottom Line: Do we need to be concerned about lectins in beans? Maybe. Beans have huge health benefits if you're not one of the people who responds badly to them. But if you're someone who has unexplained symptoms possibly related to food or gut health, it might be worthwhile to look into where lectins might be hiding in your daily diet, and to avoid beans till you figure out exactly what's going on. And if you do eat beans—soak them first!

[*] http://www.dadamo.com/txt/index.pl?1007

[†] https://www.ncbi.nlm.nih.gov/pubmed/10884708

[‡] https://www.ncbi.nlm.nih.gov/pubmed/16183566

[§] https://www.sciencedirect.com/science/article/pii/S0304383509003450

[**] https://www.ncbi.nlm.nih.gov/pubmed/8402638; http://www.jbc.org/content/280/11/10614.full

[††] Personal communication, 2018.

[‡‡] Personal communication by email, Jan. 6, 2019.

[§§] https://tonic.vice.com/en_us/article/mb49gq/what-are-lectins-and-are-they-bad-for-me

Why do those symptoms suddenly become more noticeable once you're on a healthier diet? According to Kresser, it's because they were being hidden by poor eating habits.

Consider what happens when you stop smoking. Many people feel a lot of anxiety. But that anxiety was present before—you just didn't notice it as much *because you were smoking.* Smoking was *compensating* for that anxiety, an attempt to "self-medicate." Well, according to Kresser, the exact same thing is true here. Maybe you had low stomach acid, so you unconsciously "compensated" by eating fewer foods that require lots of stomach acid in order to digest them properly; maybe you had low enzyme activity (enzymes are critical for breaking down food, and we make less as we age), but maybe you never noticed because your diet was front-loaded with a bunch of simple, empty carbs. Or maybe due to your low-fiber diet, you never noticed that you have chronic inflammation in the gut. ("Consuming large amounts of insoluble fiber when your gut is inflamed is a little bit like rubbing a wire brush against an open wound," says Kresser.)

So, in a way, your unhealthy choices were doing the same thing for you that cigarette smoking does—preventing you from "noticing" things (like anxiety, inflammation, or digestive problems), things that were there all the time. That doesn't mean those unhealthy choices were good ones. It just means they were successful in suppressing the overt symptoms of your underlying problems.

Kresser points out that gut problems like low stomach acid, decreased enzymes, and gut inflammation have several causes, and only a couple are directly related to diet. Parasites, bacteria, fungi—all can cause low-grade inflammation. The Paleo Diet won't necessarily eliminate these problems, and they should be addressed with the help of a good health practitioner.

To be fair, there's a counterargument to be made here. Denise Minger points out that many of the symptoms we're talking about *are* actually new and didn't just go "unnoticed" before. These symptoms may result from the increased amount of insoluble fiber consumed on paleo, which can cause shifts in the gut microbiome that increase gas production or indigestion. Moreover, she adds, since you're eating very few grains (if at all), the drop in soluble fiber could change stool bulk and possibly increase constipation. Finally, a sudden increase in fat intake might require more bile acid production, all of which could lead to brand-new symptoms.

That said, these temporary symptoms might be worth enduring for the benefits you gain shortly after you switch to a non-processed-food diet.)

David Katz, MD, director of Yale's Prevention Research Center, recently reviewed many popular diets in an attempt to find out if they had anything in common. They did. "The best [diets] push real foods that are minimally processed or direct from nature," he says. (This comment is particularly interesting because Katz has gone on record as being opposed to the Paleo Diet, yet "real foods that are minimally processed or direct from nature" is precisely what the Paleo Diet "pushes"!

And at the end of the day, paleo is about real food. Food your grandmother's *grandmother*—and her grandmother before her—would have recognized as food.

That, after all, is the basis of every healthy diet ever invented.

It's a hard prescription to argue with.

How Much Fat Should I Consume?

Although paleo and keto have many "core values" in common, one of the biggest differences is in the percentages of fat, carbohydrate, and protein that they advocate.

Remember that the ultimate purpose of any keto diet is to get you into nutritional ketosis—which only happens when you restrict carbs. That's precisely why it's hard to quantify exactly what *percentage* of your diet should come from carbs on a keto diet. (Ten percent of calories might seem like a really small percentage, but for an athlete eating 5,000 calories a day, that still comes out to 250 grams of carbs per day, which will keep anybody out of ketosis.) That's the reason that keto diets tend to be defined by the *number* of grams of carbs you can consume, not the *percentage* of carbs in your overall diet.

Dr. Jeff Volek—one of the best-known and most respected researchers on the subject of ketogenic diets—defines keto diets as typically having 50 grams of carbs or less, with "proportional increases in fat and protein."[9] Other experts will offer exact percentages, but they range all over the map. In the 1920s, when the ketogenic diet began to be used for treating seizures, it was defined as a diet in which 90% of calories came from fat, 6% from protein, and just 4% from carbs.[10] A more recent study investigating the the impact of keto on epilepsy used a diet of 80% fat, 15% protein, and 5% carbs.[11] The KetoConnect website—an excellent portal for all things keto—says that *in general*, keto diets will have anywhere between 60% and 80% of calories coming from fat, 15–35% from protein, and 5% or less coming from carbs.[12] (For someone eating 3,000 calories a day, 5% of calories from carbs would come out to 37.5 grams of carbs, right in the sweet spot of "under 50" that Jeff Volek talks about in his research.)

The limitation on carbs for paleo isn't nearly as strict as it is for keto, which is why you typically won't be (and don't need to be) in ketosis on a paleo diet. While the two ways of eating can and do overlap, paleo programs *tend* to be more protein-friendly, while keto programs are decidedly more fat-friendly. (You can see this in the first modern commercial Paleo Diet book by Professor Cordain, reviewed later in the chapter—there's a strong emphasis on "lean protein" and "low-fat," neither of which you'll see in the keto community.)

Definitive paleo macro ratios are also hard to come by. (Fat, carbohydrate, and protein are all considered *macro*nutrients, while vitamins and minerals are called *micro*nutrients. When the low-carb crowd talks about "macros," they're talking percentages of carbs, fat, and protein.) Early humans did not eat a totally consistent mix of protein, fat, and carbs day in and day out, season in and season out. It's likely that they alternated times of feasting with times of fasting. "In simple terms," says Robb Wolf, author of *The Paleo Solution*, "the paleo diet is built from modern foods that (to the best of our ability) emulate the foods available to our pre-agricultural ancestors: Meat, fish, fowl, vegetables, fruits, roots, tubers and nuts." Wolf has an excellent article on his website about why he does *not* make recommendations for exact macronutrient percentages.[13] That said, reliable estimates of paleo macros tend to cluster in the range of 20–35% calories from protein, 20–40% from carbs, and 25–45% from fat.[14]

Meanwhile, Dave Asprey's Bulletproof Diet—a kind of hybrid model of keto and paleo—takes what his website accurately calls "a loose approach to macros." As a general recommendation, you'll get 50–70% of calories from healthy fats, up to 20% from protein, up to 20% from vegetables, and up to 5% from fruit or starch.[15] (Bulletproof is considerably harder on fruit than paleo is.) In addition, Bulletproof recommends intermittent fasting, periods of keto dieting, cyclical carb meals, and something called *protein fasting*, all covered in the Bulletproof section later in the chapter.

The point is that the boundaries between these programs are somewhat fluid.

Confused? No problem. I'm going to reveal to you the deep, dark secret about macronutrient ratios, which—I promise you—will make you feel better.

The Deep, Dark Secret About Macro Percentages

I've been in health and fitness for 29 years, as of this writing, and I've interviewed an awful lot of big players in the diet and exercise world. I've also gone to dinner with more than a few of them, including many of the researchers, docs, nutritionists, and other health professionals mentioned in this book. So I have a pretty good idea of how they eat.

And I can safely tell you this: Never have I seen a health guru sit down at the table, take out a food scale, and start to calculate their macros. Not once. Sure, many of us have done that once or twice in our lives,* and there are always the wonderfully obsessive bio-hacker types who self-monitor everything about their physiology 24/7 (hats off to Dr. Peter Attia and others like him). But honestly, everyone else is just guessing and estimating, at least for the majority of their meals and probably for 100% of the meals they eat out. I've eaten dinner with people whose public recommendations about the percentage of fat, protein, and carbs in the diet differ by double-digit percentages, but guess what? In real life, they were pretty much eating the same thing at the buffet.

I mention this not to make the point that macro recommendations are meaningless, but rather to assure you that you don't have to worry about them as much as you probably do. You don't have to weigh, measure, and compute everything so that you can adhere to some "perfect" ratio of carbs, fat, and protein. Relax. Even the gurus spend a lot of time approximating and guessing.

The 15-Second Elevator Speech

Keto and paleo (and Bulletproof, for that matter) are overlapping and sometimes intersecting takes on the same theme: a concentration of whole food that your great-grandmother would have recognized as food, as similar as possible to the food we had before processing methods were invented, maybe even as similar as possible to the food we had before agriculture. And that does not include "low-fat" versions of anything.

Perhaps, even more important than exact macronutrient proportions is the basic notion common to paleo and keto:

---

* I spent an entire month in 1989 recording every morsel of food I ate and every minute of exercise I completed. I calculated percentages of protein, fat, and carbs; I tracked my body fat; and I monitored my weight. At the end of the month, I had a pretty good idea of the number of calories I needed to maintain my weight and how they needed to be proportioned among the three macros. (Interestingly, years later, when I calculated the number of calories I needed using sophisticated equations, the number was amazingly close to what I had come up with back in 1989.) I'm all for self-experimentation, and all for the whole "know thyself" thing. I'm just saying that most people don't do that kind of thing very often, if at all, and certainly not at the buffet table at the American College of Nutrition conference!

Eat from the "Jonny Bowden Four Food Groups":
Food You Could Hunt, Fish, Gather, or Pluck

The following diet was the first commercially available popular diet book to lay out the principles of paleo. Loren Cordain, professor emeritus at Colorado State University, is widely acknowledged as one of the world's leading experts on the natural human diet of our Stone Age ancestors. He's authored more than 100 peer-reviewed scientific articles and abstracts, and his research into the health benefits of Stone Age diets for contemporary people has appeared in the world's top scientific journals.

This review focuses on the first edition of *The Paleo Diet*, published in 2002. The book was fully revised in 2010, and then again in 2011 with *The Paleo Answer*. He's modified his position on a couple of the things I took issue with originally, including the ban on saturated fat, for example. If you're curious about where he started, the theoretical underpinnings of paleo, take a look at my original review of the Paleo Diet®, below. If you're not particularly interested in how his thinking has evolved and just want the highlights of his current approach (taken from his website, circa 2019), the sidebar on page 203, is a good summary.

And following is my review of the book that started a movement: Cordain's original *Paleo Diet*.

6. THE PALEO DIET
LOREN CORDAIN, PHD

WHAT IT IS IN A NUTSHELL

All the lean meat, poultry, fish, and seafood you want, plus unlimited fruits and non-starchy vegetables. No dairy, cereals, legumes, or processed foods.

About the Paleo Diet

The Paleo Diet is perhaps the most sophisticated example of the "Stone Age" or "caveman" type of diet book, and Dr. Loren Cordain is one of the best-known researchers in the field of what might be called "nutritional anthropology" or "Paleolithic nutrition." The general theory behind the Paleo Diet—and others like it—is this:

- Being fat comes primarily from eating a diet that is *completely unsuited* to our ancient genes and digestive system.

- The human genus spent a couple of million years adapting to and functioning on a diet *entirely* different than the one we eat today.

- Our digestive systems—identical to those of our caveman ancestors—are simply unsuited for the staples of today's diet: dairy, refined sugar, fatty meat, and processed food.

- By returning to the diet that humans lived on for the vast majority of their time on earth, we can correct a great many of the problems in human health, including but not limited to obesity.

The argument for this position is pretty strong. DNA evidence shows that genetically, humans have hardly changed in the 2.5 million years the genus has been on the planet. The human genome has changed less than 0.02% (one fiftieth of a percent) in forty thousand years. Most of the diseases of modern civilization—cancer, obesity, diabetes, and heart disease—have happened at the same time that we've experienced a sea change in our diet, and the modern diet is completely different from the one humans have lived on for the overwhelming bulk of our time on the planet.

Through fossil records and research on contemporary hunter–gatherer societies, we have a pretty good idea of what Paleolithic peoples ate—and it didn't look like anything you'd find at a fast-food joint.

Consider the diet of our Paleo ancestors, before the invention of modern foods: they ate no dairy (how easy would it be to milk a wild animal?) and no cereal grains; they didn't salt their food; the only sweetener they used was honey, which they ate rarely (when they could find it); wild-animal foods dominated their diet (so protein intake was high and carb intake was low); and since all carbs came from wild fruits and non-starchy vegetables, fiber was very high.

Beginning to get the picture?

On the other hand, the average modern American diet contains

- 31% calories from cereals

- 14% calories from dairy

- 8% calories from beverages, especially sodas and fruit juices

- 4% calories from oils and dressings, especially processed oils and omega-6s

- 4% calories from sweets like candy, cookies, and cake

That means 61% of calories in a modern diet come from foods that were largely unknown before the adoption of agriculture (a drop in the time bucket as far as evolution is concerned), and *most* of them weren't even available until a couple hundred years ago, when food processing became the norm. The remaining 39% of our calories come from animal foods, but ones that are very different from those of our caveman ancestors. The animal foods that the average American is likely to consume are mostly hot dogs, fatty ground beef, bacon, and highly processed deli meats. (When looked at in this way, is it any wonder there are studies linking "meat" consumption in industrial societies to a number of health issues? Maybe meat as a category has gotten a bum rap, and it's the *kind* of meat we eat that's the problem!)

Cordain claims that a return to the diet of our ancestors—what I've described earlier as eating what you could hunt, fish, gather, grow, or pluck—is the answer not only to obesity and overweight, but to a multitude of other health problems. Though it seems like he stresses protein as the most important component in the diet, in actuality he makes it clear that protein *alone*—without fat or the alkalizing influence of tons of vegetables and fruits—is a big problem. Add those and the problem disappears: "There is no such thing as too much protein as long as you are eating plenty of fresh fruits and vegetables," Cordain says. And he is pretty flexible about the possible balance among them, pointing out that some hunter–gatherer societies that survived into the twentieth century lived healthy lives free of chronic disease while getting 97% of their calories from animal foods (the Inuit of Alaska), while others got the majority of their calories (65%) from plant foods (the !Kung of Africa). Most paleo societies fall somewhere between these two extremes. No paleo peoples, however, ate refined sugar. On the Paleo Diet, fully 50% to 55% of your calories come from lean meats, organ meats, poultry, fish, and seafood. The rest come from vegetables (except for starchy ones like potatoes and yams) and "healthful" fats (more about these in Jonny's Lowdown). It's simple and easy. There is no calorie-counting, no protein-gram counting, no fat-gram counting, and no carb-gram counting.

THE PALEO DIET PREMISE*
(PROFESSOR LOREN CORDAIN, 2019)

Principle One: Eat more protein. According to Cordain, the average amount of protein in hunter-gatherer societies was between 19% and 35% of calories, whereas it's only about 15% in the average Western diet.

Principle Two: Eat fewer carbs and make them low-glycemic. Carb calories on paleo don't come from cereals and pasta; they come from fruits and vegetables, both starchy and fibrous. And all high-fiber fruits and vegetables are naturally low-glycemic (meaning they digest slowly and won't spike blood sugar).

Principle Three: Get more fiber in your diet. And you do not need to get fiber from grains—in fact, they're not a particularly good source, notwithstanding a ton of marketing from the cereal companies to lead you to believe otherwise. Non-starchy vegetables have eight times more fiber than whole grains and 31 times more than refined grains.

Principle Four: Get better fat. Cordain is a big fan of monounsaturated fat (such as that found in olive oil), as well as of omega-3. He sees trans-fat as the enemy and the overabundance of pro-inflammatory seed ("vegetable") oils as a major problem. The Cordain of 2019 has softened his position on saturated fat, noting on his website that "recent large population studies known as meta analyses show that saturated fats have little or no adverse effects upon cardiovascular disease."

*http://thepaleodiet.com/the-paleo-diet-premise/

By staying within these guidelines, Cordain claims you will:

- have built-in protection against overeating because protein (and fiber) naturally feels more satiating

- enjoy the increased metabolic activity (and increased calorie-burning) that protein provides (see chapter 3 for studies that show this)

- control insulin and reduce insulin resistance, making weight loss a breeze

IS RICE MAKING A COMEBACK?

Ever since I entered the field of health and fitness, the one thing just about everyone agreed on was that white rice was horrible. (Everyone remembers the "don't eat anything white" mandate and all the endless lectures from dietitians about how brown rice had fiber and nutrients, while everything good had been bleached or processed out of white rice.)

Later, when the low-carb movement really took off, all rices (and potatoes, and starches in general) were pretty much off the table, whole-grain or otherwise. There was an emphasis on controlling blood sugar (and therefore insulin, and therefore weight). And the truth of the matter was that whole grains and refined grains weren't all that different when it came to raising blood sugar.

Now, however, rising out of the ashes like a forgotten teenage idol, white rice is making a comeback.

You see, white rice actually has a few things going for it.

Number one: it's *really* easy to digest, which is a big selling point for people with digestive disorders, leaky gut, or gut dysbiosis. (Remember, along with bananas, rice is one of the go-to foods for nausea and upset stomach.)

Number two: it's got zero fructose. And number three: it's available everywhere, and it's cheap.

Now, it's true that it has zero fiber and zero micronutrients. But every food we eat isn't necessarily consumed for its micronutrients—some of our best oils have no micronutrients either. As Paleo Leap puts it, "we don't eat these foods because they're packed with vitamins and minerals; we eat them because they're clean-burning sources of energy!"

Many programs now cycle in periods (or meals) of high-carb consumption for a variety of reasons we'll explore more in the Keto section (page 225). (My own Metabolic Factor program does precisely this.) For those high-carb meals or periods, white rice is making more appearances precisely because of how easy it is to digest and how unlikely it is to trigger food sensitivities.

If, over the next few years, you start hearing more and more about how white rice might have a place in healthy eating, now you know why.

The Paleo Diet itself allows "cheating." There are 3 levels of commit-ment, with level 1 allowing you three "open" (read: cheat) meals a week, level 2 permitting two such meals, and level 3 only one.

Many people not previously familiar with the material in chapter 3 of this book will find Cordain's passionate argument against grains surprising, as we have been so conditioned to think of grains, especially whole grains, as wonderful foods. Cordain is particularly expert on this subject, having written the seminal paper "Cereal Grains: Humanity's Double-Edged Sword,"[16] and what he has to say on the subject is worth considering even if you don't adopt this particular dietary program.

The Problem with Grains

Here's the synopsis: the agricultural revolution began about ten thousand years ago in the Middle East. Dwindling food resources—especially wild game—and rising populations gave birth to the need for smarter, more efficient ways for people to support themselves and their families. Some enterprising people figured out how to sow and harvest wild wheat seeds. Then they tried barley. Then legumes. Livestock—sheep, goats, and pigs—wasn't far behind. Later, cattle. Domesticated farm animals were milkable. Over time, there was a complete change in the diet of most of humanity.

Without the agricultural revolution, we would not have civilization as we know it. Our ability to farm—to domesticate animals for dairy products, to raise cattle, and especially to grow and cultivate grains—was responsible for allowing us to live in denser conditions and encouraged towns and cities to develop. It allowed us to become independent from our original food source—hunted game.

But this new lifestyle came with a price. Early farmers were shorter in stature than their forebears had been. Examination of their bones and teeth showed more infectious diseases and shorter life spans. Egyptian mummies frequently reveal obese bodies. There were more cases of osteo-porosis, rickets, and vitamin- and mineral-deficiency diseases, in large measure because of cereal-based diets (whole grains and legumes contain "antinutrients," pyridoxine glucosides and phytates, that respectively block absorption of B vitamins in the intestines and chemically bind iron, zinc, copper, and calcium and block their absorption). And the skulls of those living on modern foods revealed teeth filled with cavities and jaws that were misshapen and too small for the teeth, as seen in the pictures included in Dr. Weston Price's seminal 1939 book, *Nutrition and Physical Degeneration.*

Then came fermentation and salting. Grains were fed to livestock, mak-ing them fatter but also changing the quality of their meat and their fat.

(Interesting, isn't it, that grains are the food of choice for fattening livestock and yet are still recommended by the dietary establishment as the foundation food of a weight-loss program!) Meat was preserved by pickling, salting, and smoking. Two hundred years ago, things got even worse. We now had ways to refine sugar and flour and to can foods, almost always with the addition or creation of trans-fats, sugar, refined oils high in omega-6s, and high-fructose corn syrup, not to mention additives, preservatives, emulsifiers, and other toxins.

As Cordain says, imagine paleo man with a Twinkie or a pizza. He wouldn't even recognize them as food.

Cordain is one of the few writers to talk about something called the acid–base balance. Briefly, it goes like this: everything reports to the kidneys as either an acid or an alkaline (base). When there is too much acid, the body needs to neutralize it with alkaline substances like calcium. Meats are one of the top five acid-producing foods; but the other four—grains, legumes, cheese, and salt—were rarely or never eaten by our paleo ancestors, who buffered the acid load of their meats with plenty of fruits and vegetables. The main "buffering" compound in the body is calcium, and the main storehouse for calcium is the bones; this is how high-protein diets got their (false) reputation for causing bone loss. Cordain correctly points out that this loss of calcium does not happen when there are plenty of fruits and vegetables in the diet, and especially when other acid-producing foods (like cereal grains and dairy) are absent.

The objection to grains isn't all about the carbs, either, although it's easy to assume that is the reason. Paleo Leap—a paleo-centric website with some very good resources, including an excellent program for beginners—explains that the objection to grains is that they contain various anti-nutrients and gut irritants that humans aren't designed to digest. (These compounds are great for protecting the plant from things like sunlight and insects. But they're not so great for people who eat the plants that contain them.) Paleo Leap refers to carbohydrate-dense foods that *don't* contain these compounds as "safe starches," which include potatoes (even the white ones!), sweet potatoes, plantains, and bananas.

The Paleo Diet as a Lifestyle: Who It Works For, Who Should Look Elsewhere

The straightforward simplicity of the Paleo Diet—all you want of *these* foods, none at all of *those*—makes it pretty easy to follow and a good choice for those who are put off by counting grams, calories, and carbohydrates, figuring out protein allowances, or computing food blocks. But that same lack of rigidity makes it a poor choice for those who need more structure. And although it restricts nearly all of the usual problem foods for carbohydrate addicts, the unlimited fruit could easily be a problem for those who are insulin-resistant. In addition, since it is not primarily a weight-loss diet, it may be frustrating for those whose main focus for the immediate future is on losing fat.

JONNY'S LOWDOWN

Cordain's version of the Paleo Diet is a frustrating program to rate. On the one hand, you have to give tremendous credit to a no-grain diet that eliminates sugar, dairy, and trans-fats and recommends tons of vegetables. How bad can that be? Most people—especially those who eat the typical American diet—are going to reap such enormous benefits from this program that I want to rave about it just for that reason alone.

On the other hand, there are some major problems. For one thing, Cordain completely buys into the cholesterol–heart disease hypothesis; I believe that this hypothesis, in its current form, is less than a decade away from being dumped on the pile of scientific flotsam and jetsam. He also accepts the dogma that all saturated fats are bad, largely because they raise cholesterol (some do; many don't; and ultimately it may not matter much). Cordain puts eggs on the "avoid" list for their cholesterol content (something we now know is completely irrelevant, since dietary cholesterol has virtually no impact on serum cholesterol) and warns against such natural traditional fats as butter and cream, which he puts in the same category as such trans-fat nightmares as nonfat dairy creamer and frozen yogurt. He recommends canola oil (I don't agree; see chapter 10). He puts sweet potatoes—a "good" starch by almost anyone's standards—in the same class as French fries and tapioca pudding. He makes the somewhat problematic statement that "fruit won't make you fat on this diet, even in unlimited amounts." And he sometimes misrepresents low-carb diets, saying that they call for complete restriction of all carbohydrates.

That said, Cordain is a giant—a sincere and responsible scholar whose overall recommendations will propel a person eating the average American diet light-years ahead in his quest for good health. Done with care, Cordain's diet may also make you lose weight.

The following two diet programs are not in direct conflict with Cordain; they just represent slightly different approaches with somewhat different emphases. Cordain was a mentor to Robb Wolf, author of *The Paleo Solution*, and Cordain generously refers readers who want a good intro to the principles of paleo to either his own site, Wolf's website, or Mark's Daily Apple, the popular website of *Primal Blueprint* author Mark Sisson. All these guys are friends and colleagues and appear to have the deepest respect for one another. You can think of these programs as different takes on the same material—like when three different world-class conductors all perform a Beethoven symphony. It's the same symphony, but each conductor offers a slightly different interpretation.

7. THE PALEO SOLUTION
ROBB WOLF

WHAT IT IS IN A NUTSHELL

The Paleo Solution *is a program based on our ancestral diet of protein, vegetables, and fat. It is accompanied by one of the best and most complete descriptions of how the modern high-carb diet works to promote obesity, diabetes, and virtually every other disease of civilization.*

About The Paleo Solution

Desperate times call for desperate measures.

I imagine that's what Robb Wolf—the author of this first-rate book—might have been thinking when he first started his journey back to health. He had been a strapping 180-pounder, a teenage state champion in power lifting with an amateur kickboxing record of 6–0. Then, in an attempt to get "healthy," he went on a vegetarian diet for several years. Many giant plates of steamed rice, tofu, and veggies later, he found himself a sickly and emaciated 140 pounds with sky-high triglycerides (over 300), hypertension, and an A–Z catalogue of digestive disturbances including constant gas and bloat—all this at the ripe old age of 26.

Long story short: this young man—armed with a degree in biochemistry and gifted with both a passion for learning and an excellent built-in BS detector—went on a mission to figure out what had gone wrong. He found the solution, regained his health, and this book is the result.

"You can walk into your doctor's office with horrible blood work, all the while eating a low-fat, high-carb diet of whole grains," he writes. "You can then shift to an ancestral way of eating that involves lean meats, seafood, seasonal vegetables, and fruit. Walk back into your doctor's office with perfect blood work, yet he will not believe that eating more protein and fat is what fixed your broken blood work."

The "ancestral way of eating" to which Wolf refers is the core of the Paleo Solution Diet. It worked for Wolf, and it may well work for you. "We are not genetically wired for a 50 percent carbohydrate, bran muffin diet, despite what the USDA, AMA, and FDA have to say on the topic," says Wolf. "*Capisce?*"

Yes, Robb. We capisce.

For the purposes of this review, I'll concentrate on the fat-loss résumé of *The Paleo Solution,* but you should know that there's a lot more in this book than just a prescription for weight loss. This book could easily be used as a modern-day primer on basic endocrinology for the intelligent reader who is not a professional nutritionist. It's very strong on subjects like grains and fats, offers some excellent information on cardiovascular disease, and contains a terrific discussion of cholesterol. Wolf is excellent at describing exactly what all the hormones do, how they "talk" to each other, and how their messages are jumbled by the modern high-carb diet. This is great information, and he presents it with a rare combination of accuracy and humor.

Now let's get to the fat-loss part.

The Hormonal Effect of Food (Redux)

Virtually every diet discussed in the book you are reading—including my own—talks about the hormonal effect of a diet too high in sugar or carbs. If you've sampled any of the diet reviews—or read my own explanation of what happens when you eat excess carbs—you already know all about insulin and its fat-storing action. But Wolf brings up some other, lesser-known hormonal effects of excess carbs, one of which is of great importance in the weight-loss equation. Here's how it works.

You may recall from high school biology that glycogen is the storage form of glucose. When the glycogen stores in your liver are filled up, the excess glucose (sugar) is converted to fat, specifically a short-chain saturated fat called *palmitic acid.* The palmitic acid (PA) is combined with a glycerol molecule and made into triglycerides, which are packaged together with proteins and cholesterol into a molecule called a VLDL (very low-density lipoprotein). These VLDLs, with their rich PA content, move all around the body, but they *really* come alive once they are in the brain. And guess what PA does in the brain? It decreases our sensitivity to *leptin,* the hormone that tells us our stomachs are full.

When there's too much PA in the brain, we literally become "leptin-resistant." Leptin is a hormone that sends a "satiety" signal to the brain, essentially saying "Hey guys, we're full, no more food needed, stop scarfing it down." When the brain stops "listening" to leptin, appetite no longer works correctly. Your body produces more and more leptin in a futile attempt to get the brain to "know" that you're full, but the brain isn't paying attention. You remain hungry despite the fact that your blood sugar is high, your belly is full, and your leptin is shouting at you to stop eating. It's like one of those horror movies where someone is screaming a warning at you that the monster is right behind you, but the train is roaring into the station and you can't hear them! Leptin is screaming "stop," but your brain can't hear it 'cause it's so full of carb-created VLDLs!

There's more. Your liver is converting sugar into fats and VLDLs at such a high rate that some of this fat begins to accumulate in the liver itself, leading to non-alcoholic fatty liver disease (NAFLD). (NAFLD is the main focus of one of the other excellent diets discussed in this book, the Eadeses' *6-Week Cure for the Middle-Aged Middle.*)

If this weren't bad enough, consider that the pace at which all this happens is sped up considerably by fructose, a known driver of NAFLD. Fructose turns up the glucose-transport molecules in the liver, making the liver, in Wolf's words, "hungry for sugar." This in turn leads to increased PA production, which leads to—you guessed it—even greater leptin resistance.

As Wolf puts it, "The wheels are seriously falling off the wagon by this point."

So now we've seen at least two ways in which a high-carb diet makes you sick and fat. First, the high carb intake is driving your blood sugar through the roof, which in turns drives your insulin levels through the roof. Unless you're very, very lucky, this scenario turns into full-blown insulin resistance, which makes it fiendishly difficult to lose weight and sets you up for metabolic syndrome, diabetes, obesity, and heart disease. And second, the high level of carb intake puts a huge burden on your liver, leads to an overproduction of triglycerides and VLDL, and ultimately leads to leptin resistance, meaning the brain no longer listens to the hormone signal that tells you to stop eating. You keep eating, you get fatter, insulin and leptin resistance get worse, and—from a health perspective—you're pretty much out of luck.

Wolf also brings something we've discussed earlier in this book into the picture: the nasty little molecules appropriately nicknamed "AGEs." AGEs (advanced glycation end-products) are the products of a reaction between proteins in our body and sugars. The sugar gloms on to some normally slippery, healthy proteins and makes them sticky and less able to travel through the bloodstream. AGEs damage proteins, DNA, enzymes, and even receptors for both insulin and leptin, which is the very last thing you need. They "age" the body and are implicated in many degenerative diseases. (Our old friend fructose is seven times more effective at forming AGEs than glucose. Just sayin'.)

The point is that all this damage—and the weight gain that goes along with it—comes from the ridiculously high amount of carbohydrates in our diet, which we are in no way genetically prepared for.

According to Wolf, this loss of hormonal sensitivity—particularly for insulin and leptin—leads to a host of health problems, of which overweight is just one. Controlling these hormones is the key to losing fat, but—as he himself found out—it's also the key to healing.

So, What Can I Eat?

The ancestral diet that Wolf advocates is really very simple: meat, poultry, seafood, vegetables, and fat (and a little fruit). No dairy, no grains, and no legumes. This prescription shares a lot with the original Paleo Diet, written by Wolf's acknowledged mentor, Professor Loren Cordain. But there are a few differences, one of which has to do with fat.

Wolf takes a much more reasonable position on saturated fat than Cordain took in *The Paleo Diet*. (One of the only things I strongly disagreed with in Cordain's book was his agreement with the position that "saturated fat is the devil." Wolf's is much closer to my own position, so, naturally, I like his view more. "Saturated fat has historically been implicated as a causative factor in everything from CVD to cancer," Wolf writes. *"However, closer analysis has shown this assumption to be largely inaccurate."*) He also points out that the ratio of omega-6 to omega-3 fats is of far more importance in disease progression than saturated fat. This, too, is a position I wholeheartedly agree with. No wonder I'm such a fan of this book!

Wolf's "day job" is that he owns one of the best gyms in the country (voted in the top 100 by *Men's Health*), so it's no surprise that his section on exercise is the best I've ever seen in a low-carb diet book. It's thorough, intelligent, and nothing like the cursory boilerplate stuff that often gets tagged on as an afterthought in so many diet programs. There are programs for different levels of fitness, and they are well designed and intelligent. Of course, you could choose to follow the diet and do your own thing in the exercise department, but you can't go wrong following any of the exercise programs carefully described (and illustrated with photos) in this book.

This is not a "diet" book in the conventional sense. The program is more like a philosophy of eating and health, and rather than give you a specific menu to follow, Wolf gives you a shopping list. He does give you a 30-day meal plan, but it functions like training wheels, providing a suggested guide for meal planning based on the ingredients he's included. What you learn from this book is what to put on your shopping list and what to leave off. He himself has a list of fifteen meats, fifteen veggies, five fats, and twenty herbs and spices, all easily available from your grocery store, which you can combine in thousands of ways. He suggests you pick five meats, five veggies, five fats, and as many herbs and spices as you can carry. "If you take one item from each of these columns and consider that a meal, you have 22,500 meal options," he says. The eating prescription is simplicity itself:

"Put some oil in a pan, start browning meat, add herb or spice, and then add a vegetable. Cook for five to ten minutes. Eat." Try for 30 days.

The Paleo Solution as a Lifestyle: Who It Works For, Who Should Look Elsewhere

Let's be honest: this is a pretty drastic departure from the way many people have eaten all their lives. In paleo world, dairy, grains, and legumes are definitely off the menu, and even some foods considered acceptable on most low-carb plans have cautions attached, especially for people with autoimmune or inflammatory issues. Even fruit is minimized, especially at first, thought it's not totally banned. "There is no nutrient in fruit that is not available in veggies, and fruit may have too many carbs for you," he says. But Wolf is not a zealot, and even has some suggestions for "easing into" the paleo lifestyle, one meal at a time.

Still, this is also not the kind of program where you're taken by the hand and treated like a baby. This is like the Marine Corps of diet books— it's not for the faint-hearted, and you'd better be ready to say good-bye to a lot of familiar foods (or, more accurately, "food products"). It seems to me to be particularly suited to those rugged, individualistic types of both sexes who don't need to have everything spelled out for them and are perfectly capable of constructing their own meals from a clear, basic shopping list. If that's you, you should give this program a go. It's particularly suited for those with multiple health issues who haven't gotten a lot of help from the conventional medical system and are ready to take an *un*conventional—if historically sensible—approach. According to Wolf, the ancestral diet solves a lot of problems, and weight is only one of them.

The program is definitely not vegetarian-friendly, though if you're really committed, you might be able to make a go of it. Vegans, don't even bother.

JONNY'S LOWDOWN

This is one of the best low-carb diet books I've ever read, and it's hard to think of a situation in which it wouldn't produce a huge benefit in your overall health. You can keep this book on your shelf as a reference on digestion, hormones, and the effects of carbohydrates on your health. It has the best and most thorough exercise program of any diet book I've ever seen. He's got some excellent, albeit technical, information in here, but it's presented in a highly readable and often very funny manner, and he never talks down to the reader. I recommend this book wholeheartedly.

8. THE PRIMAL BLUEPRINT
MARK SISSON

WHAT IT IS IN A NUTSHELL

The Primal Blueprint is a high-fat, moderate-protein, low-carb, paleo-type diet that is smart and sensible and incredibly effective. It's a bit more flexible than some of the other Paleo-oriented diets, especially when it comes to dairy, but it shares a lack of love for grains and legumes. The emphasis is on lifestyle, not diet, and it's very user-friendly. The author holds that if you follow the basic template 80% of the time, you will get the results you want.

About The Primal Blueprint

The story of how *The Primal Blueprint* came to be published and went on to become an Amazon best seller and an Internet sensation is an interesting one. Mark Sisson is a former world-class marathoner and Ironman tri-athlete with a bachelor's degree in biology who describes himself as "an athlete, a coach, and a student, on a lifelong quest for exceptional health, happiness and peak performance." He's the founder and publisher of MarksDailyApple.com, the leading "paleo" blog on the Internet. But when he tried to get his book published, door after door slammed in his face. "Mark, you're not a doctor," he was told. "You have no credibility. You need a celebrity attached or it won't go anywhere. Ditching grains? Eating more fat? Making workouts slower or shorter? It just won't fly with today's reader."

Except it did. Sisson published the first edition himself, and it sold over 130,000 copies in six printings and climbed to the top of the charts on Amazon. Deservedly, I might add.

The basic premise of *The Primal Blueprint* is similar to other "paleo-centric" programs: *We are genetically adapted to a diet of foods that we could hunt or gather.* For Sisson, like the other "paleo-ists," being overweight and sick is a direct consequence of our reliance on foods and "food products" that are processed, man-made, and introduced relatively recently into the human diet. To Sisson, a return to the caveman way of eating—or a reasonable facsimile of it—will restore us to health (and to leanness).

What's not to like?

On the Primal Blueprint, you'll eat meat and other protein sources, as many vegetables as you can possibly consume, and all the fat you like. For those who like visuals, there's a terrific "Primal Blueprint Food Pyramid," at the base of which is *meat, fish, fowl,* and *eggs.* These foods constitute the bulk of your dietary calories. Next up on the pyramid is *vegetables,* with an emphasis on locally grown and/or organic. The next level consists of *healthy fats,* which includes saturated fat. Butter, coconut oil, avocados, coconut products, olive oil, and macadamias are all mentioned as good fats. (In my view, the fact that saturated fat is *not* demonized—as it is in the original Paleo Diet—gives this program additional credibility.)

Moderation foods are the next level of the pyramid. These include locally grown, in-season, high-antioxidant fruits like berries, high-fat dairy (preferably raw, fermented, and unpasteurized), starchy tubers, quinoa, wild rice (for athletes), nuts, and seeds. The small triangular peak of the pyramid contains herbs and spices, *sensible indulgences* (such as red wine and dark chocolate), and supplements.

For anyone who might be skeptical that such a simple program can work, I suggest looking at the before-and-after pictures of some of the Primal Blueprint success stories. They're nothing short of stunning. I was particularly impressed with the women in this section, since "meat-centric" programs so often appeal to men. The pictures of the women who have followed the Primal Blueprint should forever put to rest the idea that

Paleo diets are just for men. Both sexes seem to do equally well on this program, and the photographic proof is right there.

Sisson is very clear from the beginning that this is not a "diet" program in any conventional sense. "The Primal Blueprint is a lifestyle with some important but extremely flexible eating guidelines," he writes. He starts the book with the "Ten Primal Blueprint Laws," of which only two have anything to do with food:

1. Eat plants and animals.

2. Avoid poisonous things.

3. Move frequently at a slow pace.

4. Lift heavy things.

5. Sprint once in a while.

6. Get adequate sleep.

7. Play.

8. Get adequate sunlight.

9. Avoid stupid mistakes.

10. Use your brain.

Sounds simple, but it's about as smart a set of guidelines as you could come up with if you want to be lean and healthy.

A Word About Exercise

Sisson is no fan of long, drawn-out, strenuous aerobic sessions for either weight loss or health. Law number three (above) is to move frequently at a slow pace, law number four is to lift heavy things, and law number five is to sprint from time to time. Taken together, this means an exercise program that's a blend of frequent low-intensity energizing movement (e.g., walking, hiking, easy cardio); regular, brief strength-training sessions; and occasional all-out sprints. He explains why and how in detail in the book. Did I mention that he's on the money on this one? No? Well, he is.

He's also on the money about a whole lot more. The section on heart disease ("How to Sneeze at Heart Disease") is superb. He dismisses the cholesterol hypothesis and advances the position that heart disease is caused by oxidation and inflammation (a view cardiologist Stephen Sinatra, MD, and I also take in our book, *The Great Cholesterol Myth*). His discussion of fat is excellent, clear, and accurate. So is his discussion of sleep and play.

In fact, there's hard to find much in this book that *isn't* terrific.

The temptation—for me—is to tell you about *all* of the positive aspects of this book, but I'm going to resist that temptation and just give you one example: what Sisson calls "The Carbohydrate Curve." He writes: "Your body composition success is overwhelmingly dependent on controlling your carbohydrate intake and hence, your insulin output." A graph in the book plots "grams of carbohydrate per day" against outcomes like *burn more fat, maintain body comp, store more fat,* and *obesity and illness.* Eat in the 100 to 150 gram "maintenance zone" and you won't gain fat. Eat in the 40 to 100 gram "sweet spot" zone and you'll lose body fat. It's simple, easy to follow, and—best of all—it works.

Conventional Wisdom versus Primal Blueprint

Even if you don't want to read this book in full, I suggest you pick it up and at least study the chart in the very beginning of the book, comparing "conventional wisdom" to "Primal Blueprint." Sisson details the conventional wisdom on a variety of categories, including cholesterol, eggs, fiber, meal habits, strength training, cardio, weight loss, sun exposure, footwear, prescription drugs, and goals, accurately summarizing the "wisdom" of the authorities and then contrasting it with the principles of the Primal Blueprint. As you would expect, the two columns present very different points of view. If the surprising contrasts on these pages speak to you as much as they did to me, you'll understand what's in store for you if you go "primal."

The Primal Blueprint as a Lifestyle: Who It Works For, Who Should Look Elsewhere

It's hard to think of someone for whom this program would not work. It's also very hard to take issue with the principles on which it's based, principles that are rock-solid and very smart indeed. The only question is whether you'll be able to follow the program, since—like all paleo-centric eating plans—it pretty much eliminates most of the "comfort" foods we consume daily, and many of the foods we've been taught are universally healthy (like grains).

This is definitely not a "quick-fix" diet. The author is scrupulous about stressing the lifestyle aspects of the program, and only one (possibly two) of the "Ten Primal Blueprint Laws" has anything to do with food. That said, weight management is an almost-guaranteed "side effect" of living Primal (or Paleo, take your pick). But it's not for those looking for instant gratification. Following this excellent program is going to take some readjustment and some rethinking of your beliefs about what's healthy and "necessary" in the human diet and about what's causing all the problems (hint: it's not fat!).

If you're willing to do this kind of fundamental reassessment and you're prepared to give this plan a trial for the recommended 21 days, you will undoubtedly become a convert to this way of life.

Since the program is pretty heavy on protein and fat, vegetarians will have a problem with it. If you're a vegetarian for health reasons, you owe it to yourself to read the book. If you're a vegetarian for ethical or moral reasons, the book is probably not going to change your way of thinking, and you'll be happier elsewhere. Vegans, don't even bother.

JONNY'S LOWDOWN

When at first I combed through this book trying to find something to disagree with, I came up empty-handed. It's pitch-perfect on just about everything. I particularly like the way Sisson presents the material—even if you've seen this stuff before, you'll love the way he lays it out. At the beginning of each chapter, he tells you what the chapter is going to cover, and at the end he summarizes the important points. There's a ton of tips sprinkled throughout the book, and a wonderful "Primal Approved: At A Glance" section that summarizes what foods you should eat, what foods you should avoid, what exercises work, and what lifestyle changes matter.

All in all, this is one of the best of the new crop of diet/exercise/weight-loss books, and I recommend it without reservation.

9. THE AUTOIMMUNE PROTOCOL DIET (PALEO AUTOIMMUNE PROTOCOL)

SARAH BALLANTYNE, PHD

WHAT IT IS IN A NUTSHELL

A stricter version of paleo designed for people with autoimmune diseases. Also known as AIP.

About the AIP

The AIP diet is a kind of super-strict version of paleo specifically designed for people who are dealing with the challenge of autoimmune disease. If you had to describe it in an elevator, you'd probably say "It's like paleo— only harder."

Autoimmune expert Dr. Sarah Ballantyne offers a much more complete description: *AIP is a specialized version of the Paleo diet, with an even greater focus on nutrient density and even stricter guidelines for which foods should be eliminated.*[17]

First things first. AIP stands for autoimmune protocol, also referred to as paleo autoimmune protocol (they mean the same thing). You start with basic paleo principles: no gluten, dairy, beans, legumes, sugar, or alcohol. (Yes, there's some division in the paleo world over dairy, and some paleo programs do allow it, but no matter—on AIP, it's off the menu.)

The autoimmune protocol goes one step further than paleo, banishing foods that may be absolutely healthy but that have been found, at least anecdotally, to provoke inflammation in a lot of folks. (How many folks? Who knows. The Autoimmune Protocol takes a "just in case" approach, banning these foods because they are known triggers for an awful lot of people, particularly those with autoimmune challenges.)

Take nightshades. Members of the *Solanacea* family of plants, they include a lot of paleo-friendly foods like bell peppers, tomatoes, and egg-plants. Nightshades contain a substance called *solanine* (an alkaloid), and therein lies the problem.

If you ask the Arthritis Foundation—and other major mainstream medical groups—they'll say there's no solid evidence that the solanine in nightshades causes inflammation or worsens arthritis pain. That may be true in an epidemiological sense, meaning that if you look at studies of hundreds of thousands of people, you may not see a statistically significant impact of nightshades on overall arthritis pain at the population level. But studies like that don't tell you much about what's going to happen with any given individual—like *you*. And there is little doubt that many people subjectively report a significant worsening of symptoms when they consume nightshades. Whether it's the solanine—or something else in the nightshade family—these foods cause problems for many, especially folks with autoimmune disease. Hence, they're gone on the autoimmune protocol (at least in the beginning. More on that in a moment.)

More importantly, studies are now being conducted to test the AIP diet in humans, and the results are confirming what we would expect: it works! A trial of adults with active inflammatory bowel disease (IBD) found that a six-week AIP elimination diet, followed by a five-week maintenance phase, improved IBD symptoms and intestinal inflammation. In fact, by the end of the elimination diet, 73% of the IBD patients were in remission from their disease and stayed in remission throughout the maintenance phase of the study.[18]

Another food that's eliminated is eggs, one of nature's most perfect foods. Eggs are off the menu because certain proteins and enzymes—particularly one called *lysozyme*—seem to be able to penetrate the gut wall and create quite a bit of mischief and inflammation, at least for some people, which may (or may not) be the reason that eggs are one of the top allergenic foods in the diet. (Eggs are one of the eight foods responsible for the vast majority of allergic reactions in the general population.[19]) If you want to really nerd out on the science of how this all works, there's no better resource than medical biophysicist Dr. Sarah Ballantyne (aka PaleoMom), who explains it beautifully on her website.[20] Eggs also contain arachidonic acid, a fatty acid that is sometimes inflammatory.

Nuts and seeds—also paleo and low-carb staples—are also gone, due to anti-nutrients like phytates and lectins. And fruit is limited to a couple of servings a day, as fructose can be irritating to the gut. The AIP is also no fan of food additives like guar gum and carrageenan (thought to potentially contribute to leaky gut), and NSAIDs (non-steroidal anti-inflammatories like ibuprofen). NSAIDs should be discussed with your health provider—lots of autoimmune protocols make use of NSAIDS, which aren't necessarily the best thing for the gut even if they may be effective for pain.

I mentioned that many of these foods are taken out of the diet "at least in the beginning." That's because AIP has a built-in mechanism for reintroduction, much as the Atkins diet does. Some popular articles have counseled people to carefully reintroduce some of the otherwise healthy foods one at a time and monitor carefully for reactions—anything from bloat to brain fog. That's a good general description. A much more detailed description of reintroduction—and also one more likely to be successful—comes from Dr. Ballantyne, who suggests you wait *at least* 3–4 weeks before trying to bring back foods you had eliminated. She notes that this protocol is adopted from the same procedure used to challenge food allergies and sensitivities. This is how Dr. Ballantyne herself describes the process:

1. Select a food to challenge. Be prepared to eat it two or three times in one day, then avoid it completely again for a few days.

2. The first time you eat the food, eat half a teaspoon or even less (one teensy little nibble). Wait fifteen minutes.

3. If you have any symptoms, don't eat any more. If you don't have symptoms, eat one teaspoon of the food (a small bite). Wait fifteen minutes.

4. If you have any symptoms, don't eat any more. If you don't have symptoms, eat one and a half teaspoons of the food (a slightly bigger bite).

5. That's it for now. Wait two to three hours after eating those small amounts and monitor yourself for symptoms.

6. Now eat a normal-sized portion of the food—either by itself or as part of a meal.

7. Do not eat that food again for five to seven days and don't reintroduce any other foods during that time. Monitor yourself for symptoms.

8. If you have no symptoms during the challenge day or at any time in the next five to seven days, you may reincorporate this food into your diet.[21]

Autoimmune diseases can be triggered by a number of things, not just foods. These triggers include stress, for example, or environmental toxins. Those with autoimmune diseases frequently suffer from hormonal dysregulation (hormones being out of whack), gut dysbiosis (an imbalance of good and bad microbes in the microbiome), leaky gut, and micronutrient deficiencies. That's why the four major focuses of the paleo autoimmune protocol are:

1. **Nutrient density.** Many people with autoimmune diseases have micronutrient deficiencies, hence the emphasis on the most nutrient-rich foods possible. (Organ meats are very popular.)

2. **Hormone regulation.** A running theme of this book is that food has a hormonal effect, and hormones are frequently out of whack for those with autoimmune disease. (Just think about the effect that carbs have on insulin!) Hormones are impacted not only by what foods we eat but by whether we get enough sleep and how well we manage stress. All are focuses of the AIP.

3. **Gut health.** The notion that all health starts in the gut may seem like a new idea,[22] but it actually goes back to Hippocrates, the father of modern medicine, who famously said "All disease begins in the gut."[23] Healing leaky gut is a prime target of the paleo autoimmune protocol and with good reason.

4. **Immune system support.** It's all about the microbiome. *"Immune regulation is achieved by restoring a healthy diversity and healthy amounts of gut microorganisms, restoring the barrier function of the gut, providing sufficient amounts of the micronutrients required for the immune system to function normally, and regulating the key hormones that in turn regulate the immune system,"* writes Ballantyne.[24]

ARGUMENTS AGAINST PALEO
(Complete with Rebuttals)

1. My doctor says there's no research on it.

Your doctor is wrong. For starters, conduct an online search for the following titles, all published in peer-reviewed journals:

- "Paleolithic and Mediterranean diet pattern scores and risk of incident, sporadic colorectal adenomas"
- "Paleolithic nutrition improves plasma lipid concentrations of hypercholesterolemia adults to a greater extent than traditional heart-healthy dietary recommendations"
- Long-term effects of a Palaeolithic-type diet in obese postmenopausal women: A 2-year randomized trial"
- "A Paleolithic diet is more satiating per calorie than a Mediterranean-like diet in individuals with ischemic heart disease"

- "Paleolithic diet decreases fasting plasma leptin concentrations more than a diabetes diet in patients with type 2 diabetes: a randomised cross-over trial"
- "Paleolithic and Mediterranean diet pattern scores are inversely associated with all-cause and cause-specific mortality in adults"
- "The Paleo Diet and diabetes"

That's just a smattering of the studies that have been done as of this writing (2019), and the number of published papers is likely to be significantly higher by the time this book is published. Dr. Ballantyne maintains a useful list of studies on her site—search "Sarah Ballantyne Paleo Diet Clinical Trials and Studies."

2. Paleo folks died young, even if they ate such a healthy diet. And if our diet sucks, how come we live so much longer?

Stone Agers—dare we nickname them "Stoners"?—did indeed die young; 30–35 years was roughly the average life expectancy at birth of preindustrial populations. The biggest factor pulling down that average was the number of babies who died in childbirth. Average life expectancy in Paleo times was short because infant and childhood mortality rates were sky-high! This significantly lowered the average life expectancy, just like your grade point average would be significantly lowered if you had a bunch of Ds. Our civilization isn't healthier than Paleolithic folks; we just know how to keep babies alive better than they did, so our "average" life expectancy is naturally higher.

A second factor: if you survived childhood in a hunter–gatherer society, your death was overwhelmingly likely to be due to infectious diseases, most of which we now have under control. Older hunter–gatherers almost never died of coronary artery disease or diabetes. The aerobic fitness of the average Paleo person was in the range of what's "athletic" for modern Western populations, and diabetes prevalence was very low.[25]

3. The reason you don't see much diabetes and heart disease among Stone Agers is that they didn't live long enough to manifest those diseases!

Chronic diseases kill people in their later years, so yes, if there aren't a ton of people around in their eighties, you're not going to see as many diseases of "old age" (such as cognitive impairment and heart disease). But these chronic diseases don't just begin in old age—there are early signs, sometimes even appearing in childhood. It's very easy to compare young members of industrial societies with age-matched members of hunter–gatherer societies. When you look at biomarkers of "developing abnormality," such as insulin resistance, rising blood sugar and blood pressure, and obesity, you find that they are common in the former and rare in the latter. As Eaton and Konner point out, about 20% of hunter–gatherers lived to 60 or later; but even in this age bracket, most chronic degenerative diseases (with the exception of arthritis) are almost completely absent among hunter–gatherer or technologically primitive groups. This strongly suggests that it is our Western lifestyle that promotes those "afflictions of affluence," not our chronological age.

4. **Humans are capable of genetic adaptation! Our environment is very different from that of our Paleo forefathers, but we humans are very adaptable.**

It's definitely true that since modern humans left Africa somewhere between 50,000 and 100,000 years ago, genetic evolution has continued, especially in the past 10,000 years since agriculture was invented. There have been changes in the pigmentation of our hair, skin, and eyes, and adaptive defenses against microorganisms.

But respected paleoanthropologists[26, note 25], geneticists[26, note 24], evolutionary theorists[26, note 27], and biologists[26, note 26] all agree that genetically speaking, we're not all that different from our Stone Age ancestors. The core fundamental physiological and biological processes of being human are the same. "No one proposes that genetic adaptations could have caught up with dietary and lifestyle changes over the past 2 centuries," say Eaton and Konner.

No one denies that our capacity for physical and cultural adaptation allowed humans to adjust—and even thrive—in a host of different environmental settings. If we couldn't adapt to changing environmental conditions, I wouldn't be sitting at a computer writing this book, and you wouldn't be reading it. Instead, we'd both be in loincloths (at best), hunting for mammoths or gathering roots and berries. But the fact that we can adapt to certain circumstances doesn't necessarily mean that those circumstances are ideal. Managing to survive and adapt under a number of environmental conditions hardly guarantees that our biology is running at top efficiency in any particular environment. "As a rule," write Eaton and Konner, "biological organisms are healthiest when their life circumstances most closely approximate the conditions for which their genes were selected." In other words, you can keep a lion alive in a zoo on chocolate chip cookies—but you won't be getting a lion at the top of his game.

What's more, some things take longer to show their harmful effects than others. Deprive someone of oxygen, and you'll see in a couple of minutes where they're headed. But scurvy doesn't develop until months of vitamin C depletion; osteoporosis takes decades. And lung cancer doesn't happen to someone after they smoke the first pack—or even the twentieth or two hundredth. "Many individuals appear outwardly healthy well into middle adulthood and even beyond," write Eaton and Konner.

But there's a "but."

"If preagricultural lifeways are truly those for which humans remain genetically programmed, we can expect that, despite our adaptability, most of us will eventually have to pay the piper," they write. "The evolutionary hypothesis proposes that chronic degenerative diseases are the price."

5. **There was no single "paleo" diet or universal ancestral lifestyle pattern, so how can the Stone Age experience provide a model for health recommendations in modern times?**

Right you are. The fourteen communities studied by Dr. Weston Price differed substantially from one another in terms of their diets, as did the folks in the Blue Zones studied many decades later. We already know that there was wide variance in those Stone Age diets that have been studied. As mentioned earlier, estimates of meat and vegetable intake ranged from 35% meat and 65% vegetable to as high as 80% meat. All of that does indeed make the argument that there's no one perfect diet suited to every human on the planet.

But concentrating on the very real differences between people who receive, say, 35% of their calories as meat and those who receive, say, 75% of theirs can distract us from something far more important—the similarities among all these versions of paleo, and the differences between paleo diets and our modern industrialized diet.

In *all* hunter–gatherer diets *ever* studied, there were no processed foods. Vegetables and fruits were what grew naturally and in the wild and were not doctored or bred to increase their sugar content. Speaking of sugar, there was none—or at least none that was manufactured. If you wanted something sweet, you'd shimmy up a tall tree and grab some honeycombs. Sodium intakes may have varied from group to group, but potassium intakes were uniformly high. Protein sources like caribou and mammoths were not contaminated with antibiotics, steroids, and hormones.

Rather than concentrate on the minor details of difference in the various paleo diets of yore, let's focus on the big picture. Processed foods vs. unprocessed. Starchy-carb "staples" vs. meat and vegetables. Convenience-store snacks vs. rare raw honey. Sugary breakfast cereal vs. tubers and roots. Those are the distinctions to concentrate on when we talk about the advantage of the "ancestral diet."

The rest is just details.

III. THE KETO REVOLUTION

The first time most Americans heard the word ketosis was in 1972, when the first edition of *Dr. Atkins' New Diet Revolution* (aka the Atkins Diet) was first published. Atkins, you may recall, described ketosis as "delightful as sunshine and sex," an almost magical state in which fat literally melted off the body. Ketosis—or, more properly, nutritional ketosis—is simply the state in which the body is making measurable amounts of ketones, by-products of fat metabolism the presence of which virtually guarantees that your body is indeed "burning" fat.

But in the original Atkins diet, you only stayed in ketosis for a little while before moving on to the next phase in the diet, in which you gradually added carbohydrates back. The major difference between Atkins and the keto diets of today (the keto "revolution") is that the keto diets of today are about *staying in* ketosis, not just using it as a steppingstone to a diet that ultimately includes carbohydrates. Today's keto dieters believe—not without reason—that there are specific and measurable benefits to ketosis, and they don't see any particular reason to leave that state just so they can have the dubious pleasure of eating a little bread.

Since ketosis is a state—not a program per se—it's hard to classify it with other diet programs. You're basically in ketosis when you're producing measurable levels of ketones (measurable in the blood, urine, or breath), and it doesn't much matter how you get there—the proof is in the testing. And since people differ in their ability to get into ketosis—some folks will need to reduce carbs to almost zero, while others may be able to get into ketosis with 50 grams a day—it's almost impossible to give precise proportions of recommended carbs, protein, and fat. The basic formula is to reduce carbs to the level at which your body is now producing ketones. Period. How you do that is up to you. (For those who insist on a percentage breakdown, it usually looks something like this: 5% carbs, 60% fat, and 35% protein.)

Some special branded diets—like Bulletproof or Metabolic Factor—flirt with ketosis or use it as a tool, while others simply try to maintain ketosis whenever possible. And some keto-friendly diet book authors have devised keto diets with special emphases like Dr. Will Cole's vegetarian and vegan-friendly version of keto that he calls Ketotarian (see page 268).

We'll explore some of the more interesting takes on keto in the following section.

If you've read this far, you're probably wondering what all the fuss is about regarding ketosis. Some of you, truth be told, might not be 100% sure of what the term actually *means,* while many others might be wondering why people even want to get "into ketosis" in the first place! A few of you might already be convinced that a ketogenic diet is for you but are confused about how to do it in the most effective way.

I hope this section will answer all your questions.

To paraphrase an old Virginia Slims commercial, ketosis has "come a long way, baby." From being demonized as a dangerous state to be avoided, it's gone on to become the darling of the health world in both the diet community and the research community. As of this writing, you'd be hard-pressed to find a medical or nutritional conference that didn't include research on the ketogenic diet and its potential for positively affecting a whole variety of conditions, from Alzheimer's to multiple sclerosis.

But it doesn't end there. Athletes are using ketogenic diets to enhance performance. Ben Greenfield, an elite tri-athlete with a substantial Twitter following and a popular podcast, follows a ketogenic diet because he believes it optimizes his athletic performance. Vinnie Tortorich, a legendary Hollywood trainer and resident fitness expert on *The Adam Carolla Show,* believes that his keto diet helps his cancer stay in remission (which it's been for almost a decade). The integrative neurologist and bestselling author of *Grain Brain,* Dr. David Perlmutter, eats a ketogenic diet most of the time and thinks it's the best one for the brain, stating that ketosis is the "original and most-optimal state of metabolism." At the University of Tampa, Dr. Dominick D'Agostino's lab is conducting research on keto diets in conjunction with the U.S. Navy for potential applications with the Navy SEALs.

And then of course, there's weight loss, which is probably the reason you heard about ketogenic diets in the first place.

There's certainly plenty of research supporting the use of ketogenic diets for weight loss. In fact, if you search the PubMed database, you'll see that low-carb diets in general perform well in weight-loss trials, and keto diets—a stricter version of low-carb—perform very well indeed, particularly for people with lots of weight-loss resistance, prediabetes or diabetes, or other metabolic dysfunctions. The studies are so plentiful and easy to find at this point that I'll limit myself to recommending that you go to PubMed and put "ketogenic diet" and "weight loss" into the search engine. You could also search for the published research of Jeff Volek, PhD; Stephen Phinney, MD, PhD; and Eric Westman, MD, MPH.

Before I get into some of the research, let's define our terms and talk about what nutritional ketosis actually *is*, what it *does*, and why you should (or should not) consider one of the variations of keto diets discussed later in the chapter.

In the absolutely simplest sense, a keto diet is a diet that literally forces your body to burn fat. When you hear about keto diets being "fat-burning" diets, that description is actually accurate—"fat burning" is the colloquial way to say what ketogenic diets actually do: They metabolize and oxidize—i.e., "burn"—fat.

Since "burning fat" is the goal of every weight-loss plan ever invented, it's easy to see why ketogenic diets caught the attention of everyone looking for "the next big thing" in weight loss. Of course, keto diets have been with us since the beginning of time and are hardly "the next big thing but they certainly seem to be on their way to becoming mainstream. And why not? Keto diets force you to burn fat, and weight-loss diets are all about burning fat—it's a match made in diet heaven!

So, how does it work? How can a diet "force" your body to burn fat?

How Keto Forces You to Burn Fat

It's actually quite simple. It's a matter of available fuel.

See, the only four things in the world that provide calories are carbohydrates, fats, protein, and alcohol. Your body is always burning a mixture of these fuels. Let's assume that alcohol is not a major fuel source for your

WHY DO SO MANY LOW-CARBERS USE INTERMITTENT FASTING?

Jason Fung isn't the first person to talk about intermittent fasting—but he's become the go-to guru on the subject for many of those in paleo/ keto/low-carb communities. Here's how that happened.

Jason Fung is a nephrologist—a kidney doctor—and the overwhelming majority of his patients were diabetics. (Type 2 diabetes is by far the biggest cause of kidney disease.) He treated his diabetic patients in all the conventional ways, often with drugs like insulin that had the potential to make things even worse by causing more weight gain.

"I'd give them insulin, I'd give them drugs," he told me in an interview. "And in the end, the diabetics still got kidney disease. It wasn't like anything was getting better."

The solution was obvious. "If type 2 diabetes is causing kidney disease, then the solution is to get rid of the type 2 diabetes."

And that meant controlling blood sugar and insulin.

If you haven't yet read the previous chapters and don't know (or don't remember) the story of insulin, here's a quick recap. Insulin is the hormone that rises precipitously in the presence of high blood sugar. Its job is to get that sugar out of the bloodstream and deposit it into cells. But when you eat too much sugar, the system breaks down. (Did I mention that insulin's nickname is "the fat-storing hormone"?)

When blood sugar and insulin are constantly being driven to high levels—as they are with the standard American diet—insulin's ability to regulate things starts to diminish. You develop a condition called *insulin resistance*, which we now know plays a role not only in diabetes and obesity, but in heart disease and Alzheimer's.

Ever since Robert Atkins introduced his eating plan, controlling insulin has been the raison d'etre for low-carb diets. That's what led Dr. Fung to investigate ketogenic diets, since, as you've seen, keto diets are far more carb-restrictive than their paleo brethren. He liked what he saw with his patients and started to dig into the published research. He became an advocate for keto because of that strict limit on sugar, and he became an advocate for intermittent fasting because it was another way to limit the amount of time that the body spends in a high-insulin state.

No wonder he's a friend to low-carb. Low-carb diets are *all about* staying out of high-insulin states. In case you've forgotten why that's important, insulin resistance is strongly linked to a number of diseases besides diabetes and obesity, including:

- *Heart disease*

- *Stroke*

- *Alzheimer's disease*

- *High blood pressure*

- *Nonalcoholic steatohepatitis fatty liver disease (NAFLD)*

- *Polycystic ovary syndrome*

- *Gout*

- *Atherosclerosis*

- *Gastroesophageal reflux disease (GERD)*

- *Obstructive sleep apnea*

Intermittent fasting has a ton of benefits and has been incorporated into a lot of the programs you're reading about in this section. Bulletproof recommends intermittent fasting. Many of the keto programs use it. "Like caloric restriction," says Dr. Michael Eades (coauthor of *Protein Power*, page 165), "intermittent fasting reduces oxidative stress, makes animals more resistant to acute stress in general, reduces blood pressure, reduces blood sugar, improves insulin sensitivity, and reduces the incidence of cancer, diabetes, and heart disease." Eades points out that in animal studies, intermittently fasted animals greatly increase their levels of *brain-derived neurotrophic factor* (BDNF), a substance that not only increases the growth of new nerve cells in the brain but also protects against stress and toxins. "*If you buy into the idea that the Paleolithic Diet is the optimal diet for us today because it is the diet we were molded by the forces of natural selection to perform best on, then you should probably also buy into the idea that a meal timing schedule more like that of Paleolithic mean would provide benefit as well,*" says Eades.* "*I would think that the optimal way to go would be to follow an intermittent fast using low-carb foods during the eating periods. One would get the best of all worlds healthwise this way.*"

Because there are a ton of ways to do intermittent fasting and it's easy to find terrific info about it online, we won't go into the various ways to do it here. Fung's book with Jimmy Moore, *The Complete Guide to Fasting*, is a great guide to the current state of the art.

*https://proteinpower.com/drmike/2006/09/13/fast-way-to-better-health/

daily activities, which leaves protein, carbs, and fats—the big three, also referred to as "macronutrients." The body prefers *not* to use protein as a fuel except in dire emergencies like starvation. It prefers to save protein for things like building muscles and neurotransmitters and teeth. That leaves dietary carbs and dietary fats, which, after being broken down by the body, respectively become *glucose* (sugar) and *fatty acids* (fat), the two basic fuels for human metabolism.

In a perfect world, we'd all have a nice flexible metabolism capable of burning any particular mix of fuel at any particular time in an efficient way but—well, we don't. When we eat a diet high in sugar and starch, high in processed carbs and grains—in other words, the diet we've been eating for the past 40 to 50 years—our metabolisms become far more acclimated to running on sugar than they do on fat. After all, sugar is constantly coming down the pike in one form or another, and the body can just grab that out of the bloodstream and use it for all its immediate needs. When it runs out, it sends a message to your brain, telling you you're starving, which is why you feel you need to eat every two hours.

You've got the textbook example of a sugar-burning metabolism. You're good at sugar burning, but you're probably *lousy* at fat burning. Which makes perfect sense. Why would your body go to the metabolic trouble of opening up those fat stores locked in the adipose tissue on your butt, thighs, and belly and use valuable enzymes to break them down into fuel when it's already got plenty of "fuel" coming in from the snack you just grabbed at the corner store?

This is the situation in which hundreds of thousands of people find themselves, and it can be summed up in one phrase: *weight-loss resistance.* Your fat stores sit there mocking you, like a huge savings account that you don't have the ATM code for.

Ketogenic diets have been breaking through weight-loss resistance for a long time. You may remember William Banting, the corpulent undertaker from chapter 2. The diet recommended by his doctor, which was basically composed of meat and vegetables, was probably a ketogenic diet. (It wasn't called that at the time, because no one knew what ketones were nor how to measure them; but had that technology been available, it's a good bet that Banting would have been in nutritional ketosis.)

Do they work for everyone? Absolutely not. Are they the solution to every medical ill? Of course not. Are they *necessary* for weight-loss success? No, because people have lost weight (and failed to lose weight) on any diet you can name that was ever invented *ever*.

Nonetheless, ketogenic diets have enormous promise, not just for breaking through weight-loss resistance but also for performance enhancement, both mental and physical.

The method by which ketogenic diets help break through weight-loss resistance holds the key to why they may be good for so many other health conditions: Ketogenic diets lower insulin resistance. Insulin resistance, as you've read, is at the foundation of just about every cardio-metabolic disorder on the planet and may even be at the foundation of Alzheimer's disease. To understand why ketogenic diets are terrific for insulin resistance, let's remember what happens when we eat a diet high in sugar and processed carbs like grains.

If you're like many people, eating a high-carb meal causes two things to happen immediately. One, your blood sugar jumps sky-high; and two, so does your insulin. Here's the big metabolic joke on us: high insulin essentially turns off the fat-burning process. Metaphorically speaking, insulin locks the doors to the fat cells. Fat can't be "burned" or released into the bloodstream to any significant degree in the presence of insulin.

Since sugar is the first source of energy used by the body, someone with a weight problem eating a high-sugar, high-grain diet will get all the "fuel" they need for living (and plenty for storage as fat in addition), but their insulin levels will be so constantly high that they'll never be burning fat! (Remember, those are the folks who have to eat every two hours because their blood sugar is always crashing!)

Think about it: If we could tamp down insulin for a while and prevent it from rising so frequently or to such high levels, our cells would gradually become more *sensitive* to insulin (since there'd be less of it!), and insulin *resistance* would begin to go down. Because our insulin levels decrease to a healthy level, the fat cells would no longer be locked and they could release their goodies into the bloodstream where they can finally be used for energy!

That's exactly what ketogenic diets do. They stop your blood sugar from rising high (and staying high for a long time), which in turn keeps your pancreas from having to secrete a ton of insulin in a desperate attempt to fix the condition. Your insulin levels go down, and you can start to burn fat. Your metabolism shifts from that of a sugar-burner to that of a fat-burner. That's why people make a big deal out of getting into "nutritional ketosis."

Now let's talk about exactly what ketones are, how the ketogenic diet produces them, and why it matters.

HOW DO WE MAKE KETONES?

Normally, carbs are broken down into glucose, and then into pyruvic acid, and finally into a substance called *acetyl-CoA*. Fats are broken down into their component parts—fatty acids and glycerol—and then *further* broken down (by a process called beta-oxidation) into two carbon fragments that *also* combine to make acetyl-CoA (see the illustration on the following page).

On a "normal," high-carb diet, two things happen to the acetyl-CoA. First, some of it gets broken down in the liver into ketone bodies. It's important to remember that this is a *normal* part of metabolism. You are making ketone bodies right now while you sit there, reading this book. The liver is *always* producing ketone bodies. Ketones aren't a toxic substance, nor is their presence in your bloodstream evidence that you're starving.

Ketosis was initially misunderstood by conventional doctors because ketones are indeed made by the body when you are starving, and, as everybody knows, starving is not a good thing. If you didn't think about it very clearly, you could reverse the order and assume that since ketosis is one of the reactions to something bad, ketosis itself must be bad. That's like assuming that umbrellas cause rain.

Ketosis is one of the metabolic adaptations to starvation—because when you're starving, your body can still make and use ketones for fuel. And ketosis in starvation is very, very different from nutritional ketosis in the ketogenic diet. Why? In starvation, the body is breaking down muscle because there's no dietary protein coming in! The body literally has to eat its own muscles to get amino acids it can use for fuel. In the low-carb diet—even the high-fat, moderate-protein kind—dietary protein is plentiful, and that prevents the loss of muscle that occurs with true starvation. The loss of protein is actually what causes death from starvation. When you supply sufficient protein in the diet—as you always do on a low-carb regimen, this simply doesn't happen.

Ketones are a normal physiological substance that plays many important roles in the human body. (This, of course, did not stop Jane Brody of the *New York Times*—one of the biggest apologists for the high-carbohydrate/low-fat diet in America—from calling ketones "toxic compounds that can damage the brain" and "pollute the blood." None of that is true.)

THE PRODUCTION OF KETONES

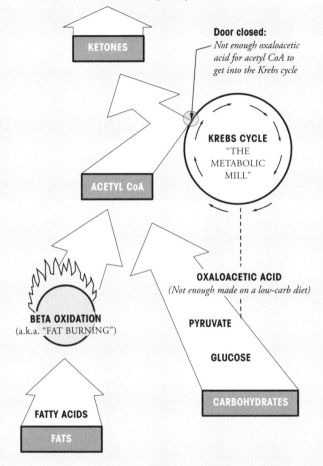

Sent out as fuel for the tissues, heart, brain

KETONES

Door closed:
Not enough oxaloacetic acid for acetyl CoA to get into the Krebs cycle

KREBS CYCLE
"THE METABOLIC MILL"

ACETYL CoA

BETA OXIDATION
(a.k.a. "FAT BURNING")

OXALOACETIC ACID
(Not enough made on a low-carb diet)

PYRUVATE

GLUCOSE

FATTY ACIDS

FATS

CARBOHYDRATES

So, let's review: the liver makes ketones—which are essentially by-products of fat metabolism (specifically the breakdown of acetyl-CoA)—*all the time*. That's the first thing that happens with the acetyl-CoA.

What's the *other* thing that happens with it?

Well, on a diet with plenty of carbohydrates, the acetyl-CoA combines with a by-product of *carbohydrate* metabolism called *oxaloacetic acid*. When acetyl CoA combines with oxaloacetic acid, it enters an energy-production cycle called the Krebs cycle. (This is what is meant by the old '80s saying "Fat burns in a flame of carbohydrate.")

Without the carbohydrate necessary to produce oxaloacetic acid, acetyl CoA can't gain admission to the Krebs cycle and be burned.)

Those are the two pathways that acetyl CoA can take: Go to the liver and help make ketones, or combine with oxaloacetic acid from carbs, enter the Krebs cycle, and be burned up for energy. As long as you're eating enough carbs to keep churning out oxaloacetic acid, that's exactly what happens.

But what happens when you're *not* consuming a lot of carbohydrates?

Now, all of a sudden, there is not enough carbohydrate (glucose) coming down the pike to produce the oxaloacetic acid necessary to bind up with acetyl-CoA and do-si-do right into the Krebs cycle. What happens *then*?

Well, the acetyl-CoA *accumulates* in the liver. The liver promptly breaks it down into more ketones (also known as ketone bodies). There are three of these ketone bodies, and their names are *acetoacetate*, *beta-hydroxybutyrate*, and *acetone*. Of the three, beta-hydroxybutyrate appears to be the most important one. Meanwhile, it's the release of acetone that gives you that "fruity" breath.

What determines whether the liver just goes about its business, producing a relatively small amount of ketones, or whether it springs into overdrive and produces enough ketones to put you into nutritional ketosis? One thing only: how much sugar is stored in your liver. (Stored sugar in the body is known as *glycogen*.) In a low-carb diet, there's just not a whole lot of glycogen around. That means the path to the Krebs cycle is closed.

So now virtually *all* of the acetyl-CoA—including what would have normally skipped along the yellow brick road to the Krebs cycle—winds up going down the ketone-production road. *Now* your body's making ketones in sufficient quantities that you can detect them in the urine. Or the blood, or the breath.

As mentioned, ketones are the product of fat burning in the body. It's also possible to get ketones from outside the body. They're called exogenous ketones, and we'll talk about them later. If you're producing a lot of ketones, you can be sure you're burning fat, because this is the major way to produce ketones. You're "in ketosis" when your ketones reach a certain level as measured on an instrument, such as a blood test, a breath meter, or a urine strip. Once you're "in ketosis," you are officially burning (or *oxidizing*) fat.

Measuring Ketones

There are three ways to measure ketones: in the urine, in the breath, and in the blood.

The easiest and cheapest way is to test the urine with strips that are available at every drugstore. These are particularly good in the beginning of a keto diet, because your body hasn't learned to make the shift from sugar to fat yet, so a lot of the ketones you just started making wind up getting excreted in the urine because your body hasn't yet become what we call "fat-adapted" or "keto-adapted." During this time, seeing the urine strips turn color can be quite motivating.

Whether they're the most accurate way of measuring once you get going is another question. Many people think that once you're "keto-adapted" and are good at using fat and ketones for energy, fewer ketones escape into the urine, making the strips less accurate for keto-adapted people. Regardless of whether you use them forever, urine strips are a great place to start. Just follow the directions and look for changes in color that indicate you're in ketosis.

A better and more accurate way to measure ketones is in the blood, but it's more expensive and a lot less convenient. Many advocates of keto diets who are really trying to get every last health benefit from the diet use blood meters, originally developed for people with type 1 diabetes, for more accurate monitoring.

If you do use blood, here are the numbers to use. They come from one of the great keto specialists in the world, the wonderful Dr. Andreas Eenfeldt, a Swedish medical doctor and low-carb expert whose Diet Doctor website is one of the best and most reliable sources of information about all things keto and low carb. Here's what he says about blood measurements:

"Blood ketones are best measured on a fasted stomach in the morning (before breakfast, that is). Here are pointers on how to interpret the result:

- Below 0.5 mmol/L is not considered "ketosis." At this level, you're far away from maximum fat-burning.

- Between 0.5 and 1.5 mmol/L is light nutritional ketosis. You'll be getting a good effect on your weight, but not optimal.

- Around 1.5–3 mmol/L is what's called optimal ketosis and is recommended for maximum weight loss.

- Values of over 3 mmol/L aren't necessary. That is, they will achieve neither better nor worse results than being at the 1.5–3 level. Higher values can also sometimes mean that you're not getting enough food."[27]

Always remember that ketones are benign products of normal metabolism, and the fact that you can actually detect their presence in your urine (by the use of ketone test strips), blood, or breath merely means that your body is breaking down fat for energy in measurable amounts.

What Does the Research Say?

Evidence that ketogenic diets can help combat obesity is abundant: a meta-analysis of 13 different randomized controlled trials found that ketogenic diets are significantly more effective than low-fat diets for long-term weight loss.[28] (And compared to those on low-fat diets, patients on ketogenic diets typically saw greater improvements in HDL cholesterol, triglycerides, and blood pressure.) Ketogenic diets show great promise in the treatment of diabetes—not surprisingly, since obesity and diabetes are so closely related as to be commonly referred to as "diabesity." For example: A diabetes trial found that a ketogenic diet significantly lowered HbA1c levels (a measurement of long-term average blood sugar) and *quadrupled* the number of patients who could discontinue their diabetes medications.[29]

Ketogenic diets are also being carefully studied in cancer treatment. In some kinds of cancer, such as gliomas (which account for 80% of all malignant brain tumors), combining cancer therapy with the ketogenic diet was able to slow tumor progression—and, in some cases, even induce prolonged cancer remission.[30] Ketogenic diets have also shown promise as adjuvant treatments for malignant brain tumors.[31] More research in humans is needed before we can tell for sure how ketosis affects other forms of cancer, but there's reason to be hopeful. Cancer cells need glucose (sugar) to survive—it's what they live on. This has prompted some experts to suspect that ketogenic diets could essentially *starve* cancer cells.[32]

Ketogenic diets appear to have a therapeutic role for a variety of neurological conditions, including Alzheimer's disease, Parkinson's disease, autism, and brain trauma.[33] Dale Bredesen—an internationally recognized expert on neurodegenerative diseases and the author of *The End of Alzheimer's*—uses a version of a ketogenic diet in his ongoing research on Alzheimer's disease. Dr. Terry Wahls, noted for her TED lectures and her program, The Wahls Protocol, uses a ketogenic diet in her research on multiple sclerosis.

Finally, ketogenic diets have been used as treatments for childhood epilepsy for more than 70 years. They are currently used at 78 centers in the United States alone, including the Johns Hopkins Children's Center.

KETONES FOR ALZHEIMER'S?

In Alzheimer's disease, some brain cells have difficulty metabolizing glucose, the primary source of energy for the brain. Deprived of fuel, some of these valuable neurons may die.

That's why having an alternative source of fuel for the brain would be such a big deal.

Enter ketones.

Ketones are such good fuel for the brain that a Colorado biotech company called Accera developed an oral liquid that helps the body produce more of them. The drug—brand name Axona®—is marketed as a potential adjunct (i.e., additional or complementary) treatment for Alzheimer's. It's worth pointing out that the prescription-only drug Axona is actually a proprietary form of MCT oil (MCT stands for *medium chain triglycerides*—a group of four fatty acids). Many people in the keto community already know that MCT oil can effectively convert to ketones, and ketones are a wonderful alternative fuel for the brain. This is precisely why MCT oil is the "fat of choice" in childhood epilepsy programs that use the ketogenic diet.

The patients enrolled in the original trial of Axona showed significant improvement in memory and cognition,* but then again, improvements are seen with MCT oil, which is *not* prescription-only.†

---

* https://www.biospace.com/article/releases/accera-inc-release-experimental-drug
-ketasyn-tm-ac-1202-treats-alzheimer-s-as-diabetes-of-the-brain-/

† https://www.alzheimersanddementia.com/article/S1552-5260(17)30901-9/fulltext

---

Also worth mentioning is the grassroots-level interest in keto as a performance-maximizing diet for elite athletes. Well-known endurance athlete Ben Greenfield has long touted keto diets and credited them for his own physical accomplishments. And even a cursory Google search of keto diets and athletic performance will yield a plethora of advice for serious athletes wanting to experiment with keto for better performance. Early studies by Stephen Phinney, MD, PhD, indicated that elite cyclists would adapt to a keto diet and be achieving their previous levels of performance within a month. It's definitely worth keeping an eye on this interesting development in the world of athletic performance.

If Keto Is So Great, Why Doesn't Everybody Do It?

Great question, complicated answer.

First let it be said that many people *do* stay in ketosis all the time, or at least most of the time. But many don't. For some, it's monotonous. Some people hit plateaus that they just can't seem to break through. Some people just don't feel it works for them. Some people have a version of the APOE gene (APOe2) that makes it very difficult for them to absorb and digest fat, while others have a version of that same gene that makes them feel great on a high-fat diet. (This might explain why some people feel better on keto than they have at any time in their whole lives, while others feel positively lousy on it.) Some people like the idea of keto but don't think they can do the diet without eating a ton of meat (untrue).

Wherever you stand on "all keto, all the time," it's still worth thinking about different ways you can incorporate what I call "keto wisdom"—my name for *insulin sensitivity training*—into your own particular regime.

There are vegan keto programs (see Ketotarian, page 268), keto programs for female athletes, keto cycling programs, carb cycling programs, keto "light," keto for athletes—and there'll probably be more variations by the time this book is published. (Just as I was writing this, I received a review copy of *The Hormone Fix* by my friend Dr. Anna Cabeca, who uses a version of keto she calls "keto-green," which is keto with a heavy emphasis on quality vegetables.

You can think of keto diets as falling into one of three groups:

The Standard Ketogenic Diet

The Standard Ketogenic Diet (SKD) is the basic keto diet, the most popular and common. This is what was used in the Induction Phase of the Atkins diet. It's roughly 5% carbs, 15–20% protein, with the rest of your calories (75–80%) coming from fat. Intermittent fasting is very popular among advocates of the SKD, and some people make it a regular part of their keto plan.

The High-Protein Ketogenic Diet

The High-Protein Ketogenic Diet is exactly what it sounds like—a higher-protein version of keto. Carb consumption is still kept extremely low. Higher protein versions of keto are controversial in the "keto" world because protein *can* be converted to glucose via a metabolic process called gluconeogenesis. That *could* keep you out of ketosis. If your number one objective is to stay in ketosis, protein is definitely something you'd want to monitor, though many people are able to stay in ketosis—or flirt with ketosis—using higher amounts of protein than might be found in the "standard" keto diet.

Cyclic Ketogenic Diets

Cyclic Ketogenic Diets are eating plans that periodically cycle in periods of "carb refeeding." The carb refeeding can be anything from one high-carb meal (as recommended by the Metabolic Factor, see page 253) to two days of carb loading, depending on what you're going for. Carb-cycling programs of the latter kind are often used by bodybuilders and athletes, while programs like Metabolic Factor—which was designed for ordinary people who are trying to lose weight—incorporate much more moderate and targeted carb feasts.

Some folks use the term "cyclic ketogenic" to refer to cycling a period of ketogenic—say every month—into your regular eating plan. One of my friends does four keto months every year, cycling them in once every season. Another does keto one or two days a week.

The point is that there are many ways to do keto, and lots of excellent guides available, both in print and online. I always recommend that beginners start with the book *Keto Clarity* by Dr. Eric Westman and Jimmy Moore, which is a book-length version of this section and a great keto resource. A quick search for "keto for beginners" will yield a cornucopia of good books and online options. (Hint: You can't go wrong with Mark Sisson's *The Keto Reset Diet*.) There's also absolutely wonderful material on the Diet Doctor website of Dr. Andreas Eenfeldt, including a complete video course called "A Ketogenic diet for beginners."[34]

A ketogenic diet should not be used by three groups of people:

(1) uncontrolled type 1 diabetics;

(2) pregnant or nursing women (not because higher levels of ketones in the blood are dangerous, but just because we don't know for sure whether they have any effect on the baby); and

(3) people with existing kidney disease (see myth #5 for a full explanation of the connection between protein and the kidneys).

If you are not in one of the three groups I just listed, the ketogenic diet is *perfectly and utterly safe.*

KETO OBJECTIONS

1. Are Ketones Dangerous?

Hardly. They're a perfectly good source of energy. Drs. Donald Voet and Judith Voet, authors of a popular medical biochemistry textbook, say that ketones "serve as important metabolic fuels for many peripheral tissues, particularly heart and skeletal muscle."[35] A paper coauthored by a number of distinguished researchers, including one from Harvard Medical School, stated that ketones provide an efficient source of energy for the brain and that mild ketosis could have a wide range of benefits for conditions ranging from Alzheimer's to Parkinson's.[36] The integrative neurologist and bestselling author of *Grain Brain*, Dr. David Perlmutter, says, "I believe a low level of ketosis is actually the natural and most optimal state of metabolism for humans."[37]

Ketones are not dangerous—quite the contrary: They are therapeutic in a wide variety of settings.

Many conventionally trained medical doctors still believe that ketones are somehow toxic. That's because some continue to confuse *ketosis* with *diabetic ketoacidosis*. Diabetic ketoacidosis is indeed a life-threatening condition. But it has zero to do with nutritional ketosis. In diabetic ketoacidosis, insulin is sky-high, blood sugar is sky-high, and ketones are off-the-chart high. In nutritional ketosis, both insulin and blood sugar are at healthy low levels, and ketones are mildly elevated. The two conditions are completely different.

2. Keto diets are high-fat diets. What does that do to my heart?

Contrary to what the naysayers would expect, ketogenic diets routinely show up as *beneficial* when it comes to heart health. One study in the *Journal of Nutrition* looked at the effects of a 6-week ketogenic diet on risk factors for cardiovascular disease.[38] The study found *improvements* in triglycerides and insulin levels, plus a slight *increase* in HDL cholesterol (the "good" kind). Most importantly, the *type* of LDL ("bad" cholesterol) tended to change from the kind that's dangerous (pattern B) to the kind that's not (pattern A). And when it comes to long-term ketogenic dieting? More good news for the heart! One trial placed obese patients with high cholesterol on a ketogenic diet for 56 weeks and found that total cholesterol, HDL cholesterol, triglycerides, and blood sugar had all decreased significantly by the end of the trial, while beneficial HDL increased significantly.[39] This suggests that even over longer periods of time, ketogenic diets are not only *not* harmful to the heart, but can actually improve known risk factors for heart disease.

What's more, it's high time we questioned the "high fat diets cause heart disease" narrative entirely! A famous meta-analysis published in the *American Journal of Clinical Nutrition* found that when 21 different studies were pooled, there was no significant evidence for the claim that saturated fat is linked to higher risk of cardiovascular disease.[40] An even more recent meta-analysis concluded the same thing (along with finding *no* link between saturated fat and all-cause mortality, ischemic stroke, or diabetes).[41] Trans-fats, however, *were* associated with total mortality and heart disease in this meta-analysis, highlighting the importance of the *type* of fats we eat rather than just the quantity.

3. What about fiber? There's no fiber in protein and fat!

This is an objection to ketogenic diets that's harder to dismiss, and there's quite a bit of controversy around it. When I recently moderated a panel of medical doctors who were strongly supportive of the keto diet, I asked this very question, prefacing it by saying that I thought the lack of fiber was the Achilles heel of the ketogenic diet. I was surprised by the almost-unanimous reaction of the panel, which was basically, "We don't need no steenkin' fiber!" I'm exaggerating—but it was clear that the panel did *not* seem to think that fiber was as big a deal as I did. Indeed, a quick check online reveals that there are indeed some folks out there questioning "the fiber hypothesis" (that we need a ton of fiber for optimal health) and asking for a reevaluation of some of the conventional wisdom on fiber. And they're not all nut-jobs. These folks argue that studies showing that high-fiber diets reduce cancer may not be as robust as we might think, and that some of the benefits of high-fiber diets may be exaggerated. They also (rightly) point out that many of the foods we've been told to consume for their fiber intake have so many negatives (like sugar and high-glycemic starches) that any benefit isn't worth the cost.

On the other hand, there is an exploding amount of research on the microbiome confirming that gut health is important for almost every aspect of health you can imagine. It has long been a basic tenet of functional medicine that fiber is essential for gut health. Period. Colon cells feast on prebiotic fiber (soluble fiber), creating important substances like butyric acid that act as fuel for the gut. So it's kind of hard to accept that fiber is of little importance.

On the other hand, we're at the very dawn of the age of the microbiome, and the discoveries about individual variations in gut ecology, not to mention the influence of genetics, may make any conclusions we draw about the role of fiber in a ketogenic diet premature. It's entirely possible that the microbiome of people eating high-fat, low-fiber diets may adapt in such a way as to not create the problems we might anticipate seeing from a low-fiber diet.

Finally, it's worth mentioning that a keto diet does not *have* to be low-fiber. You can certainly load up with high-fiber, low-starch vegetables, and even with an allowance of only 50 grams of carbs a day you'd still do pretty well. Take raspberries: A cup of raspberries has 14 grams of carbs, but 8 of those come from fiber! Other high-fiber, low-carb foods include bell peppers, avocados, blackberries, spinach, and collard greens.

Anything we say "definitively" now about the fiber–keto connection is likely to be obsolete before this book gets published. So let's agree to leave this one issue unresolved. Right now, the overwhelming epidemiological evidence points to the importance of fiber in the human diet, but epidemiological evidence has been misleading before. The best we can say about this particular objection to keto is "We just don't know the answer yet." Stay tuned.

4. What about Keto Flu?

One of the famous "downsides" of keto is the notorious "keto flu," a period of adaptation in which you feel, frankly, like shit. The symptoms are often flu-like—hence the name—but also can include fogginess, fatigue, and a general "out-of-sorts"-ness.

The keto flu is a by-product of your body's attempt to get used to a different fuel source and become, as they say, fat- or keto-adapted. And this can take a few days or even a week or more. Hang in there. It's no worse than having the sniffles at work for a few days. It passes, you become fat-adapted, and it's smooth sailing after that!

10. THE BULLETPROOF DIET
DAVE ASPREY

WHAT IT IS IN A NUTSHELL

A cyclical ketogenic diet, with a high emphasis on food quality.

About the Bulletproof Diet

In 2014 I was giving a talk at an event in southern California. Outside the lecture hall, vendors were giving out free samples of some new kind of coffee. I went over to get some and was greeted by an enthusiastic young man named Josh who explained to me that this wasn't just ordinary coffee: Instead, it was something called "Bulletproof Coffee."

With a name like that, how can you not be intrigued?

Bulletproof coffee is the brainchild of Dave Asprey, a Silicon Valley heavyweight with an MBA from Wharton who ran the Internet and Web Engineering program at the University of California, Santa Cruz and built an impressive résumé of executive positions at major tech companies. But he wasn't just a metaphorical heavyweight in the sense of being an IT genius—he was *literally* a heavyweight. He weighed 300 pounds, suffered with Hashimoto's thyroiditis, and was generally in poor health.

But that was then.

Asprey decided to approach his own health as if it were an IT project, "hacking" his own biology. (Asprey was partly responsible for the introduction of the word "biohacking" into the performance lexicon. Biohackers study how to tap into their body's own biology and biochemistry in order to improve performance, longevity, and well-being.) Years later, the results speak for themselves. Asprey is lean and muscular, has a six-pack, looks twenty years younger than he is, and has vowed to live to 180 years old. Many around him believe he'll do it.

The idea for Bulletproof Coffee—the original product that launched the empire that became Bulletproof 360 and spawned the Bulletproof Diet—came to him when he was hiking in Tibet in 2004. He was 18,000 feet above sea level and it was −10°F (−23°C); not surprisingly, his energy was bottoming out, and he was exhausted. He stopped at a guesthouse and was offered a creamy cup of tea made with yak butter.

Yak butter. Remember that. We'll come back to it.

For people who live and work in such rugged terrain, the high-fat yak-butter tea is a necessity. After all, fat is the densest source of calories, and fat is your body's preferred source of energy. (As the world-famous ultramarathon runner Stu Mittleman once told me during the low-fat craze of the 1980s, "You gotta *eat* fat if you want to burn fat.")

Asprey drank the tea and experienced near-instant rejuvenation. He promptly started researching why the tea had made him feel so good.

As Asprey experimented with high-fat morning beverages, he eventually substituted mold-free organic coffee for the tea, and grass-fed butter or organic ghee for the yak butter—and voila, the recipe for the original Bulletproof Coffee was born. Later, a fat called Brain Octane™ Oil (more on this later) was added to the recipe.

Bulletproof Coffee morphed into the Bulletproof Diet and ultimately became part of the multimillion-dollar Bulletproof empire, which includes Bulletproof Radio, one of the top-rated biohacking podcasts in the U.S. Bulletproof is not just about weight loss and not even just about good health: It's about being a super-performer, hacking your own biology to find ways to turbocharge your brain and body. And it's very tech-heavy—Asprey is a huge fan of stuff like cryotherapy (extreme cold for high performance) and a $15,000, 5-day neurofeedback program called 40 Years of Zen.

And the foundation of all this is, of course, the Bulletproof Diet.

The Bulletproof Diet is a particular flavor of ketogenic diet that's starting to be referred to as "cyclical keto"—it recommends eating keto for 5 or 6 days a week, and then having a "carb refeed" day. (Full disclosure: My own program, Metabolic Factor, on page 253, is a cyclical keto diet as well, but it uses the "carb refeed" technique in a very structured, targeted way.)

According to Asprey—and to other advocates of cyclical keto diets—refeeding on sweet potatoes, squash, or even white rice once a week is a hedge against some of the downsides some people experience with long-term full-on keto diets, including—in my experience—plateaus.

Asprey says that one of the Bulletproof Diet's distinguishing features is its emphasis on vegetables. This emphasis may not be unique to Bulletproof, but Asprey does make a bigger deal about vegetables than some other versions of keto do. He also restricts fruit a lot more than paleo diets do, which is not surprising. Too much fruit can keep some people out of ketosis, but since ketosis is not a goal of the paleo diet, paleo folks don't usually limit fruit.

The Bulletproof Diet also strongly emphasizes the healthiest possible version of the foods it recommends—100% grass-fed meat, for example, and wild-caught salmon. That's partly because Asprey himself suffered with autoimmune disease and is particularly aware of the need for a toxin-free,

THE RECIPE FOR BULLETPROOF COFFEE

As of 2019, this is the current, official recipe for Bulletproof Coffee, taken directly from Asprey's blog, at https://www.bulletproof.com/blogs/recipes/official-bulletproof-coffee:

- 2½ heaping tablespoons ground Bulletproof Coffee Beans

- 1-2 tablespoons Brain Octane Oil (see page 246)

- 1-2 tablespoons grass-fed butter or organic ghee

Asprey's own health problems were partly connected to mold, hence the emphasis on mold-free coffee; but you can make your own generic version of this without using Bulletproof-branded products—just use coffee and butter, or coffee and MCT oil.

nutrient-dense diet that is fundamentally anti-inflammatory. (The emphasis on extreme nutrient density and on anti-inflammation is something Bulletproof shares with both the AIP protocol and Whole30.)

Intermittent fasting is also built into this program. (See sidebar on page 228.) You'll get the fastest results on the Bulletproof Diet if you incorporate it every so often by eating your calories for the day in a shortened window of time—say, 6 to 8 hours starting in the afternoon. Boom. That's all there is to it. Intermittent fasting works amazingly well in tandem with ketogenic diets, because ketones provide steady energy for your body—no crashes, no hangry feelings, no distraction, no slumps.

Asprey is the first to admit that switching from a standard American diet to the Bulletproof Diet—or any other low-carb, keto-friendly program—is a very big overhaul. He offers a cool step-by-step way to get into it gradually.[42] Even if you just complete the first couple of steps, you should notice a difference in your energy and general well-being.

Here's an overview of Asprey's blueprint for getting into the Bulletproof diet and lifestyle, one step at a time.

1. Eliminate sugar.

This includes fruit juice, sports drinks, and even sauces. And yes, it even includes natural sweeteners like honey or maple syrup. Sorry.

SO, WHAT'S THE STORY WITH BRAIN OCTANE?

To understand what Brain Octane is, we need to have a quick discussion about something called MCT oil.

MCT stands for "medium-chain triglycerides," a particular family of fats (or, more correctly, fatty acids). All fatty acids are formed from chains of carbons; chains are typically about 2 to 24 carbons long. When a fatty acid has 6 or fewer carbons in the chain, it's called a short-chain fatty acid; when it has more than 12 carbons, it's called a long-chain fatty acid. The chains from 6 to 12 carbons long are said to be "medium-chain triglycerides" and are sold as a supplemental oil as MCT oil.

MCT oil is known to act somewhat differently from other saturated fats. Bodybuilders on calorie-restricted diets for contest preparation frequently use MCT oil as an added source of energy, since it tends to be burned for fuel rather than stored as fat. There are four fatty acids that are technically considered MCTs. They are defined by the number of carbons in their chain. Caproic acid is the "shortest" MCT, with 6 carbons (C-6). Caprylic acid (C-8) has 8 carbons in its chain, while capric acid (C-10) has ten, and lauric acid (the predominant fat in coconut oil) has 12 (C-12).

C-6, being the shortest of the MCTs, converts to ketones the quickest; but, as Asprey observes, it has the unfortunate characteristic of smelling like goats. (In fact, caproic acid comes from *capra*, the Latin word for—you guessed it—goat!) On the other side of the spectrum, the longest MCT, lauric acid (C-12), behaves more like a long-chain fatty acid and converts to ketones slowly, if at all. (Lauric acid is, however, anti-viral, making it a very desirable fat for reasons having nothing to do with making ketones.)

That leaves C-8 and C-10, which Asprey considers the two "best" of the MCTs. Of those two, Asprey considers C-8 to be the best of the best. Brain Octane is 100% caprylic acid (C-8), and, according to Asprey, converts to ketones within minutes, "making it very powerful for suppressing hunger and fueling your brain in a way that other MCTs do not."[*]

Asprey also manufactures a second MCT product, Bulletproof XCT Oil, a blend of both C-8 and C-10, but notes that while it's cheaper than pure C-8, you don't get as high a ketone spike. As a fat for making ketones, however, he says, "It still beats coconut oil and generic MCT oil!" (Note that another reputable company—Perfect Keto—makes an excellent product called Pure MCT oil that is 70% C-10 and 30% C-8. I personally alternate between Bulletproof's Brain Octane and Perfect Keto's Pure MCT oil.)

*https://blog.bulletproof.com/the-definitive-guide-to-mcts/#ref-1

2. Replace sugar with the right fats.

Here's where you can see the difference between Asprey and the keto-advocates and Cordain's original Paleo Diet. The classic Paleo Diet would tell you to keep fat relatively *low* and to make sure most of it is *un*saturated. Asprey tells you to include fats like grass-fed butter, ghee, and MCT oil. His program is definitely not friendly to the theory that "saturated fat is the demon." (Like most folks in the low-carb tent, he is bullish about removing inflammatory fats like corn oil, canola oil, and other high omega-6 processed oils.)

3. Switch to 100% grass-fed meat and wild-caught fish.

One of the distinguishing things about Asprey's program is that it's not really focused on weight loss at all. Remember, Asprey is a biohacker who's openly declared that his goal is to live to 180. The emphasis of his program has *always* been on health, not just weight loss. Hence the insistence on grass-fed meat and wild salmon, which, for reasons too long to go into here, are by far the preferred way to consume those foods. (CliffsNotes version: Grass-fed meat is not treated with antibiotics, steroids, and hormones, and wild salmon is not raised on an artificial, pro-inflammatory diet of grain.)

4. Remove grains and gluten.

Asprey, along with many others in the low-carb keto space, believes that modern grains cause an awful lot of problems, not the least of which is inflammation. He's anti-gluten. If you want a more thorough understanding of why he and others feel this way, check out two of the foundational books in my resource section: *Wheat Belly* by Dr. William Davis, and *Grain Brain* by Dr. David Perlmutter.

5. Get rid of synthetic additives, colorings, and flavorings.

Asprey suggests avoiding things like aspartame, monosodium glutamate (MSG), and dyes. "Even 'natural flavors' on the ingredient label is questionable," he writes. "Hundreds of ingredients fall under the 'natural flavor' category—some create havoc in your body. Know what you're eating."

6. Eliminate legumes.

If this step sounds like it came right out of the paleo playbook, that's because it does. As with paleo, the objection to beans and legumes has to do with lectins and Asprey's belief that they cause inflammation (which they *can*—but not always—see "Lectins: The Bad, the Ugly . . . and the Good?" page 194).

7. Remove all processed, homogenized, and pasteurized dairy.

Why?

For one reason, dairy contains casein and lactose which, as Asprey notes, can cause digestive distress for a lot of people. Grass-fed butter has much lower casein and lactose because of the churning process. Asprey says that "most people feel a lot better removing milk, cheese, and other dairy products." (I am not among them, so I question whether this applies to everyone, though there's no doubt that some people respond better to a diet that doesn't include dairy.) Asprey says if you *want* to keep dairy in your diet, make sure it is raw, full-fat dairy from grass-fed cows. (I completely agree.)

8. Switch to organic fruits and vegetables.

Again, this guideline is about toxic load. "Avoiding insecticides and herbicides goes a long way," Asprey says.

9. Cook your food gently, if at all.

High-heat cooking, especially barbecue with a roaring flame, can cause the production of carcinogens called heterocyclic amines. This hardly means that all food has to be eaten raw (there are actually a number of problems with that approach), but I agree wholeheartedly with Asprey that we'd be better off with slower, lower-heat cooking in general.

10. Limit fruit consumption to 1–2 servings per day.

I don't necessarily endorse this notion, but it comes from the idea that fruit can provide a fair amount of sugar, which for many people can be problematic, even when that sugar comes from whole, natural foods like fruits. One reason for his concern is that fruits contain fructose. While I'm no fan of high-fructose corn syrup—which I've frequently referred to as metabolic poison—I've always believed that fructose, in small amounts, found in fruit—alongside all the other great things in fruit—is much less of a problem than that same fructose that's extracted from fruit, concentrated, and added to practically every packaged food on the planet from hamburger buns to hot dogs.

BULLETPROOF PROTEIN FASTING

The Bulletproof Diet recommends a practice called the Protein Fast. It's one full day per week with virtually no protein. On that day, Asprey recommends that you keep your protein intake to less than 15 grams (an extraordinarily low amount, particularly in the low-carb neck of the nutrition woods).

Just for comparison, the government recommends .8g of protein per kilogram of body weight, a figure that's hotly debated because many clinicians and practically all athletes think it's too *low* for most people. Yet even that formula works out to 36 grams a day for someone weighing only 100 pounds, and it goes up from there. Less than 15 grams of protein per day would be a serious protein deficiency by even the most Spartan protein formulas, and would cause enormous health problems (see kwashiorkor (a debilitating and deforming disease of protein malnutrition)).

Asprey knows this, of course, and is careful to point out that we are not talking about restricting protein as a lifestyle. But remember that Asprey is first and always a biohacker. He believes that a protein-free day is a great biohack for stimulating autophagy.

Autophagy functions as a kind of cellular housecleaning that is seen in creatures ranging from yeast cells to humans, though it gets much more complicated in big, multicellular organisms such as us. It has an important role in maintaining health. The word autophagy literally means "eating self," but don't worry, it's definitely a good thing. Autophagy is like the cell world's own personal cleaning crew, salvaging the good parts and removing "metabolic trash."

The biochemistry of autophagy is—trust me—not for the faint of heart, guaranteed to put all but the most dedicated science nerds to sleep. (If you want to take a deep dive into each metabolic step, I recommend *Autophagy in the Pathogenesis of Disease*, published in the journal *Cell, Volume 132 No. 1*, which you can find online at *Science Direct*.) Meanwhile, here's what you really need to know.

Autophagy is the cell's adaptive *response to starvation*. But just because it's one of many adaptive responses to starvation doesn't mean it's a bad thing. (Ketones are also produced as a response to starvation.) This breakdown process actually keeps you alive. By "digesting" its own parts, the cell can get rid of junk proteins and cellular trash and can recycle the good stuff into new, healthier proteins. That's probably why the scientist who won the Nobel Prize in 2016 for his research on autophagy titled his Nobel lecture "Autophagy—An Intracellular Recycling System."

Asprey recognizes that the number one way to turn on autophagy is to not eat for 24 or more hours. He also recognizes that fasts are hard. · He came up with the Bulletproof Protein Fast as a biohack meant to accomplish the same thing. "It turns out there's an even better way to turn on autophagy, and that's by occasionally limiting protein consumption. When you do this, you force your cells to find every possible way to recycle proteins. In their search, they bind and excrete toxins that were lurking in your cell's cytoplasm, the gel-like substance enclosed within the cell membrane. It's like taking your car to the car wash and having it deep cleaned."*

*https://blog.bulletproof.com/what-is-protein-fasting-bulletproof-diet/

The Bulletproof Diet as a Lifestyle: Who It Works For, Who Should Look Elsewhere

I think Bulletproof is a program that will appeal to a huge variety of people. It's really not terribly complex, it makes intuitive sense, it's relatively easy to follow, and it stresses whole foods and intermittent fasting. What's not to like?

And Asprey is the perfect ambassador for the Bulletproof way of life. He has an interesting story, overcame enormous health challenges, and every time I see him he looks five years younger than he did the last time I saw him. It's hard to go wrong with Asprey.

JONNY'S LOWDOWN

This is one of those "go-to" programs I find myself recommending a lot to people who want to experiment with a healthy diet free of processed foods and high in nutrient density.

When an Uber driver tells me he wants to change his diet, lose weight, and feel better—but doesn't know where to start, I'll almost always tell him to start with Bulletproof. And that's about the best endorsement I could give!

DOES KETO MESS UP WOMEN'S HORMONES?

One of the big Internet rumors about keto is that it can really mess up a woman's hormones, particularly thyroid. (Clearly, men have thyroid hormones also, but women are particularly "thyroid-sensitive"—they're 5 to 8 times more likely than men to have thyroid problems, and 1 in 8 women will develop a thyroid disorder over the course of her lifetime.) That's one reason Asprey recommends the carb feast, which may indeed be a great idea. But I'm not completely convinced about the connection between keto diets and thyroid problems.

There is some research showing that levels of T3, one of the two main thyroid hormones, can decrease on keto diets, but, as Dr. Anthony Gustin points out,* a low T3 level is not the same as hypothyroidism (low thyroid). The actual *active* thyroid hormone is T3, which is made in the body from T4. Hypothyroidism is typically diagnosed with a high level of TSH (thyroid-stimulating hormone) and a low level of T4.

"Not only do we see T3 lowering independently of normal thyroid function, but lower levels of T3 actually show benefit for being anti-catabolic, preserving muscle mass and improved longevity," says Gustin.[†]

Sara Gottfried, MD, a functional-medicine physician who specializes in women's hormones, says that keto can promote fat loss for many people. She occasionally prescribes it for fat loss and help with specific hormone imbalances involving insulin, as well as for obesity, weight-loss resistance (assuming the thyroid is healthy), metabolic syndrome, and PCOS (polycystic ovary syndrome) with weight gain and insulin resistance.

"Aside from these specific health conditions, I believe we have to tweak the keto diet a little more for success in women," Gottfied writes.[‡] "We are not simply smaller versions of men, and our hormones require more support."

* https://dranthonygustin.com/no-ketosis-does-not-ruin-womens-hormones/

† http://online.liebertpub.com/doi/abs/10.1089/ars.2010.3253; http://avmajournals. avma.org/doi/pdf/10.2460/javma.2002.220.1315; http://onlinelibrary.wiley.com/ doi/10.1196/annals.1396.037/full; http://www.sciencedirect.com/science/article/pii/ S0197458006001084; http://jcem.endojournals.org/content/91/8/3232.long

‡ https://www.saragottfriedmd.com/the-ketogenic-diet-for-women/

CLEAN KETO VS DIRTY KETO: WHAT'S THE DIFFERENCE?

First, I'd like to give a personal shout-out to whoever invented the labels *dirty keto* and *clean keto*. I've been talking about this concept for a decade, but I never had a name for it. Now I do, and it doesn't only apply to keto.

Let me explain.

For years, when we nutritionists talked about lowering insulin resistance with a higher-fat, moderate-protein, lower-carb diet, we emphasized the effect of macros (protein, carbs, and fat) on hormonal health. We knew that fat was the macronutrient that had the least impact on the hormone insulin (also known as "the fat-storing hormone"). We also knew that it didn't much matter where the fat came from, at least as far as insulin was concerned, whether its source was crummy damaged fats, margarine, or pro-inflammatory processed oils like canola and soybean. Insulin ignored good fat, bad fat, ugly fat—all fat. And ditto with protein. When we talked about protein in the early days, few of us bothered to distinguish between 100% grass-fed meat and McDonald's, because the body's hormonal response would be the same. Protein is more satiating, regardless of where it comes from, and is less likely to produce spikes in insulin than carbohydrates (though *more* likely than fat).

But while it may not matter *hormonally* where your food comes from, it matters enormously when it comes to overall health. This is where the notion of "dirty" versus "clean" comes in. For example, when low-carb started to reach critical mass in the early 1990s, everyone seemed to be interested in one metric and one metric only—*how many grams of carbs does it have?* As I pointed out many times, it was the wrong question to ask. Gasoline doesn't have *any* carbs at all, but that doesn't mean I want to drink it. We have to look at food *quality*, not just at macro percentages.

And that's what dirty versus clean keto is all about.

You can go into nutritional ketosis via "Dirty Keto" (i.e., junk protein and junk fats) or you can do it via "Clean Keto," the healthiest versions of those foods that it's possible to find.

Obviously, the latter is the preferable way to go. And that's true whether you're doing a keto diet or any other diet. For overall health, food quality probably matters far more than macro percentages.

11. THE METABOLIC FACTOR
JONNY BOWDEN, PHD, CNS

WHAT IT IS IN A NUTSHELL

A cyclical ketogenic program designed to change your metabolism from sugar-burner to fat-burner in 22 days. The program is basically keto, interrupted by strategically placed "carb feasts," timed for maximal metabolic and weight-loss benefits.

About the Metabolic Factor

The Metabolic Factor is a program by Jonny Bowden, PhD, CNS. Hopefully you can see the challenge in writing about it here.

Obviously, I believe in this program, which represents my current best thinking about how to get on the path to metabolic, hormonal, physical, and mental health, and lose a bunch of weight in the bargain—all in 22 days. I wanted to include it because it's out there, I'm proud of it, it's worked for thousands of people, and I wanted you to know about it. At the same time, I didn't want to be "that guy," using my book to "promote" my own program over any of the other excellent ones I'm writing about.

This section will be relatively brief. I'll outline the structure of the Metabolic Factor program and the basic rationale behind it, point out how it fits with the principles in this book, and share some of the benefits I've seen for thousands of people who have tried the program since the first version of it appeared online a few years ago. If you want more details—and I hope you will—you can access the program from the Metabolic Factor link on my website (jonnybowden.com), get more information, and take advantage of the no-hassles, no-questions-asked 30-day free trial.

Meanwhile, here are the basics. Metabolic Factor is a *cyclical ketogenic* program. You cycle in and out of keto, breaking your routine with strategically placed high-carb meals that are built into the program and used in a very targeted way. We call these meals "carb feasts." The insertion of these meals into the program at very specific times helps you avoid some of the pitfalls we've seen with all-keto all-the-time programs, such as monotony, compliance, and plateaus.

With Metabolic Factor, you spend the first 10 days eating what's essentially a keto diet, although we don't call it keto and there's no requirement that you measure ketones. On the tenth day, you indulge in a *carb feast*, a meal in which you can eat anything you like. And yes, you read that correctly—and yes, "anything" *does* include whatever food you were just wondering about, including chips. On the eleventh day, you return to the original keto-friendly program, which you interrupt again by a carb feast meal on the fourteenth, eighteenth, and twenty-first days. Rinse and repeat for the *next* 22 days, *or* stop and modify it for your specific needs. We show you exactly how to do that in the program, with the goal of giving you maximum metabolic flexibility.

The promise of the program is to take you from being a "sugar burner" to being a "fat burner," or at least get you well on your way to fat-burner status, in 22 days. As you'll learn during the program, transitioning to a fat-burning metabolism is great for shrinking the size of your belly, but a fat-burning metabolism has a lot of other health advantages too: Fat is a "clean-burning" fuel. When you burn fat, it doesn't produce as many of the chemicals that cause inflammation and oxidative damage as burning sugar does. These chemicals are at the core of virtually every degenerative disease we know of. In fact, they're at the core of aging itself.

That's why moving from a sugar-burning to a fat-burning metabolism not only helps you burn fat and stay looking and feeling young, it also reduces your risk of the following:

- Pre-diabetes/metabolic syndrome/type 2 diabetes
- Heart disease
- High blood pressure
- Cancer
- Quicker aging—more wrinkles, declining skin condition and appearance, etc.
- Exhaustion, fatigue, and lack of energy and endurance
- Low sex drive and/or stamina
- Poor mood—depression, anxiety, anger
- Hormonal imbalance
- Loss of lean muscle mass

Fat is precisely and exactly the perfect fuel to power our cellular machinery. Fat is what we want our cells to run on. Your body can store about 69 gazillion calories of fat in your fat tissues (triglycerides), but only about 1,800 to 2,000 calories of sugar (as glycogen). That's because sugar should only be used sparingly—in emergencies.[*]

---

[*] There are a few cells that run exclusively on sugar. These are nerve cells, red blood cells, and the adrenal medulla.

Sugar is the perfect fuel if you need a quick burst of energy lasting under 30 seconds, because the body can use that sugar instantly, while it takes up to 20 minutes for the body to mobilize a significant amount of fat.[43]

Sugar is great in a pinch—but when you're *primarily* a sugar-burner, you stay fat, sick, tired, and depressed. For sustained energy, you're much better off being able to use fat as your primary fuel. Nature knew what she was doing when she gave you an endless supply of fat.

The question is, how do we access these storage tanks of fat that seem to pile up in the last places we need them on our body? It feels like our fat stores—which cling stubbornly to all the places we don't want them to cling—are like a giant store of fuel in a tank with a locked gas nozzle. What if we could unlock that gas tank of metabolic energy and start to actually burn the fat that takes up space on our butt, thighs, and hips? Wouldn't that be wondrous?

The Metabolic Factor program helps you do just that by following the three laws of metabolism. The program itself goes into great detail about these three laws, and how to use them to your advantage, but here's a brief introduction:

1. The Law of Metabolic Compensation

One of the easiest ways to conceptualize your metabolism is to think of it like a seesaw. A push in one direction is always matched by a pull in the other. If your metabolic machinery says "hungry," it'll be matched by a response ("eat!"). The metabolism is always adjusting to different circumstances. Anything that stimulates it in one direction is ultimately met with a response in the opposite direction. The body is always seeking that state where the seesaw is evenly balanced, a state known in science as *homeostasis.*

Now, it should be easy to understand what happens when you eat less and exercise more, which has been the standard weight-loss advice in this country for decades. The metabolism responds to this "deprivation" state with more hunger, lower energy, increased cravings, and a slower metabolic rate. Those changes stack the deck against you being able to maintain that deprivation state—you'll soon end up eating more and exercising less. You'll regain any lost fat, and possibly a few more pounds just for good measure. That's metabolic compensation. You've got to use it to your advantage, or it will just keep "compensating," and you'll stay at the same weight.

2. The Law of Metabolic Multitasking

An awful lot of people have come to me for weight loss when they're at the end of their rope and nothing else has worked. These folks have done particularly badly on programs that start them out with a whole new way of eating and a whole new exercise program. In my experience, that's a recipe for failure. We don't do that on Metabolic Factor, and here's why:

When you eat less and exercise more, you may burn fat, but you also break down muscle. The result is you get smaller but flabbier, a condition often referred to as "skinny fat." Exercising more and eating more protein may build or maintain muscle, but it does very little to burn fat. This results in a bigger, more bulky appearance. Gaining muscle over a layer of fat is like putting on a form-fitting jacket over two ski sweaters. Of *course* you look bulky.

The body likes to be burning *or* building—it's not a fan of doing both at the same time; and frankly, it's not very good at it. In Metabolic Factor, we focus on unlocking your fat stores *first*, so we can begin burning them. Building and shaping muscle will come later. Most people make the mistake of trying to do everything at once.

3. The Law of Metabolic Individuality

When it comes to finding the sweet spot for health and fitness, balance is the name of the game. It's what we call the Goldilocks effect—not too *much*, not too *little*. You want it *just right*.

And here's the real secret: There *is* no one-size-fits-all diet. I've been saying this ever since my first book in 2001, and I'll probably be saying it for as long as I'm writing and teaching. Listen carefully, because this is a core truth: *You are not like every other person on the planet.*

You are like *some* other people in some ways, completely *different* from those same people in other ways, and completely *unique* in still other ways. You're unique metabolically, you're unique psychologically, you're unique hormonally, and you're definitely unique in your personal preferences.

One of the best pieces of advice that I (or any other health "guru") can give you is this: *stop studying programs and diets and start studying you!* That's the only way on earth to really find out how, for example, eating carbs affects *your* body. Who really cares how they affect your mom, your neighbor, your hairdresser, Beyoncé, the people in a magazine's weight-loss issue, or the super-fit people at the gym?

Metabolic Factor is all about giving you the tools to do your own tinkering so that at the end of the day, the right plan for you will evolve from your own experimentation, a plan that you can sustain *and* that actually works for *you.*

Earlier I mentioned something I called metabolic flexibility. That's one of the most impressive benefits we're seeing in people who go through the program. After all, you want your metabolism to be able to effectively handle any fuel that comes down the pike. You want your metabolism to be able to dig into your fat stores and use those fats for energy on a regular basis, but you *also* want to be able to handle a piece of birthday cake once in a while. Metabolic flexibility is the goal of the Metabolic Factor.

One thing I've noticed during my 30-year career is how many health professionals who started out in the diet world (like me) are talking less and less about what you eat and more and more about how you live. That's not because nutrition isn't important—obviously, nutritionists like me wouldn't be passionate about what you should eat if we didn't think nutrition mattered! But what all of us are realizing—and I think I can speak for just about every functional-medicine practitioner I've ever met here— is that health is about a lot more than what's at the end of your fork. It's about the condition of your gut (your microbiome), how you digest and absorb nutrients, how you sleep, how you manage stress, how your body handles toxins, how strong your relationships are, how much (and what kind of) exercise you get, and even—or maybe especially—how much you love.

Most weight-loss programs that don't address these vitally important factors are doomed to long-term failure, because every single one of the things I just mentioned—sleep, stress, diet, exercise, detoxification—impacts your waistline. The Metabolic Factor addresses each of these pathways to health and gives you specific steps you can take to improve them.

I hope you'll check it out from the link to The Metabolic Factor on my website, or from any other link that you may see in a health-oriented mailing list that has promoted it (thanks, everyone!). I hope you'll read more about it—and, if you're interested, take it for a trial spin.

The Metabolic Diet as a Lifestyle: Who It Works For, Who Should Look Elsewhere

I was frankly surprised by the wide range of people who have been helped by Metabolic Factor and have written to us to describe their successes, many of which have been nothing less than remarkable. The carb feast seems to give people a much-needed sense of security about trying keto—because they're never more than a few days away from any food they want to consume. So compliance on this program was higher than any other program I've ever written.

If you're willing to eat differently for a while—i.e., a high-fat, moderate-protein, very–low-carb diet—the cyclical nature of Metabolic Factor makes it a much lighter lift for keto experimenters. The dropout rate has been vanishingly low, and the vast majority of people who've tried it have continued on it well past the initial 22 days.

Every author likes to believe that the audience for their books is "everybody," and every diet-book author wants to believe that their diet is perfect for everybody—but neither is so, ever. That said, Metabolic Factor seems to appeal to a huge variety of people in all stages of weight-loss resistance, including many who have failed multiple times on other diet programs. It may not be for everybody, but it sure can benefit a whole lot of people.

JONNY'S LOWDOWN

I've written approximately 4 weight-loss programs in my 30-year career, beginning with Diet Boot Camp back in the 1990's. Each program after that has incorporated the best of what I had done prior, and expanded on it.

Metabolic Factor is the latest version, and it incorporates everything I've learned about dieting, compliance, metabolism, weight loss, and overall health. I'm very proud of it, and am clearly not objective, but I believe it's one of the finest and safest and most scientifically sound of the weight-loss programs available.

IV. NEW AND NOTABLE
(OR THE REST OF THE GANG)

Here are some programs that don't fit neatly into any of the previous categories, but have certain shared principles with many of the programs discussed so far, such as their emphasis on "no low-fat" as a failed philosophy. They all have interesting quirks and distinctions, and appeal to different people at different times for different reasons.

12. WHOLE30
MELISSA HARTWIG

WHAT IT IS IN A NUTSHELL

A balls-to-the-wall, take-no-prisoners 30-day program in which you eat NOTHING but whole, unprocessed foods.

About Whole30

Whole30 is the ice-bucket challenge of diets.

Just imagine what you might eat on one of those weight-loss-as-entertainment shows with an ex-marine sergeant as the trainer. The kind of trainer that holds you 100% accountable, accepts no excuses, and takes no prisoners. On this program, when a food is "forbidden," it's *forbidden*. There are no gray areas. The rules are black and white.

That's the kind of program we're talking about.

And that's the "bad" news. The "good" news is that it only lasts 30 days.

The program was born as a kind of self-experiment—a "hack" before "bio-hacking" made its way into the popular lexicon. Melissa Hartwig, an ex-addict who turned her life around with fitness and owned a strength-and-conditioning facility, was talking one day with the original cofounder of Whole30. The two had just finished a brutal workout and were trying to figure out what they could do to improve. How could they better their performance? How could they improve their recovery?

They decided—wisely—to focus on reducing inflammation. Since chronic inflammation is a contributor to or promoter of every single degenerative disease on the planet—and since athletes are frequently sidelined by it—targeting inflammation made a lot of sense.

A certified sports nutritionist, Hartwig began by removing the foods that were at the top of every food sensitivity list or at least were known anecdotally to cause problems for a lot of her clients: dairy, grains, sugar, alcohol, and legumes.

Through her blog, she invited 200 people to participate with her new eating plan: Completely eliminating all the foods or food groups in the above list for 30 days. People reported the elimination of cravings, and the disappearing of symptoms (such as bloating, brain fog, depression, and anxiety). They also noted improved sleep, more energy, and, incidentally, weight loss. The "30-day challenge" went viral, and Whole30 was born. Ten years after its initial inception, the Whole30 empire now claims six *New York Times* bestsellers, a website that, as of 2019, serves 2 million unique visitors a month from over 100 countries, and a social media base of more than 2 million fans.

This very popular program doesn't even pretend to fit into the categories we're discussing in this chapter. And to be clear, its founder takes umbrage at the notion that her program is even a "diet" (more about that in a moment). It's definitely not a ketogenic diet, and it splits with paleo on a number of details. Unlike paleo, for example, there is absolutely no alcohol allowed on Whole30, nor are there any sugars, including the unrefined, natural ones.

We're discussing the Whole30 program here because if we were to draw a Venn diagram of dietary approaches, we'd see a lot of areas where keto, paleo, and Whole30 overlap. Though Whole30 is by no means a "low-carb" diet (you can eat as much fruit and vegetables as you like), it shares with most low-carb programs a less-than-welcoming attitude to cereal, grains, breads, and pastas. Our hypothetical Venn diagram would also show a huge overlap between Whole30 and the clean-eating movement, embraced by many people in both the paleo and keto communities. (See the discussion of "clean vs. dirty keto," page 252). Like keto (and some paleo programs), Whole30 has no restriction on saturated fat, nor does the program forbid meat. The ban on grains and dairy is certainly nothing you'd find in "conventional" diet programs (which is why conventional dietitians and doctors tend to dismiss Whole30), but these bans are quite at home in the keto and paleo worlds. And if you think getting precise macronutrient distributions for paleo or keto is hard, it's downright impossible with Whole30. Whole30 doesn't even talk about macros.

What it *does* talk about is the quality of the food. The basic mandate is that if it comes in a package, has unpronounceable ingredients, was processed in a factory, contains sugar, or looks like something your great-grandmother wouldn't recognize as "food," you can't eat it. Period.

In that sense, the program does have a lot in common with paleo— and, indeed, some pundits have characterized Whole30 as a stricter and less-forgiving version of paleo. It's easy to see why. Both avoid sugar, grains, legumes, and dairy, but Whole30 goes further by completely eliminating "natural" sugars like honey and typical "paleo treats." If it's a natural, unprocessed, or minimally processed food, it's okay to eat on Whole30. That includes pasture-raised animals (including organ meats), wild-caught fish, every vegetable and fruit on the planet, and a wide variety of healthy, natural fats (including saturated fats from healthy sources like grass-fed beef), coconut oil, Malaysian red palm oil, and of course seafood.

Oh, and one more thing: no dessert. One of the rules of the program is the following: "Do not consume baked goods, junk foods, or treats with 'approved' ingredients." There's even an acronym for this kind of thing— being compliant with the *letter* of the law but not the spirit. [In Whole30 World, it's called SWYPO—sex with your pants on.] "Recreating or buying sweets, treats, and 'foods-with-no-brakes' (even if the ingredients are technically compliant) is totally missing the point of the Whole30 and will compromise your life-changing results," says Hartwig. She points out that a pancake is still a pancake, even if it's made with coconut flour. Basically all waffles, tortillas, biscuits, muffins, cupcakes, cookies, brownies, pizza crust, cereal, and ice cream are off the menu. Whole30's mantra is "when in doubt, leave it out."

If you're thinking this is tough love, you're right. "*Don't you dare tell me this is hard,*" writes Hartwig.[44] "Fighting cancer is hard. Birthing a baby is hard. Losing a parent is hard. Drinking your coffee black. Is. Not. Hard. You've done harder things than this, and you have no excuse not to complete the program as written. It's only thirty days, and it's for the most important health cause on earth—the only physical body you will ever have in this lifetime."

Hartwig is adamant that Whole30 is not a diet. It's not something that's meant to be done all the time, and it's not even something that you're meant to return to time and time again. It's meant to act as a "reset" for your body and your mind, a way to understand your own hunger cues and identify your personal food triggers—foods that set you up for overeating, binging, or cravings, or create identifiable symptoms like brain fog or fatigue. It's about experiencing what your body actually feels like when it's functioning at its highest level and cultivating a whole new relationship with food and with your own body.

"I honestly think that's [what] differentiates us from every other program out there," says Hartwig.[45] "If you don't have access to the foods you would otherwise reward yourself or show yourself love with, you're forced to find other, healthier ways to show yourself self-care. And it's an enormous learning opportunity that stays with you after your Whole30 is over."

Does it work? Well, it's never been scientifically studied in the way that, for example, keto diets have been studied, with peer-reviewed papers in scientific journals. All we have is "anecdotal" evidence. But the anecdotal evidence is pretty impressive and the program has millions of diehard fans. On the face of it, I can't think of a single reason why someone eating a 100% no-junk diet and consuming nothing but whole foods for 30 days would be anything but good. My only consideration is how lasting the change would be.

But What About U.S. News and World Report?

Whole30 and keto occupied the last two places in *U.S. News and World Report's* "best diet" rankings for 2018. (Paleo didn't do much better.) This is more a statement about *U.S. News and World Report* than it is about the programs themselves. With few exceptions, the panel is composed of mainstream academics, and the standards by which they judge tend to fall in line with the talking points of conventional dietitians. Any diet that doesn't limit saturated fat is going to lose points, and any diet that "cuts out major food groups" (like grains) is going to go to the bottom of the pile. The *U.S. News and World Report* panel tends to give high marks to commercial diets that hawk processed foods (like Jenny Craig), love diets that limit fat and sodium (like the DASH diet), and consider anything that isn't in line with government guidelines a "fad" diet. (For those who might have forgotten, we're talking about the same government guidelines that gave us the food pyramid.)

Whole30 as a Lifestyle: Who It Works For, Who Should Look Elsewhere

I think this is a great plan if you're into challenges. If, for example, you signed up for the 30-Day Butt Challenge or the 100-Pushup Challenge, you're going to find Whole30 right up your alley. It takes a lot of dedication and commitment, and it's not easy. But if you are the type to really put your mind to something for 30 days and commit to it 100%, this program will undoubtedly reward you.

If you're not that person . . . look elsewhere.

JONNY'S LOWDOWN

This is a hard program to evaluate, since it's really more of an experience than a diet. (Now you know why I compared it to the ice-bucket challenge.) The foods are great, and the goals are admirable (who couldn't use a new relationship with food?).

My issue is with what happens afterward.

With the Atkins diet, for example, you know exactly what to do after the initial (potentially difficult) "induction" period—you add back carbohydrate foods methodically and carefully in measured portions. You monitor both your weight and how you feel so you can decide how much of these foods to include. With Whole30, you're on your own after 30 days, at least as far as program specifics go. There's no formula that tells you what you can add back and when. I think this would make it difficult for a lot of people. By the same token, there's absolutely no reason why you can't do the Whole30 challenge and then move to a more sustainable way of eating that's a little more forgiving.

I would lump Whole30 into the class of experiences that include sweat lodges, jumping out of an airplane, marriage retreats, ayahuasca ceremonies, and the Landmark Forum. They're powerful, one-time experiences that have the potential to be life-changing if you find a way to incorporate the lessons you've learned doing them into your everyday life. If you can do that, more power to you. If Whole30 helps you to be more conscious about food, more in touch with your own triggers, and more able to successfully navigate the toxic food environment we all live in, then all I can say is a resounding "Right on, brother!"

13. THE CARNIVORE DIET
SHAWN BAKER

WHAT IT IS IN A NUTSHELL
An all-meat diet.

About the Carnivore Diet

I'll be honest. When I first set up an interview with Dr. Shawn Baker to discuss his Carnivore Diet, I assumed he was a pretty crazy dude. Granted, I had never met him, but I knew that his *diet*—which can be summed up as "eat meat, drink water"—was about as far-out and extreme as you could get in the nutrition world.

And I—like many of the people who are now converts to the carnivore way of life—had a lot of questions.

For example: What about vitamin C? In fact, what about *all* the vitamins and polyphenols and anti-inflammatories and antioxidants found in fruits and vegetables? And what about fiber, for goodness' sake? How do you even go to the bathroom?

I figured this guy had to be one of those wild-man-in-the-woods Ted Nugent types who goes bow-hunting for wild caribou, an interesting character, no doubt, but certainly—from a nutritional point of view—pretty off the wall.

Now, I'm not so sure.

Let's get the basics of the diet out of the way, because this is just about the simplest plan ever invented. You eat nothing but animal products. That's it. As one Internet pundit put it, "eat meat when you're hungry, drink water when you're thirsty." And though it's not really limited to red meat—you can also eat dairy and eggs—it *is* limited to animal products.

The other thing to know about the carnivore diet is that there's basically no research on it—at least, not the kind of research there is on, say, the Mediterranean Diet, or the Ketogenic Diet. (Extremely attentive readers may recall the 1920s experiment discussed on page 26, in which the explorer Vilhjalmur Stefansson spent time at Bellevue Hospital in New York being observed and monitored by a team of doctors while eating nothing but meat and fat. We'll come back to Vilhjalmur in just a minute.)

So, most if not all of the info we have on the carnivore diet is what's known as "anecdotal" evidence. It comes from the experiences of people we hear about, know about, read about, follow on social media—but not from peer-reviewed, scientifically conducted studies. While scientists consider anecdotal evidence unreliable, we should remember that anecdotal observations—especially when those observations happen frequently in a wide variety of settings—are the best material for forming and testing hypotheses. This is why anecdotal evidence shouldn't be ignored.

Vilhjalmur Stefansson's experience in the Arctic, eating the way the Inuit did—a virtually all-animal-food diet—was anecdotal. He did it, he wrote about it, he apparently thrived on it, and he became quite the "zero-carb" advocate, though they didn't call it "zero-carb" at the time. While the Bellevue experiment was an attempt to look at this experience scientifically, it was still the experience of just one man.

Even back then in the 1920s, eating an all-meat diet was nutritional heresy. Doctors were recommending that you eat plenty of vegetables, and Stefansson's advocacy of meat (with plenty of fat, mind you) flew in the face of everything that was (and still is) believed by most nutritional experts. (For those who want to read more about Stefansson, I recommend "Adventures in Diet Part 1" from the November 1935 issue of *Harper's Monthly Magazine*, written by Stefansson himself,[46] or "The Arctic Explorer Who Pushed An All-Meat Diet" from *Atlas Obscura*, available online.[47]

Fast-forward almost a hundred years, to Dr. Shawn Baker.

Now, the first thing you notice when you see a picture of Shawn Baker—go on, look him up, I'll wait, I'm sure you're curious—is that he looks like the guy a Hollywood director would pick if he had to cast a superhero to fight against a villain played by Vin Diesel. Baker is just under 6 feet tall, around 240 pounds, and would be right at home shirtless on the cover of *Muscle and Fitness*. He's also a world-class athlete who holds or set world records in the deadlift (772 pounds) and Concept 2 Indoor Rowing. In addition to his medical credentials—he's an orthopedic surgeon who was chief of orthopedics at Bagram Air Base in Afghanistan—he also won first place in the Texas Strongest Man competition and fifth place in the USA Strongest Man competition. He's been a drug-free athlete all his life.

When a guy like this talks about nutrition and performance, you tend to pay attention.

Baker doesn't make any universal claims for his diet. He doesn't say it's for everyone, and—when you talk to him—you get the feeling he's *almost* as surprised by the results as you are. He told me that most of what we know about nutrition is population-based. Looking at hundreds of thousands of people over many years, eating vegetables tends to be associated with greater health. While data like that yields some good "public-policy" generalizations ("eat your vegetables"), it tells you nothing about how any given *individual* is going to do on any given diet. Baker—who was clearly focused on his own individual athletic performance and general health—simply found what worked for him, and is sharing that info with other people.

What he does *not* do is proselytize. "I am absolutely certain of only one thing," he told me, "and that is that I'm wrong about something."

Baker has meticulously documented his own personal journey online, frequently putting up his own lab results. He calls what he's doing an "N of 1" study. (In scientific studies, N refers to the number of subjects; an "N of 1" means you're basically documenting the results of one individual.) That said, there are a fair number of people online doing the same thing. I was surprised to see how many "zero-carbers" are documenting their results, complete with lab tests. And I was equally surprised to find out how well they're doing. Baker himself told me that his inflammatory markers (including homocysteine and interleukin-6) are vanishingly low. He has no vitamin deficiencies, and he feels great.

"I just figure that if I'm getting leaner, if my body composition is getting better, if my joints stop hurting, my digestion gets better, my mental health gets better, my libido improves, my sleep improves—well, most people can see that's a good result," he told me in a recent interview. "I think we need to drop the dogma about how we get there and just focus on the results. That's ultimately what this diet is about."

Baker points out that some of the benefits of his diet—and of keto or very–low-carb in general—come about because of what you're *not* eating, what you're getting rid of. "There's really no junk food on a carnivore diet," he says. The question of junk factory-farmed meat came up. While Baker knows grass-fed is better, he also knows it's not practical or affordable for a large number of people. "It's a big picture/small picture thing," he said. "A grain-fed steak still beats a box of cereal."

Asked about the voluminous literature linking fruits and vegetables and fiber with good health outcomes, he points out that this is still based on mostly epidemiological evidence. "There's not a great, robust bunch of literature looking at randomized control trials with fruits and vegetables showing a great benefit," he told me. "And there are many compounds in plants that are just flat-out deleterious, particularly as the dosage gets higher and higher." He pointed out oxalates, phytates, phytic acid, lectins, and gluten as examples. "I think that everyone's tolerance is a little different," he said. "I know for me, personally, removing these fiber foods from my diet has tremendously improved my digestive health, and I think that, if nothing else, it has been a great benefit."

It's really important to understand that even though this kind of eating may be referred to online as an "all-protein" diet, and might even *sound* like an "all-protein" diet, it is decidedly *not* 100% protein. (If it were, you would die from a condition known as "rabbit starvation.") On a calorie-for-calorie basis, meat is mostly fat (unless you're consuming virtually fat-free meat like rabbit). "If I were to calorically guess what I get from fat, it's probably around 60–70% of what my diet is. The rest is mostly protein, with trace amounts of carbohydrates," Baker told me. Point taken. Do *not* try a low-fat version of a carnivore-type diet!

If you've read this far, you're probably wondering if the Carnivore Diet is a ketogenic diet. "I have never once checked my ketone levels," Baker told me. "I never cared about that. My goal with a diet is not a ketone level. It's how do I feel, how do I perform, and how do I function."

The Carnivore Diet as a Lifestyle: Who It Works For, Who Should Look Elsewhere

It should be immediately obvious that this diet is not for everyone. First of all, eating nothing but meat would be wildly unappealing to a huge segment of the population. Second of all, the quality of meat available to most of us is pretty terrible, so unless you were willing to go 100% grass-fed, it would be hard to recommend a carnivore diet since you'd be eating factory-farmed garbage. And third of all, maintaining carnivore status can be a real challenge when you eat with other people or are part of a family that's not all committed to the same program.

That said, there seems to be a certain segment of the population that thrives on this diet. To get a sense of this, do some searching on Twitter. Carnivore dieters—many of them MDs—love to post their blood tests, which are uniformly impressive and scarily counterintuitive. If that kind of rebellious contrarianism appeals to you, this might be your perfect diet.

JONNY'S LOWDOWN

This diet is obviously not for everyone. But it's hard to deny how well it works when it does work. (The celebrity psychologist Jordan Peterson and his daughter Mikhaila are converts, and Mikhaila has documented her journey online, as have other enthusiasts.[48]) Baker told me that the diet is so satiating that he often only eats one to two meals a day. One result of his diet is that he winds up doing an awful lot of intermittent fasting. And that comes with benefits of its own.

Full disclosure: when my weight is slightly up, I'll use a day or two of carnivore eating to get back on track. It almost always does the trick. (The once-popular Dukan Diet featured a similar technique called "Protein Thursday," a one-day boot camp where you ate nothing but protein and the fat that comes with it. Dr. Pierre Dukan—who became famous as the doctor who kept Kate Middleton in shape—recommended a day of protein as a kind of metabolic reset which you could use to knock off a pound or two quickly if you saw that you were gaining a little too much weight. That technique has always worked for me, personally.)

There's a notion in logic that you only need one exception to disprove an absolute. So, for example, the absolute statement "All swans are white" needs only the existence of a single black swan to disprove it. Shawn Baker—and others who are getting similar results with this diet—may be black swans. They may never be in the majority—they may even be outliers. But the fact that they exist at all—and that they are clearly doing as well as they are—disproves a lot of "absolutes" that we believe about diet, such as the notion that meat is always bad.

This diet—and the results that some people are getting with it—causes us to question some nutritional orthodoxy and reexamine some cherished beliefs about our diet. At the very least, it should serve as an object lesson in the basic principle of biochemical individuality. Everybody's different. And it's undeniable that some people—we don't know how many, but we sure know it's more than a couple—are doing spectacularly well with this diet, by any metric you care to use. And unlike a lot of anecdotal evidence, many of these folks are documenting those results with objective data like medical tests.

For those reasons alone, I think it's worth paying attention to.

14. KETOTARIAN
WILL COLE, MD

WHAT IT IS IN A NUTSHELL

A plant-centric ketogenic diet, suitable or adaptable for vegetarians and vegans.

About Ketotarian

Ketotarian is a blend of two of the most popular (and controversial) diets in modern times—vegan and keto. It's the brainchild of Will Cole, MD, a functional-medicine doctor who, along with best-selling author, podcaster, and blogger Jimmy Moore, hosts the popular podcast Keto Talk. Cole advocates a ketogenic diet for all the reasons you've read about in this section. "The benefits of this approach to eating go far beyond just losing weight," he says.

Let's start with mitochondrial function, a huge benefit of keto diets that not a lot of authors emphasize. Mitochondria are found in almost every cell in the body and are responsible for producing 90% of the energy we need to function (which is why they're often referred to as the "energy factories" of the cell). They're so important that they even have their own DNA. Loss of function in the mitochondria—often referred to as mitochondrial dysfunction—can result in excess fatigue and other symptoms that are common signs of almost every chronic disease.[49] Ketogenic diets have been shown to increase the creation of new mitochondria, a process called mitochondrial biogenesis.[50]

Cole also focuses on autophagy as another benefit of the keto diet. The word *autophagy* combines *auto* (the prefix that means "self") and *phagy* (the suffix that means "eating"). It refers to a kind of cellular cannibalism that our bodies perform to get rid of the bad stuff and strengthen the good. Because it's responsible for removing cellular debris, autophagy is believed to play a big role in longevity and optimal health. A great way to "turn on" autophagy is with a keto diet and its partner in health, intermittent fasting. "Keeping autophagy at a healthy, active level is another way to keep your inflammation levels balanced, and prevent accelerated aging and disease," Cole counsels.

Cole agrees with a point often made by keto advocates: Keto diets may help with cancer. We know for a fact that cancer cells depend heavily on sugar—it's their own version of mother's milk. (There's even a name for this—the Warburg effect.[51]) We also know for a fact that keto diets are *by definition* very, very low in sugar. The hypothesis that a no-sugar diet might be a good thing for keeping cancer at bay certainly passes the smell test. And sure enough, a number of studies have indeed shown that keto diets can help reduce tumor size and the growth of certain cancers like stomach,[52] lung,[53] prostate,[54] and glioblastoma.[55]

Then there's inflammation. "What I love about the Keto Diet is its ability to lower inflammation," Dr. Cole told me when I interviewed him for this book. He points out that studies that show that beta-hydroxybutyrate—one of the three ketone bodies produced by the body during nutritional ketosis—can help reduce proinflammatory proteins like NF-kappaB, COX-2, and NLRP3 inflammasome.

Cole highlights how the Keto Diet is terrific for controlling some of the underlying mechanisms responsible for high levels of chronic inflammation. One example: the Nrf2 pathway. Nrf2 (which stands for nuclear factor-like 2) is a protein that controls genes responsible for antioxidant and anti-inflammatory activity. When Nrf2 goes "up," inflammation goes down; conversely, when Nrf2 is low, inflammation goes up. Ketones produced during nutritional ketosis "upregulate" Nrf2, turning up the volume on its powerful anti-inflammatory actions, while "downregulating" pro-inflammatory cytokines.[56] "The keto diet is very exciting for people with chronic inflammatory issues and mitochondrial issues, which typically go hand-in-hand, and is an amazing way to improve these pathways on a positive level," Cole told me.

Of course, let's not leave out one of the strongest accomplishments on the Ketogenic Diet résumé: the reduction or elimination of insulin resistance. "Insulin resistance is at the core of blood sugar problems and ends up wreaking havoc on the body, eventually leading to heart disease, weight gain, and diabetes," the functional-medicine specialist writes. And—there's not much controversy about this—the Ketogenic Diet lowers insulin levels. It also improves the cells' sensitivity to insulin, making them *less*, not more, insulin *resistant*. Less insulin resistant—and *more* insulin sensitive—is exactly what we want our cells to be.

So far, so good. But where does the vegan part come in?

Glad you asked.

Dr. Cole noticed a few things that disturbed him about the way some people were approaching keto—not all people, obviously, but enough to worry him. Many were so concerned with macros—the percentages of protein, carbs, and fat in their diets—that they were paying no attention to micros—vitamins, minerals, and other indicators of food quality. (Remember, it's possible to get into ketosis on junk food. See "Clean Keto vs. Dirty Keto" on page 252). Many of the foods that he saw his patients consuming might be "keto-friendly," all right, but being keto-friendly doesn't necessarily make them good for you. (We're talking to you, pro-inflammatory oils like corn, canola, soybean, safflower, and other "vegetable" oils we've been told to consume more of.)

By the same token, Dr. Cole noticed that many of his patients were staying clear of keto because they believed it was all about eating meat and saturated fat. And he noticed similar misconceptions even among those committed to keto diets—the notion that vegetables had to be significantly limited, for example. "Since keto is a low-carb diet and vegetables contain varying amounts of carbohydrates, I have seen countless well-intentioned keto eaters grow fearful of consuming vegetables. Sadly, they are unwittingly missing out on the phytonutrients and prebiotic foods needed for a healthy gut microbiome," he writes.

He also noticed that many keto-eaters consume a fair amount of dairy. While he doesn't believe there's anything inherently wrong with dairy (or meat, or fish, or eggs for that matter), he does note that dairy is one of the most common food allergens. Inflammation from dairy allergens or from lactose intolerance affects millions of people and can lead to symptoms ranging from gas and bloating to joint pain and eczema. "The A-1 subtype of beta-casein—which is the sub-type of beta-casein most common in U.S. cows—can be a trigger for digestive problems and inflammation," he says. (Note: There is now a form of milk sold in supermarkets that contains only the A-2 subtype of beta-casein, which is believed to be far less of a trigger for inflammation.)

Finally, some people just don't feel as well when they eat a lot of meat. Rightly or wrongly, for better or for worse, for ethical/moral/spiritual/metabolic/digestive reasons, they feel better on a meat-free (or relatively meat-free) diet. Ketotarian is perfect for them. "[It] marries the best of low-carb diets and a plant-based way of eating, while avoiding the common pitfalls that I have seen countless well-intentioned people make with both these diets," he writes. "The Ketotarian way of eating brings together healthy plant-based fats, clean protein, and the rich, vibrant colors of nutrient-dense vegetables."

Let me say that Dr. Cole is the least doctrinaire vegan I've ever encountered. He doesn't traffic in "vegan science"—you won't hear him repeat nonsense like "there's plenty of vitamin B-12 in plant foods!" nor will he try to equate plant-based omega-3s with the kind that come from fish. And speaking of fish, he's a big fan of the wild-caught variety (hardly a typical vegan menu choice).

Cole also doesn't trash the usual whipping boys of veganism: animal products and saturated fat. He's actually not opposed to either. "I don't think that saturated fat should be demonized," he told me. "I don't think it's bad for us." And there are plenty of saturated fats in Ketotarian, notably coconut oil and even organic ghee (a type of clarified butter), which, the last I looked, was definitely in the category of "animal product." (I told you he wasn't dogmatic!) While the recipes in Ketotarian are mostly vegetarian or vegan, he's a big fan of eggs, wild-caught salmon, and even—don't fall off your chair, now—the occasional grass-fed burger! (Apparently, he's gotten quite a bit of flack on social media for this, particularly from what we'll politely refer to as the "militant vegan fundamentalist" crew.)

So, what's up with this guy?

His own particular vegan journey offers a clue. He was a *strict* vegan for years. "I had to come to grips with the fact that I was eating *healthfully* but wasn't feeling *healthy*. Something was missing." He is now what some cynics might refer to as a "recovered vegan" (my words, not his).

Cole has found that many vegans are actually "carbatarians," living on bread, pasta, greens, and vegan desserts, pointing out that all too often, grains become the staple of the modern plant-based diet. "And if they aren't breadheads, they're depending too heavily on soy for their protein, which is typically genetically modified and always high in estrogens," he explains. "I see many vegans and vegetarians with wrecked digestion and declining health, clinging to their zealous belief that this is the way people should eat and live."

Yet—according to Cole—plant-based diets can, when done correctly, provide you with the nutrients you need to thrive. While Ketotarian is definitely plant-based—and would be considered keto-vegan—it also uses what Cole calls "a few key food medicines" to give people a little more variety of healthy fats and provide some nutrients that are next to impossible to get from vegan diets unless you supplement. Cole includes in this list of "food medicines" eggs (particularly egg yolks), grass-fed ghee, and wild-caught fish and shellfish.

What comes across very clearly in reading *Ketotarian* and spending an hour talking with its author is Cole's desire to offer people who don't eat meat—for whatever reason—an opportunity to experience keto with quality foods that are plant-based. Because it's not dogmatically vegan, it should probably be referred to as a plant-*centric* diet, which is what it really is.

One of the reasons that I personally have a warm spot for Cole's book is that it shares with my own program, Metabolic Factor, an emphasis on the switch from a sugar-burning metabolism to a fat-burning metabolism. That's really what ketogenic diets are all about. In fact, it's one of the main benefits of the diet, one that Cole emphasizes throughout the book. Having a fat-burning metabolism is known as being "keto-adapted," or "fat-adapted"—and it's the holy grail of a healthy metabolism.

"Becoming fat- or keto-adapted not only gives you sustainable energy throughout the day for your brain and metabolism, but also crushes food cravings," he writes. "In terms of energy for your body, fat is like a log on a fire: slow-burning, and long-lasting."

Ketotarian: Who It Works For, Who Should Look Elsewhere

This is an absolutely wonderful program for those who—for whatever reason—choose to not eat meat (or eat very little of it). It allows you to get all the benefits of nutritional ketosis while remaining vegetarian or vegan. But vegan purists beware—Cole is no fan of dogma, and is not militant about his recommendations. If you're looking for textbook veganism and a trashing of all animal-based products, you won't find it here. What you will find is an invitation to explore the benefits of ketosis while sticking to a plant-based—or *mostly* plant-based—way of eating.

JONNY'S LOWDOWN

Considering the increasingly partisan mood in nutritional politics, what Dr. Cole has done here is truly remarkable—he's managed to put together a mostly vegan program that does not trash meat or saturated fat, nor indulge in vegan science, while making a strong case for combining the best of the plant-based world with the proven benefits of keto. I say "Bravo." If I were ever to decide to go vegan, this is the program I'd follow.

15. #NSNG
VINNIE TORTORICH

WHAT IT IS IN A NUTSHELL

A simple program with exactly two rules: No sugar, no grains. Period.

About the #NSNG Diet

#NSNG is the brain child of Vinnie Tortorich, author of the bestselling book *Fitness Confidential* and resident on-air fitness and health correspondent for *The Adam Carolla Show*. Even though #NSNG may not be as well-known as some of the other programs in this book, it's wildly popular in the Twitter-sphere, due in equal measure to the pure simplicity of the program and to the undeniable charisma of its inventor.

Tortorich is a child of the Louisiana bayou, a tough-guy athlete whose skeptical view of conventional wisdom dovetails nicely with the ethos of *The Adam Carolla Show*. He came to California to be a trainer, and he succeeded— becoming one of the top go-to people for Hollywood stars and stars-to-be. That in turn landed him on *The Adam Carolla Show*, where his no-nonsense approach, sense of humor, and ability to communicate clearly resonated with Carolla's huge audience. It helped that he is accessible; he answers just about everyone who asks him anything on Twitter. He has a terrific (and popular) podcast called Fitness Confidential. He goes around the country working the lecture circuit. And he even performs in comedy clubs, where he sometimes shows clips from infomercials and riffs on some of the more ridiculous health claims. (Full disclosure: I've seen him. He's really funny.)

The reason his program is so popular—and why I'm including it in this book—is that it's breathtakingly simple. And it works. In the diet world, where it's next to impossible to get consensus on anything and where following a "diet" can sometimes feel like a cross between a math class and a political-science seminar, anything that is both effective and truly-really-madly-I'm-not-kidding simple has an immediate advantage.

So, here are the three rules of the program.

1. No sugar, no grains.

2. No sugar, no grains.

3. No sugar, no grains

In case you hadn't decoded the name #NSNG by now, it stands for . . . wait for it . . . *no sugar, no grains!*

I'm only partly being facetious. There is something tremendously appealing about a program that accomplishes everything you want a low-carb program to accomplish with just one stunningly simple rule. When someone asks me, for example, for a "quick tip" on how to lose (fill in the blank) pounds, #NSNG is my go-to. It gets the job done. It's great for Thanksgiving conversations, when you go home for the holidays and your relatives notice how much weight you've lost and want some quick "tips" so they can do the same thing. It's easy to remember, and in 90% or more of cases it's pretty much all you need to do to see a big result.

The program—like its creator—is not especially warm and fuzzy, but its no-BS approach is a big part of its appeal. I mentioned earlier that Vinnie Tortorich answers almost everything on Twitter. Don't expect long dissertations, respect for "safe spaces," and an avoidance of "trigger words." (You'll get short, direct, and to-the-point answers. "Can I eat this?" is answered simply "No!" "What do you think of this supplement?" is sometimes answered with "It's bullshit." While we're at it, Tortorich is no friend to the vegans. And don't get him started on quinoa.)

But keep in mind that a black-and-white approach to food and health is incredibly appealing for many who have suffered through the algorithms of multiple diet programs, only to wind up back in the same old place.

Although the only "rule" of the program is no sugar, no grains, many of the people who follow Tortorich's advice stay in nutritional ketosis a big part of the time, as does Tortorich himself. A cancer survivor, he believes his ketogenic diet—to which he adheres strictly—has been responsible for keeping his cancer in remission for over a decade.

#NSNG as a Lifestyle: Who It Works For, Who Should Look Elsewhere

Vinnie's program and his personal style have a definite appeal to a certain audience—tough-minded, independent, hard-performing athletes and fitness junkies. His absolutely no-nonsense, black-and-white approach is disarmingly attractive. And in an age when diet plans can sometimes seem like they require massive computational skills (proportions of carbs, protein, fat, etc.), the two-rule program is incredibly appealing.

The truth of the matter is that if you cut out sugar and grains, you'll basically be doing most of the heavy lifting that's needed for any version of low-carb found in this book. For people who find solace in simplicity—and who doesn't?—this plan is sheer bliss.

JONNY'S LOWDOWN

About the only thing that vegans and carnivores and everyone in between agrees on is sugar and how bad it is for our metabolic health. While it may be true that grains are not as "bad" for some people as they are for others, it's still hard to see how anyone wouldn't benefit from taking a vacation from them. At the end of the day, No Sugar No Grain could wind up being the single simplest and most effective four-word mantra in the world for anyone wanting to make a significant improvement in their health.

16. THE MEDITERRANEAN DIET
ANCEL KEYS

WHAT IT IS IN A NUTSHELL

A pattern of eating associated with the Mediterranean region—especially Italy—and characterized by lots of vegetables, fruits, nuts, fish, wine, and monounsaturated fat from olive oil.

For years, the Mediterranean Diet has been making headlines for boosting heart health and extending lifespan, thanks to research showing that people eating this way tend to be much healthier than Americans. Of course, when we think of a Mediterranean diet, we don't just think of the vegetables-fish-and-olive oil thing, we also think of high-carb foods like Greek pita bread and Italian pasta—making this way of eating seem pretty incompatible with low-carbing. But is that really the case?

First, let's clear up a big misconception right out the gate: there is no "one" Mediterranean Diet. This is a term that nutrition researchers came up with to describe an eating pattern that's high in monounsaturated fat (especially from extra-virgin olive oil and nuts), vegetables, legumes, seafood, unrefined grains and starches, herbs, spices, and red wine, with moderate amounts of foods like meat, dairy, and eggs. Within that framework, there's a huge amount of wiggle room. And even though high-carb foods *do* have a history in traditional cuisines in the Mediterranean region, that doesn't mean we have to eat them ourselves! In fact, a Mediterranean eating pattern is easily modifiable to fit a lower-carb lifestyle. All you have to do is ditch the starches and keep the healthy fats, vegetables, protein foods, and delicious seasonings.

In fact, some research suggests that taking out the grains might actually make the Mediterranean diet even healthier. One study pitted the Mediterranean Diet against its grain-free cousin, the Paleo Diet, among patients with heart disease plus either glucose intolerance or type 2 diabetes.[57] The main difference between the diets was the absence of grains and dairy in the Paleo Diet, and the use of margarine in the Mediterranean Diet. The results showed that paleo did an even better job than the Mediterranean Diet in lowering blood sugar levels and insulin, independent of weight loss. On top of that, scientists have studied ketogenic versions of the Mediterranean Diet (based on olive oil, vegetables, and fish), finding that it could significantly lower body weight, waist circumference, fat mass, blood pressure, blood sugar, total cholesterol, LDL cholesterol, and triglycerides, while dramatically increasing HDL cholesterol.[58] Clearly, there are ways to fit a Mediterranean eating pattern (and all the benefits it brings) into a healthy low-carb lifestyle!

The Mediterranean Diet as a Lifestyle: Who It Works For, Who Should Look Elsewhere

A pattern of eating that includes lots of fish, vegetables, nuts, and olive oil can work for just about anybody. The "beauty" of the Mediterranean Diet is that it's not a diet. You could follow the "general" guidelines (fish, vegetables, nuts, olive oil, whole grains), or you can make it low-carb by ditching the starches and grains. You could even do a Mediterranean version of keto if you got about 80% of your calories from olive oil.

JONNY'S LOWDOWN

This is a good basic template for healthy eating that could be customized and tweaked to be less "carb-y" by adding more grass-fed meat, fewer starches and breads, and a higher percentage of fat (mostly from olive oil and nut oils). But it's really important to remember that the health of the Mediterranean people—and their lowered risks for conditions like heart disease and Alzheimer's—is not just due to what they eat. The entire lifestyle is different. Big meals midday, lots of bonding time with friends, laughter, sunlight, and naps. Impossible to say that the diet alone is responsible for the good metrics often seen in observational studies of the Mediterranean diet. Still, the eating plan is a good one.

CHAPTER 10

Frequently Asked Questions

I n this chapter, I've posed and then answered the questions that I see most often on my website, as well as those I'm asked most frequently in seminars and workshops around the country. I've also incorporated the questions that I've seen come up time and time again on Internet sites dealing with low-carbohydrate diets. The questions are organized into categories, such as Losing Weight on Low-Carb, Food and Water, and Exercise.

Losing Weight on Low-Carb

How Long Will It Take Me to Lose 10 (or 100) Pounds?

There is absolutely no way to know the answer to this question. A lot depends on how much you have to lose and how you respond to your program. Everyone is fundamentally different on a metabolic, genetic, and biochemical level, and each body responds differently. Even two people on the same program are likely to experience different amounts of weight loss on different timetables. Rule of thumb: in the first week or so of a low-carb diet, you may lose a bunch of weight—maybe even 7 to 10 pounds if you are really overweight to begin with—but eventually you should settle in to an *average* of 2 pounds of weight loss per week, more or less. Remember, this amount is an average, and actual individual results vary. A lot. Try not to "buy in" to feelings of discouragement if your weight loss is less—many other things could be going on. And if you're sure that you're losing weight too "slowly," try to remind yourself that even at the rate of 1 pound a week, you'll still lose 50 pounds a year.

Is a Low-Carb Diet for Everyone?

Memorize this and tattoo it behind your eyelids: no single diet is for everyone. The Bantu of South Africa thrived on a diet of 80% carbs, and some groups of Eskimos thrived on a diet of nearly zero carbs. However, here in America and in most of the industrialized nations, it's fairly safe to say that nearly everyone would benefit from a *lower*-carb diet than is currently the norm. And *everyone* would benefit from changing their carbs from the highly processed, sugar-laden, fiberless fare of convenience, fast, and packaged foods to what we might call "real" carbohydrates—things you could pluck, gather, or grow.

How low in carbohydrates you personally need to go must be determined by trial and error. If you are a basically healthy person looking to stay that way and weight loss is not a real issue for you, you can't really go wrong with the template advocated by Barry Sears, which is approximately 40% of your food as carbohydrates, 30% as protein, and 30% as fat. (And make sure those carbs come from good sources, not canned spaghetti!) Interestingly, this template is very close to what many of the foundational plans discussed in this book—among them the Atkins diet, Protein Power, and the Fat Flush Plan—recommend for maintenance after your weight target has been achieved. And no less a luminary than the renowned Harvard epidemiologist Dr. Walter Willett has said, without actually mentioning the Zone diet, that a diet containing 40% carbs, 30% protein, and 30% fat may well be the healthiest alternative to the moribund USDA Food Guide Pyramid's (or its updated version, My Plate's) recommendations.

Understand that the 40/30/30 template is very different from the basic starting point of keto or paleo. But for someone without major health issues who wants to get his or her feet wet in the low-carb universe without necessarily committing to something like the Ketogenic or Paleo Diet, it's a perfect place to start.

Do You Have to Be in Ketosis to Lose Weight on a Low-Carb Diet?

No. You don't.

Ketosis is wonderful for many things, but it's actually not a "requirement" for most controlled-carb eating programs. It is stressed in the early version of Atkins, and it is likely to happen (but not essential) in Protein Power, the Paleo Solution, and a few other eating plans like Ketotarian and The Bulletproof Diet. But many other low-carb programs don't even mention it. Many nutrition experts—myself included—feel that you don't have to actually be in ketosis to get the benefits of a low-carb diet. You can "flirt" with and be on the cusp of ketosis, but unless you are very metabolically resistant, you may be able to get the benefits of low-carb eating without ever worrying about your ketone levels.

Perhaps the most sober and rational summary of the Ketogenic Diet is given by my friend Chris Kresser, LaC, who says, "The ketogenic diet is a potent therapeutic tool that can produce remarkable results when used appropriately, but it's neither a panacea nor a one-size-fits-all approach."[1]

That's pretty much identical to the assessment of Lyle McDonald. In 1998, McDonald published *The Ketogenic Diet: A Guide for the Dieter and Practitioner*, which was then the definitive book on the subject and supported by the greatest assemblage of scientific references on ketosis ever seen, at the time, in one place. (McDonald is still going strong, and his classic book is still available as an e-book.) He said back then: "After years of experimenting with the [ketogenic] diet myself, and getting feedback from hundreds and hundreds of people, about the best anyone can say is that the ketogenic diet is a diet that works very well for many but not for all."

Once I Reach My Goal Weight, Can I Add Carbs Without Gaining Weight?

Posts on Internet bulletin boards respond to this type of question with the acronym YMMV, which means "your mileage may vary." Translation: everyone responds differently, so try it out. All of the classic programs basically suggest adding carbs back in a controlled and measured way until you discover for yourself the "magic" amount that allows *you* to maintain your goal weight. Be aware, though, that some of the foods you cut out—for example, wheat—may have been causing other problems in addition to weight gain, which is why so many of the newer programs do without it entirely, regardless of whether weight-loss goals have been achieved. Monitor your reactions carefully if you do start adding stuff back.

Should I Weigh Myself Regularly?

Opinions vary on this, but my opinion is yes—if you can prevent yourself from giving the scale too much power. It's just a tool. The scale is a great way for you to check in with reality, as long as you know how to use it right. You need to learn *not* to beat yourself up about the number. You need to understand that water retention can mask fat loss. You need to understand that body composition can change with weight-training exercise, and that you could be losing fat while gaining muscle (which would not necessarily show up right away on the scale). And you need to understand that everyone loses at a different rate. You may go for a period of time with no change whatsoever and then all of a sudden have a "whoosh" of weight loss. That said, the scale *will* keep you honest. It will tell you—in combination with other cues, like how you're feeling and what your measurements are—whether what you're doing is working. If you want to figure out your critical carb level, you'll have to use the scale at some point to find out whether additional carbs are slowing you down. Many people have been delighted to find out that they actually could have a few more carbohydrates than they previously thought, and that it didn't slow down their weight loss appreciably or, if they were already at their goal weight, it didn't cause them to gain. But you'll never know any of that if you don't watch the numbers.

What Are Net Carbs? What's the Difference between Net Carbs and Effective Carbs?

There is none. Net carbs and effective carbs are two different phrases for the same thing. The idea is that fiber, even though it's "counted" as a carbohydrate on food labels, isn't absorbed, so it shouldn't really be counted. To get the net, or effective, carbohydrate content of a food, simply go to the label and subtract the number of grams of *fiber* from the number of grams of *carbohydrate*. For example, 1 cup of raspberries has 14 grams of carbohydrate, but 8 of those are from fiber. Subtract the 8 grams of fiber from the 14 grams of *total* carbohydrate, and you get the number of net carbohydrate grams per cup: 6. Note that this formula only applies to whole foods (like raspberries or avocados). To calculate net carbs for packaged carb products—even the high-quality ones—see the next question.

Why is there a controversy over net carbs?

The reason for this controversy has mostly to do with sugar alcohols. Many calculations of net carbs use the formula "total carbs minus fiber carbs," which works great for whole foods. Lots of "low-carb" products also tell you to subtract the carbs in sugar alcohols, which are often used instead of sugar in low-carb products because they're believed to have no impact on blood sugar.

But sugar alcohols actually vary in their impact on blood sugar. Here are examples of the glycemic index and the insulin index for five commonly used sugar alcohols. For comparison purposes, the glycemic index and the insulin index of pure glucose (sugar) is 100, measured on a scale of 1–100, with 100 meaning the highest surge in blood sugar.

- **Xylitol:** Glycemic index 13, insulin index 11
- **Isomalt:** Glycemic index 9, insulin index 6
- **Erythritol:** Glycemic index 0, insulin index 2
- **Maltitol:** Glycemic index 35, insulin index 27
- **Sorbitol:** Glycemic index 9, insulin index 11

As you can see, the only sugar alcohol that gets a free pass as far as blood sugar goes is erythritol. The rest, especially maltitol, may raise blood sugar a bit, particularly in sensitive individuals. According to the excellent research team at Healthline.com, whose article "How to Calculate Net Carbs" is highly recommended, "*In terms of net carbs, erythritol seems to be the best choice all around.*"[2]

In light of this, it's been suggested that when computing net carbs on commercial low-carb food products that may contain any sugar alcohols, except for erythritol, you adjust the formula for net carbs by deducting fiber *and deducting 50% of the carbs found in sugar alcohols.* If erythritol is the only sweetener used, you can continue to deduct 100% of the carbs from sugar alcohols.

For example, here's how you would calculate net carbs on a packaged food product with 25 grams of total carbs, 10 grams of fiber, and 14 grams of sugar alcohols that are *not* erythritol:

Total carbs (25g)
 – Fiber (10g)
 – 50% of Sugar Alcohol carbs (7 grams)
 _____

 = 8 net carbs

Remember, this is *not* a universally agreed-upon formula. Some argue that the impact of a very small amount of sugar alcohol added to a product to make it palatable is not really worth talking about from a blood-sugar point of view. Nonetheless, for those who are super-sensitive to blood-sugar fluctuations and need to be extremely careful, subtracting 50% of sugar alcohols might be a good idea.

What Is the Minimum Daily Requirement for Carbohydrates?

Zero. There is no biological requirement for dietary carbohydrate in human beings. You would die without protein and you would die without fat, but you can live just fine without carbohydrates. I'm not suggesting that you should—just that you *could.*

Low-Carbing and the Body

Why Am I Getting Headaches During the Induction (or Keto-adaptation/Fat-adaptation) Phase of My Diet?

Headaches are a frequent side effect of switching abruptly from a high-carb to a low-carb diet. One of the reasons for this is that your body and your brain need to adapt to using fat and ketones as a primary fuel source after being accustomed to using sugar. Your brain can certainly use ketones, but it takes a few days to make the adjustment, during which some people get headaches.

One suggestion: drink more water. In fact, if you don't drink enough water, you may get a "ketone headache" even *after* your body has adapted to the diet. The other thing you can do is up your carbs by 5 to 10 grams a day until you're feeling better, then lower them gradually. Preventing some of the side effects is one reason for doing a 3-day transition from your previous way of eating into this new low-carb lifestyle.

Recent research indicates that it may not be just the "keto-adaptation" that's causing the headaches or lethargy. It might also be withdrawal. Since both wheat and sugar are now known to act on the brain in an addictive way, it's not impossible that some of your temporary discomfort may be very similar to what people go through when they stop smoking. (Visual: I'm raising my hand here. That's certainly what happened to me when I stopped smoking back in the early 1980's!) If you can somehow get yourself through it, it'll definitely be worth it.

I'm Getting Leg Cramps, Especially at Night. Why?

This is almost always due to a mineral deficiency, particularly potassium, calcium, and magnesium. Remember that insulin tells the body to hold on to salt and water. When your insulin levels fall, especially during the first week on your low-carb diet, the kidneys will release that excess sodium—and you will begin to lose a lot of water. This will usually result in a loss of potassium as well, and one of the symptoms of potassium loss is muscle cramping (as well as fatigue). Dr. Alan Schwartz, medical director of the Holistic Resource Center in Agoura Hills, California, recommends taking one or two potassium supplements (99 milligrams) with each meal, especially in the first week of your low-carb diet. Magnesium supplementation is also a good idea—I like between 400 and 800 mg a day.

Note: nuts are one of the most healthy foods on the planet, and they help prevent potassium and magnesium imbalances. But be careful if you're trying to lose weight—they contain a ton of calories and it is incredibly easy to eat too many.

Does a Low-Carb Diet Cause Kidney Problems?

No. This is one of the great myths about low-carbing, but it is exactly that—a myth based on an incomplete understanding of the facts. It is true that people with preexisting kidney or liver problems should probably not go on very high-protein diets, but it is *not* true that high-protein or low-carbohydrate diets *cause* kidney problems. If your doctor tells you otherwise, ask him or her to show you the research that confirms that finding. It's unlikely that he or she will find any—because, as of this writing, there is none. There is not even a problem with protein in the diet for diabetics, who are frequently given to kidney problems.

There's not even a problem with protein in the diet for diabetics, who are frequently given to kidney problems. "There's no evidence that in an otherwise healthy person with diabetes, eating protein causes kidney disease," says Frank Vinicor, director of diabetes research at the Centers for Disease Control and Prevention.[3] (For a more detailed explanation, see chapter 6.)

Is Low-Carbing Good for Diabetes?

It is not only good; it is *essential.* "Diabetes is a disease of carbohydrate intolerance," says physician and diabetes specialist Lois Jovanovic, chief scientific officer of the Sansum Diabetic Research Institute in Santa Barbara, California. "Meal plans should minimize carbohydrates because *people with diabetes do not tolerate [them].*"[4] [Emphasis mine.] Dr. Richard Bernstein, author of *The Diabetes Solution* and a diabetic himself, has been fighting the medical establishment over this since the 1970s. "What is still considered sensible nutritional advice for diabetics can over the long run be fatal," Bernstein writes.[5]

The American Diabetes Association's high-starch diet is so behind the curve that it's ludicrous. Jovanovic sums up the conventional high-carb advice for diabetics in one word: "Malpractice!"

Can Stress Stall Weight Loss?

You bet. Not only can stress stall weight loss, it can *reverse* it. Stress—which can come from lack of sleep, extremely low-calorie dieting, and, of course, from life itself—causes the release of hormones such as cortisol and adrenaline. These stress hormones send messages to the body to break down muscle for fuel, resulting in a lower metabolic rate. They send compelling messages to the brain to eat (e.g., the well-known "stress eating" phenomenon). Cortisol also tells the body to store fat around the middle. Because cortisol basically breaks down biochemicals in the body, chronic elevated levels of cortisol can trigger a protective reaction from the body in the form of insulin secretion (since insulin builds up structures in the body, including, of course, the fat cells). This makes chronically high levels of cortisol one possible cause of insulin resistance.

Another way stress can screw up weight loss is by its effect on serotonin. Stress *eats up* serotonin. Less serotonin is produced because stress interferes with the good, deep, restful sleep needed by the body to replenish its serotonin stock.[6] The demand for serotonin becomes greater, while the production of it is lower. Serotonin depletion is never, *ever* conducive to weight loss, as it works against you in very powerful ways.

What Is Leptin?

Leptin is a hormone involved in appetite control. Early research at Rockefeller University showed that obese mice were very low in leptin, leading to a lot of excitement about the possibility that giving leptin to obese people would somehow result in weight loss. No such luck. It turned out that obese people have plenty of leptin. What seems to be happening is that they have what might be called leptin resistance—their cells don't respond to it, in a scenario not unlike that of insulin resistance.

Leptin is produced by fat cells—when the fat cells are full, they release leptin, which sends a signal to the brain to stop eating—but this mechanism doesn't seem to work in obese people. *Less* leptin means *more* appetite; as body fat is lost, leptin levels drop,[7] which in turn sends a message to the brain telling you to eat more. This mechanism may be one of the many that make regaining weight after a diet so easy; it's as if this feedback mechanism is hard at work to preserve you at a set weight. Drugs to treat this "leptin resistance" are in development and, if they prove promising, may one day help to fight obesity.

This Is My First Week on a Low-Carb Diet. Why Do I Feel Lightheaded?

Loss of minerals could be the culprit. Remember that when you lower your insulin levels, you lose salt and water (but, in the process, lose potassium as well). This, plus the tons of water I hope you're drinking, could conceivably result in enough electrolyte loss to lower blood pressure to the point where you might feel lightheaded or even faint. Replace some of the lost salt with either salty foods or with some table salt. Try ¼ teaspoon of potassium chloride (Morton Lite Salt) and ¼ teaspoon of table salt to start, and see if that helps. Don't forget to take potassium supplements.

How Do I Know if I'm Insulin-Resistant?

The best way is with a fasting insulin test. This test tells you what your baseline level of insulin is when no food is around to spike it. If you're not insulin-resistant, you shouldn't have a lot in your bloodstream when you haven't eaten. Lab ranges will vary; your level should not be above seventeen, and the optimal level is below ten. A blood sugar test won't tell you if you're insulin-resistant. You could have blood sugar in the normal range, but it could be taking an enormous amount of insulin to keep it there.

Without a fasting insulin test, the best "low-tech" way is to look at your body's "insulin meter"—your waistline. If you're storing a bunch of fat around your middle, chances are you're insulin-resistant. And though the argument about which comes first—obesity or insulin resistance—continues to rage, the fact is that they are so often found together that for all intents and purposes, if you're extremely overweight, you can assume you are also insulin-resistant. (There are exceptions; some heavy people are insulin-sensitive, and some thin people—who usually exercise a ton and never overeat—are insulin-resistant. These are not the typical cases.)

Does a High-Protein Diet Cause Bone Loss or Osteoporosis?

No. If anything, a diet high in protein does the opposite, particularly in the presence of adequate calcium intake and plenty of alkalinizing vegetables. There are a tremendous number of studies now showing that protein is essential for healthy bones and that, indeed, low protein intake can be an obstacle to bone-building. (For a more in-depth discussion of calcium, high protein, and bone loss, see chapter 6.) It's also worth remembering that the total amount of protein consumed on the typical low-carbohydrate diet of 2,000 calories (or fewer) is in no way excessive, even if it is a higher percentage of your diet than it had been before you revised your eating habits.

Can a Low-Carb Diet Cause Gallbladder Problems?

No, but if you have been overweight and have been on a very low-fat diet for a long time, a high-fat diet can make your gallbladder problems—like gallstones—apparent. Here's why. The gallbladder basically responds to fat in the diet with contractions that release the bile necessary to digest fat properly. When you've been on a very low-fat diet, there's not much for the gallbladder to do, so it gets lazy, and sometimes deposits accumulate and form stones, kind of like sediment forming in stagnant waters. When you suddenly go on a high-fat diet, the gallbladder now has work to do—it contracts in response to the fat, and it *may* pass these stones. The high-fat (low-carb) diet didn't *cause* the stones; they were already there and most likely developed in response to your very low-fat diet! But switching to a high-fat diet could trigger an attack. The solution: a moderate-fat version of a low-carb diet will trigger gallbladder contractions that are strong enough to release bile, but not vigorous enough to dislodge any stones.

What Can I Do About Constipation?

The two main causes of constipation on low-carb diets are not enough water and not enough fiber. (You should be consuming a lot of both, even if you're not constipated.) Drink more water and make sure the vegetables and fruits you consume are high in fiber—spinach, broccoli, and raspberries are all good choices.

Consider a fiber supplement. My favorite is SunFiber®, which can be found as an ingredient in certain fiber supplements—just read the label— or purchase it under the SunFiber brand. It's odorless, colorless, and tasteless and doesn't give you gas or bloating. And you can slip it into anything—even kids don't notice. Almost no one gets enough fiber a day, so supplementing makes a lot of sense. Exercise almost always helps. And drinking hot water with a squeeze of fresh lemon juice first thing in the morning can help get things going as well.

A terrific "cure" for constipation is magnesium. Get the magnesium citrate form, start with 400 milligrams a day for a few days, and then, if needed, increase to 800 milligrams. That almost always does it. Finally, consider prunes (a very healthy fruit). There's a reason that the conventional wisdom on prunes has stood the test of time.

Cravings

Why Do I Get Cravings?

Cravings have many causes. Some are caused by nutrient deficiencies. In this case, what you crave is a clue to what's missing; for example, craving fatty foods could indicate that you're not getting enough essential fatty acids. In that case, try adding omega-3 fats like fish or flaxseed oil. Many cravings are caused by blood-sugar imbalances. The common craving for carbohydrates in the evening can be caused by not having eaten enough protein and/or fat earlier in the day. A good "transition" technique for weaning yourself off sugar cravings is to satisfy it with fruit (though you can

> I don't care how much the experts say it's harmless, I know how sugar makes me feel: crazy. I start craving it like an addict, and once I start eating it I can't stop.
>
> —Jean N.

blunt the insulin effect by adding some peanut butter or turkey, both of which go great with apple slices).

A lot of cravings are caused by low serotonin states. Eating high-carbohydrate foods in this scenario is a kind of self-medication. The problem is that it creates a vicious cycle that results in weight gain and more cravings. Some supplements—for example, 5HTP—can help boost serotonin naturally, and there are a number of lifestyle ways to boost it as well, such as having a pet, being out in the sun, and making love! You also need to understand that some cravings are simply conditioned responses to stress and are more emotionally driven than anything else. That's why "comfort foods" are so named—we have been conditioned to eat them when things aren't going well and we need a little TLC. The more you work on developing alternative behavioral responses to these situations—like taking warm baths or going for a walk—the better off you'll be.

What Can I Do to Combat Sugar Cravings?

There are two supplements that are phenomenal for sugar cravings. One is glutamine—I recommend that you take a spoonful or two of glutamine powder in water (available in health-food stores or through Internet sources). A spoonful of glutamine mixed with the sweetener xylitol and a few tablespoons of half-and-half or heavy cream blended in for good measure will knock the socks off even the worst sugar craving.

Here are the top five techniques for busting cravings:

1. Control blood sugar by eating more protein, fat, and fiber.

2. Avoid *any* junk carbohydrates made of white stuff (rice, bread, pasta), as well as those that contain highly concentrated sweeteners, even if their carbohydrate content is permissible on your program.

3. Never let yourself become famished. Carry protein-based snacks like nuts, cheese, and hard-boiled eggs with you at all times.

4. Get enough sleep. Lack of sleep increases appetite and stimulates stress eating.

5. Learn to recognize the emotional triggers for cravings, such as fear, tension, shame, anger, anxiety, depression, loneliness, resentment, or any unmet needs. Don't pretend they're not there—recognize them, accept them, embrace them, and own them. Then explore behavioral ways of dealing with them other than eating.

Supplements

Do I Need to Take Supplements?

The technology exists to give you health-protective and therapeutic amounts of vitamins, minerals, phytochemicals, antioxidants, and other compounds, many of which are simply not available from our food supply or, if they are, not in the amounts needed to make a difference to your health and well-being. You don't *need* to take vitamins, but then you don't need electricity either. The question is, why would you do without either of them if you didn't have to?

Doesn't Taking Vitamins Just Result in Expensive Urine?

If it does, then why bother to drink water? You just urinate it out at the end, right? Do you see how ridiculous this concept is? The expensive-urine comment, which is perpetuated by doctors who don't really understand nutrition and vitamins, implies that just because something eventually winds up in the urine, it didn't accomplish anything in the body. Why does a drug addict take drugs or an athlete take steroids? Drugs, both recreational and prescription, are detected in the urine, right? Does the fact that they're detectable in the urine mean that they didn't *work*? If that were the case, there's an awful lot of people wasting an awful lot of money on drugs and medications! It's funny how the same doctors who cry "expensive urine" in response to vitamin therapy never make the same remark about their prescription drugs that are just as detectable in the urine as vitamins are! (Why else would many companies insist on urinary drug tests?)

> *I definitely noticed a difference in my skin when I began to supplement with fatty acids like fish oil. My hair and scalp weren't as dry and even my fingernails got stronger.*
> *—Bernice D.*

The fact that drugs—or vitamin residues—are detectable in the urine means absolutely nothing except that those substances went through the body and did their job. They didn't pass through and accomplish nothing, or else steroids wouldn't be banned by athletic organizations! The body takes what it needs, uses it, and excretes the rest. In addition, there's no way to know exactly how much of a given vitamin a specific individual actually needs. It's a lot better to take too much (with a few exceptions that might be toxic in very large amounts over an extended period of time, such as very high-dose vitamin A or selenium) and let the tissues decide how much they need and how much is excess. As nutritionist Robert Crayhon says in answer to this question, "Hey, I *want* expensive urine! In fact, I want the most expensive urine money can buy!"

What's in Those "Fat-Burning" Formulas I See Everywhere, and Do They Help with Weight Loss?

A recent field trip to my local vitamin store to inspect a dozen of these formulas—labeled everything from "metabolism boosters" to "fat burners" to "lipotropics"—revealed a pretty standard revolving door of ingredients. Most used some combination of the following:

- bitter orange (*Citrus aurantium*), a stimulant that increases metabolism (thermogenesis)

- guarana, which is herbal caffeine

- white willow bark, which is basically aspirin and really doesn't add anything to the mix

- green tea extract, a.k.a. EGCG (epigallocatechin gallate), which *does* have some thermogenic properties (i.e., heat production and increased calorie burning). But don't count on the amount of green tea added to these formulas to make much of a difference to your waistline.

Combinations of these ingredients can definitely suppress appetite, give you the jitters, and maybe, just maybe, burn a few extra calories.

Some "fat-burners" include a mix of carnitine and chromium. They almost never contain the best form of carnitine and rarely contain more than 500 milligrams. (Most nutritionists think the minimum amount necessary to impact fat-burning in an overweight person is 1,500 milligrams. Not only that, there isn't much consensus on whether supplemental carnitine actually helps with weight or fat loss.) As far as chromium is concerned, while I *have* seen formulas with 200 micrograms (the absolute minimum needed), I saw one that loudly proclaimed "contains chromium" and actually had a ridiculously low 13 micrograms. Understand that the amount most often given to people with blood-sugar problems is in the neighborhood of 600 to 1,000 micrograms; 13 micrograms would do absolutely nothing and is only there so that the manufacturer can say "contains chromium"—a complete rip-off.

Other ingredients that show up in the formulas, especially the ones labeled "lipotropics," are inositol, an essential nutrient and relative of the B family, and choline, another relative of the B family that mobilizes fat. Both choline and inositol (plus methionine) are involved in the liver's ability to process fats, so there's reason to think that these nutrients might help the liver move fat through itself. If a sluggish liver is part of the reason you're holding on to fat, these nutrients could be helpful.

The other pair of ingredients often found in these formulas are tyrosine, an amino acid helpful for improving mood, and phenylalanine, an essential amino acid that can be converted into tyrosine. Both of these are precursors to dopamine, a neurotransmitter that makes you feel peppy and bright. Tyrosine is needed for the making of thyroid hormone, but it is highly unlikely that tyrosine will boost low thyroid, even though some supplement makers claim it does.

The important thing is to read the ingredients on the labels of the products you are considering. These formulas vary widely in their effects, depending on the amounts and quality of the ingredients included. At worst, they do nothing. At best, they'll give you a bit of a speedy feeling and maybe increase metabolic rate by a very small amount.

Ketosis

What Is Ketosis?

Ketosis is a term used to describe what happens when the body switches to fat as its main source of fuel, which is exactly what you want to happen. When fat is the main source of fuel, there is an increase in the number of ketone bodies made as a by-product of fat metabolism. Ketones can be measured in the urine by means of ketone test strips. (For greater detail, see the extended section on the Keto Diet on page 225.)

Is Ketosis Dangerous?

Absolutely not. Ketones are a natural part of human metabolism—your body is always producing ketones. When you are in benign dietary ketosis, you are just making *more* of them, because fat, rather than sugar, has become the main source of fuel for your body. A strict ketogenic diet has been very successful in treating epilepsy in children and has been used for years at the Children's Hospital of New York-Presbyterian.[8] Children have been kept on it for years at a time. If there were dangers associated with ketosis, we would have heard about it by now. (For a full discussion, see chapter 9.)

Do I Need to Be in Ketosis in Order to Lose Weight?

No. First of all, ketosis doesn't *cause* weight loss. You can easily be in ketosis eating 10,000 calories of fat a day, but you'll never lose any weight that way. Ketosis is simply a by-product of fat-burning. There have been many people who've lost weight on low-carb diets without being in ketosis, and there are many who have been in ketosis and not lost weight. Ketone loss, in the urine and the breath, accounts for only about 100 calories a day.[9] That said, there are some extremely metabolically resistant people who truly seem to do much better on Atkins-like induction plans in which they *are* in ketosis, carbohydrates are kept to very low levels (20 to 30 grams or so a day), and calories are moderately low.

> It was absolutely amazing to me when I really studied ketosis and found out that almost everything I had heard about how dangerous it was was utter hogwash.
> —Dana McG.

You may want to go into ketosis just to get started, but the vast majority of people can lose weight over time on a low-carb diet by hovering around the border of ketosis. And as we've seen, many of the programs discussed in this book—from the Zone to Whole30 to the many versions of paleo—don't emphasize ketosis at all. The point is this: if you keep your carbs low enough (and your calories reasonable), you will be lowering your insulin levels and breaking down fat. Exactly how low they have to be for you to continue to lose weight is something you will have to experiment with.

Why Don't My Ketone Test Strips Show a Positive Reading?

There are a number of reasons you may not get a positive reading, and you probably don't need to be too concerned about it. There are three ketone bodies: beta-hydroxybutyric acid, acetoacetic acid, and acetone. The strips detect only the latter two, which are less than ⅕ of the total ketones produced. Beta-hydroxybutyric acid goes completely undetected and many people in the keto world argue that it is actually the most metabolically important ketone of the three. It's entirely possible that you might not test positive on the ketone strips, yet if you performed a more sophisticated urinalysis, you'd find plenty of ketones floating around, especially if you test with a method more sensitive to detecting beta-hydroxybutyric!

Other things can influence whether the strips change color, such as how much water you're drinking. If you're drinking a lot, which you should be, that'll very likely keep the strips from turning a deep color.

Of course, the possibility exists that they're not turning color because you're just not in ketosis, probably because you are eating more carbs than you think or there are hidden carbs in your food choices.

Food and Water

How Many Calories a Day Should I Be Eating?

For weight loss, a good rule of thumb is to take your goal weight and multiply by 10. If you've got more than about 25 pounds to lose, multiply your *current* weight by 10 and then deduct 500 calories from that number. This formula doesn't work as well if you are at a relatively low weight—say 125 pounds—and are trying to drop only a few pounds. You should never, ever let your calories fall below 1,000 per day (that is, unless you're specifically doing some kind of fasting program under medical supervision).

If you'd prefer not to do any calculations, you can remember it this way: the average weight-loss diet for men is about 1,500 to 1,800 calories and the average for women is about 1,200 to 1,400.

Remember that these formulas are only approximations. Every person's situation is going to be different based on one's own metabolic and historical factors, genetics, age, hormonal profiles, muscle mass, activity levels, and so on. The calorie calculators found on diet Internet sites woefully overestimate how many calories you "need," especially for weight loss. Ignore them. And remember that calories are only part of the picture (albeit an important part); the kinds of food you eat determine what messages are sent by your hormones, and the hormones are what control the whole shebang.

I'm a Vegetarian. Can I Do Low-Carb?

Yes, depending on the type of vegetarian diet you are following. If you're a vegan, it's going to be harder, but definitely possible—see Ketotarian (page 268). If you can eat eggs and whey protein, it's definitely doable. If you eat fish (i.e., pescatarian), it's a snap. Check out the ever-expanding catalog of cookbooks for vegetarian low-carb, vegan keto, and other variations on that theme, all available online.

It's worth noting that in 2009, researchers tested an all-vegan low-carb diet that later became known as "Eco-Atkins."[10] They kept carbs to 120 grams a day and all protein and fat came from nonanimal sources. People lost weight and saw their blood lipids improve considerably.

A note on vegetarianism: if you're avoiding eating animals for spiritual, ethical, or moral reasons, I am in great sympathy with you. I myself am a believer in animal rights and animal welfare, and I get it. Those of us who have strong kinship feelings with animals have to find a way to make peace with the fact that most humans do better with some animal products in their diet.

Dr. Terry Wahls, who pioneered the Wahls Protocol for multiple sclerosis and is doing clinical studies on ketogenic diets and multiple sclerosis, has spoken of trying to resolve this very dilemma. Wahls, who has multiple sclerosis and has given an inspiring TED lecture on using her protocol to keep the disease at bay, was for years a vegetarian herself. (The Wahls Protocol is definitely *not* vegan.) She speaks of taking long meditative walks and thinking about the nature of existence.

"I spent some time reflecting on life in the wild. We all consume one another in the end. Our atoms and molecules are continually recycled. Every living thing without the benefit of photosynthesis must consume other beings—plants, fungi, bacteria and animals. And in the end, they will consume me.

"I prayed and meditated on these ideas. Humans have been eating all these things for thousands of generations, so I decided I was not committing a crime against nature if I ate meat. Perhaps I was getting even closer to nature."[11]

So if your reason for going vegetarian or vegan has to do with your feelings about animals, I understand—and I invite you to do whatever soul-searching you need to do and choose whatever path works for you. I have no argument with people who are vegetarian or vegan for reasons of personal belief, ethics, morals, or religion.

But I *do* have issues with people who are vegan or vegetarian for health reasons, and with the belief that a diet which excludes animal products is *inherently* healthier than one that does not. That's just not so. Most people do better with some animal foods, and some people do a *lot* better on a *lot* of animal foods. The way I personally made peace with this issue is by patronizing as much as possible only those who sell meat from animals that have not been factory-farmed, have been *organically* raised, and have had a good and happy life. A local place in California that meets those requirements is Novy Ranches. The terrific online services Butcher Box and US Wellness Meats deliver high-quality meat right to your door. Even my favorite place to get wild fish—Vital Choice—now sells quite a bit of grass-fed, humanely raised meat in addition to their fantastic seafood offerings. Just something to think about.

Why Is Water So Important for Fat Loss?

Drinking plenty of water is absolutely necessary for fat loss. When you're not drinking enough water, the kidneys can't work properly, so they start dumping part of their load onto the liver. The liver is the main fat-processing plant in the body, but if it has to take over some of the kidneys' work, it can't work at full operating capacity. It metabolizes less fat, so more fat remains in the body, and weight loss stalls.[12] Water is also necessary to get rid of the toxic wastes released from fat stores.

Water is also—paradoxically—the absolute best treatment for water retention. The less water you drink, the more the body perceives this as a threat and sends signals that result in holding on to as much of that scarce water as possible. Sometimes this shows up as swollen hands, feet, and legs. When you're drinking enough water, this doesn't happen. There's no more "emergency," and the body releases stored water instead of retaining it.

How Much Water Should I Be Drinking?

More than you think. "Larger people have larger metabolic loads," says Dr. Donald Robertson. "Since we know that water is the key to fat metabolism, it follows that the overweight person needs more water." Robertson recommends 3 quarts a day. Many personal trainers recommend a gallon. I think the absolute minimum is 64 ounces plus an additional 8 ounces for every 25 pounds of excess weight you are carrying.

How Can I Get More Fiber in My Low-Carb Diet?

Eat an avocado! The average California avocado has a whopping 10 grams per cup, while one from Florida has 17! Concentrate on higher-fiber non-starchy vegetables like cauliflower, broccoli, Brussels sprouts, asparagus, and the like. Though most non-starchy veggies have somewhere between 2 and 4 grams of fiber per serving, that adds up. Include high-fiber fruits like raspberries, bell peppers (yes, they're a fruit), and the aforementioned avocado. Eat some nuts. And consider an odorless, tasteless fiber supplement like SunFiber, which can help you get an extra 5 grams of soluble fiber with every spoonful you add to anything you eat or drink.

What Are Sugar Alcohols? Do They Count as Sugar?

Sugar alcohols—also called polyols—are sugar-free sweeteners that are carbohydrates but are not sugar. Common ones include maltitol, mannitol, sorbitol, and xylitol. They have fewer calories per gram than sugar: sugar has 3 calories per gram, while sorbitol has 2.6, xylitol has 2.4, and mannitol has 1.6. They don't cause sudden increases in blood sugar; instead, they are slowly and incompletely absorbed from the small intestine into the blood, and the portion that is absorbed requires little or no insulin. Since they aren't technically sugar, manufacturers are able to say "sugar-free" when they use sugar alcohols as sweeteners, but

> *Every time I drink (alcohol), my diet goes out the window and I eat way more than I ever intended to. Cutting out alcohol—at least for now —has been the best thing I ever did for my waistline.*
> —Kelley F.

they're required to include these sweeteners in the carb count on the nutrition label (though not everybody does).

Scientists call them sugar alcohols because part of their structure chemically resembles sugar and part chemically resembles alcohol. They're certainly a lot better for you than pure sugar. Xylitol actually has health benefits. (I'm also a huge fan of the sugar alcohol *erythritol*, sold under the brand name of Truvía®.) But some sugar alcohols can cause slight gastric upset for some people, like a little gas or a mild laxative effect. And you have to be careful with portion sizes—even though the food may be technically sugar-free, the calories and grams of sugar alcohol can add up. And some folks—particularly carb addicts—say that products sweetened with sugar alcohols can trigger cravings just like products sweetened with sugar.

Also note that there's some controversy about whether the carbs from sugar alcohols "count" when you calculate your net carbs. Some sugar alcohols do have a higher impact than others on both blood sugar and insulin, even though that impact is relatively low. For more on sugar alcohols and glycemic impact, see page 281.

What Are the Best Oils?

That entirely depends on what you're using them for. Extra-virgin olive oil is wonderful for drizzling and even fine for reasonably low-heat sautéing, but it's a terrible choice for frying. Flaxseed oil is great for salad dressing, but not for cooking, while MCT oil is great as a supplement but completely useless for cooking. In fact, even the greatest oil on the planet can be made toxic by heating it to the wrong temperature. Pay attention to smoke points!

For cooking below 350 or 400°F, I recommend extra-virgin olive oil. If you need to go a bit higher, use virgin olive oil. (Word to the wise: I found an amazing, authentic extra-virgin olive oil for under 10 bucks—it's called Cobram Estate®, and it's the best-kept secret in the food world! You're welcome.) Virgin *coconut* oil, especially Barlean's® 100% Organic Coconut Oil, is great, and so is grass-fed butter (I know it's not an oil, but it's fine for cooking and sautéing). Ditto for organic ghee. Even lard—from humanely and pasture-raised pork—is making a big comeback; it's very stable and stands up to high heat much better than those horrible cheap vegetable oils that restaurants replaced it with because they were so afraid of saturated fat.

I'm also a big fan of Malaysian palm oil, which can be a potent source of tocotrienols and carotenoids, and—if the oil is partially refined—stands up to heat quite well. (Full disclosure: I give a shout-out to Malaysia when it comes to palm oil because of their highly protective environmental policies and the fact that orangutans and their habitats are not harmed by Malaysia's palm-oil industry.) Peanut oil is stable and can be used occasionally for stir-fries, but it is very high in omega-6, so don't overdo. You can use organic cold-pressed sesame oil, which is very good for frying, but remember that it contains a larger proportion of omega-6s, so don't use it exclusively. Almond oil is good for baking. And avocado oil is a superb oil for cooking with a very high smoke point of 500°F!

Flaxseed oil is terrific, of course, but *never* use it for cooking. It is a great source of alpha-linolenic acid (an omega-3 fat), but for that reason it can't be heated (though it can be poured or drizzled on hot foods such as vegetables). Omega-3 fats are very unstable and become extremely damaged when heated. Other terrific new oils beginning to make an appearance on grocery shelves are chia oil and perilla oil (both plant-based fats). Because of their omega-3 content, I'd be careful about using them for cooking.

For salads, try coconut oil, extra-virgin olive oil, any of the nut oils (macadamia, hazelnut, almond, walnut), avocado oil, or sesame oil. You can also use flaxseed, chia, or perilla oil. I don't recommend canola oil.

MORE ON KETONES AND THE BRAIN

Dr. Mary Newport is the medical director of the newborn intensive-care unit at Spring Hill Regional Hospital in Florida. Her husband Steve had early-stage Alzheimer's. "I was watching my husband of 36 years fade away," said Dr. Newport.

Then she discovered coconut oil.

Dr. Newport began researching clinical trials and discovered a new medication that had shown unbelievable results in clinical trials. While generally, the best that can be hoped for with Alzheimer's is to slow the progression of the disease, this drug had produced actual memory *improvement*, something rarely seen in Alzheimer's patients. Unfortunately, her husband wasn't eligible for the trial—according to the results of a MMSE test (a test commonly used to assess cognitive impairment), he scored too low and had too great a level of impairment.

But Dr. Newport didn't give up.

She researched the active ingredient in the new medication and found an in-depth discussion of its primary ingredient, a particular form of fat called MCTs—medium-chain triglycerides.

This is precisely the kind of fat found in coconut oil.

She decided to try it.

She purchased a jar of non-hydrogenated, extra-virgin coconut oil. She started by adding a couple of tablespoons into her husband's oatmeal.

Almost immediately, her husband started showing improvements. He scored higher on the exam than he had scored in a year. More than 5 months afterward, his tremors had subsided and he had become more social and interested in those around him.

The secret seems to be in ketones.

The body converts some of the MCTs into ketones, which are an additional source of fuel for starving brain cells. No one is claiming that ketones—or MCT oil, a purified form of the fat found in coconut—will cure Alzheimer's. But this inspiring story is yet another example of the way ketones can be helpful as an energy source for the brain.

"I started using 100% MCT oil for kids with brain problems about 25 years ago," says renowned neurosurgeon Larry McCleary, MD (author of *The Brain Trust Program*). "This generates more ketones and does it faster than coconut oil (and has fewer calories for the same amount of MCTs). It was part of a vigorous nutritional support program for kids with brain issues of many sorts—tumors, trauma, drowning, hemorrhage, etc. It produced dramatic results in them and it should help older people with disorders like Alzheimer's disease."

Ketones also appear to help children with epilepsy. Eric Kossoff, MD, is assistant professor of neurology and pediatrics at Johns Hopkins and the medical director of the Johns Hopkins Ketogenic Diet program. He's been using the Ketogenic Diet for years as a treatment option for epilepsy, and in 2003 developed a slightly gentler version of the diet called the MAP—Modified Atkins Program.

"The Ketogenic Diet is not viewed as an alternative diet anymore," said Dr. Kossoff. "It's viewed as an option to meds, but most docs know it's an effective therapy for epilepsy."

To be used commercially, it has to be partially hydrogenated, refined, and deodorized, and in the process its omega-3s become a potent source of trans-fatty acids.[13] If you do use it, make sure to get organic, cold-pressed, or expeller-pressed canola oil (such as Spectrum), and only use it cold.

Oils you can say good-bye to permanently include safflower, sunflower, corn, soybean, and cottonseed. Buh-bye.

What's the Story with Coconut Oil?

Coconut oil is a good, stable, healthful fat that actually has a number of healing properties, not the least of which is that it is anti-inflammatory.[14] The original bad rap for coconut oil came four decades ago, when researchers fed animals *hydrogenated* coconut oil that was purposely altered to render it devoid of essential fatty acids. The animals that were fed the hydrogenated coconut oil (as their only fat source) naturally became deficient in essential fatty acids, and their serum cholesterol increased.[15] Early commercial coconut oil was often hydrogenated (loaded with transfats), and all the good healing stuff had been removed. That altered coconut oil *wasn't* very good for you. But *real* coconut oil is a health bonanza. The Pukapukans and the Tokelauans of Polynesia, for whom coconut is the chief source of energy, have virtually no heart disease, and research on these populations concluded that there was no evidence that their high saturated-fat intake (from coconut) had any harmful effects.[16] The saturated fat in coconut oil comes mainly from MCTs (medium-chain triglycerides), which are preferentially burned as energy and less likely to be stored as fat, making them a good choice for a weight-loss program. Coconut oil also contains a high proportion of the antiviral and antimicrobial lauric acid, as well as the antimicrobial capric acid and the potent "yeast fighter" caprylic acid.[17] Be sure to purchase the virgin or cold-pressed kind.

What Are the Good Fats?

Good fats include all the oils mentioned previously as "good" *plus* natural, undamaged fats like butter, coconut, avocado, nuts, and the fat in fish, grass-fed meat, butter, and ghee.

The dietary establishment has long fostered the myth that fats are "good" or "bad" depending on whether or not they are saturated: saturated fats = bad, unsaturated fats = good. Not so. A much better way to categorize fats is by whether they are damaged or undamaged. You can damage fats in a number of ways. One way is by overheating any vegetable oil by frying at high temperatures—this creates toxic substances known as lipid peroxides. Another is through an industrial process known as partial hydrogenation, which creates something called trans-fats, by far the most dangerous of all fats. Trans-fats are found in almost all fast foods (French fries, for example, are doused in them), most margarines, virtually all commercially baked goods (including children's cookies), and movie popcorn, and in any products containing partially hydrogenated vegetable oils (look for these in the ingredients list on the package). Trans-fats are the true demons of the fat world, and the ones we want to avoid completely, as they are associated with all the degenerative diseases common in the modern world.

Unfortunately, until recently there has been no separation in the research between saturated fats and trans-fats, so saturated fats have been blamed for a great deal of the damage to the body that is actually the fault of trans-fats.[18] As of 2006, manufacturers were required to list trans-fats in the Nutrition Facts on food packaging, which is a good thing. Unfortunately, there's a loophole:

The law allows manufacturers to say "zero trans-fats" provided there's less than half a gram per serving. This has led a lot of manufacturers to keep the "suggested serving size" listed on the label preposterously low. (You know—when you pick up a packaged cookie that says "Serving size: 1/3 cookie." Right.) Because of that loophole in the regulations, you could easily be consuming a gram or two of trans-fats from "zero trans-fat" foods. (Imagine that .4 of a gram of trans-fat was in each one of those "1/3 cookie servings"—you'd get 1.2 grams just from one cookie!)

The only sure-fire way to tell if a food has trans-fats is to read the ingredients. If it says "hydrogenated oil" or "partially hydrogenated oil," it's got trans-fats, no matter what the front-panel label says.

What About Alcohol?

Alcohol has been referred to as the "non-nutritive nutrient." That's because it provides calories—7 per gram—but absolutely zero nutritional value. The body has no way to store those calories, so all "fat-burning" is put on hold while the body burns off the alcohol. (You can think of alcohol as a fire engine roaring down an avenue—all traffic comes to a stop till the fire engine is out of the area.) Alcohol can also produce cravings, both for itself and for carbohydrates—Kathleen DesMaisons, PhD, an expert in addictive nutrition, considers alcohol an extension of sugar sensitivity.[19] She also believes that although hard liquor is not technically a sugar, the beta-endorphin effect is a powerful trigger for cravings.[20]

That said, a lot of low-carb plans permit some alcohol, particularly red wine (in 4-ounce servings), which contains about 3 grams of net carbohydrate. Do the math and see if it works for you.

What Is the Glycemic Index?

The glycemic index is a numerical way of describing how carbohydrates in foods affect blood-sugar levels (an even more accurate measure is the glycemic *load*; see next question).[21] The index measures how quickly a 50-gram serving of a particular food converts to sugar. Foods with a high glycemic index cause a dramatic rise in blood sugar (and subsequent demand on insulin levels). That's why all low-carb diets suggest that you eat *low-glycemic* carbohydrates; these carbs (green vegetables, for example) have a much lower impact on your blood sugar and insulin. Don't get too hung up on the glycemic index, though. The glycemic load is a much better metric for measuring the impact of food on your blood sugar. (See the next question.)

What's the Difference between the Glycemic Index and the Glycemic Load?

The glycemic load is a more accurate predictor of what's going on with blood sugar and insulin than the glycemic index, because actual portion size is part of the calculation. The glycemic index is calculated based on a "standard" 50-gram net-carb serving of the food, but the actual "serving" you eat of real food is all over the map—see the carrots-and-pasta example below. It tells you the impact that a 50-gram serving of a particular food will have on your blood sugar. The glycemic load, on the other hand, also takes into account the amount of carbs actually in the food. Its formula factors in your actual portion size rather than just using an unrealistic "50-gram" serving as its standard. If I want to know the impact of a particular food on blood sugar and insulin, I need to know two things: the glycemic index and how much of that food I'm going to eat!

The carrots-versus-spaghetti problem is a great way to illustrate the problem of depending exclusively on the glycemic index. White spaghetti, boiled for 20 minutes, has a glycemic index of 58, which is considered "moderate." (The pasta publicists love to point out that pasta gets an unfair rap for being high glycemic when it's really only in the middle of the range.) Well, sure—if you eat a 50-gram portion. But *nobody* eats 50 grams of spaghetti (just look at the "serving size" on any box of pasta—it's 200 grams, and believe me, that's a fraction of the size of a restaurant portion). The average glycemic *load* of one cup of spaghetti provides 44 grams of net carbs. That calculates to a very high glycemic load of 25.[22] And that's just for a *one-cup* serving. If you ordered pasta in a restaurant and got served a one-cup serving of pasta, you'd complain! Under typical conditions, pasta *is* a high-glycemic food, despite its "moderate" glycemic index. Now let's contrast that with carrots.

Carrots suffered from a bad rap for many years in the low-carb community, largely because they were believed to have an extremely high glycemic index. In fact, the glycemic index of carrots varies depending on whose table you use, but let's use 71 for purposes of this example.[23] Carrots do indeed have a high glycemic index. Remember however, that the glycemic index is based on a 50-gram net-carb portion. Know how many net carbs there are in a carrot? Around three, if it's a big one. You'd have to consume a bushel of them to get the effect predicted by the glycemic index. Consume a half cup of carrots, and you'll be ingesting about 7 or 8 grams of net carbs. Plug that into the glycemic-load equation, and you're left with an awesomely low glycemic load of about 6. In many versions of the glycemic-load tables, carrots have an even lower rating, between 1 and 4! As Dr. C. Leigh Broadhurst once said, "Nobody becomes diabetic on peas and carrots."

In 2016, scientists from the Jean Mayer USDA Human Nutrition Research Center on Aging (USDA HRNCA) at Tufts University found that the glycemic index of a given food could vary as much as 25% among individuals, and a whopping 20% within the same individual tested at different times![24] I actually didn't find that study surprising. Years ago, a great friend of mine—Dr. David Leonardi, of the Leonardi Executive Health Institute in Denver—used to test his own blood sugar along with his wife's. "My wife and I would eat the exact same portion of the exact same food, and my blood sugar would skyrocket while hers would barely move," he told me then. All of which is to say that glycemic index and glycemic load are useful tools—but they're not perfect predictors. Remember, as with all things in diet and nutrition, YMMV—your mileage may vary! Individual differences always trump broad-based generalizations.

What is the Insulin Index?

The insulin index is like the glycemic index; but instead of measuring *blood sugar response* to a fixed quantity of food, it measures your actual *insulin response*. This can be very useful, because some foods raise insulin levels more than what you would predict from their carb content. Some protein-rich foods, for example, raise insulin despite the fact that they contain essential zero carbohydrates. (Beef, for example, has a glycemic index of 21 but an insulin index of 51.) Conversely, some products—like baked goods—raise insulin even higher than you would expect, given their glycemic index or load.

To complicate matters further, there's also something called the satiety index. Researchers arrive at the *satiety index* by feeding subjects a fixed amount of the food they're testing and then observing how much food the subjects eat when let loose at a buffet. A higher satiety index means the food was more filling, since folks who ate it wound up choosing a lot less food at the buffet than those who ate a food with a low satiety index. Satiety indexes in one test ran from a low of 47 to a high in the 300s. Croissants earned the lowest rating of 47, but in a total head-scratcher the winner of the satiety sweepstakes with a score of 323 was potatoes![25]

What's the Best Type of Protein Powder to Use?

I'm a big fan of grass-fed whey, though some of the better collagen protein powders and high-quality blended protein drinks that use a variety of protein sources also work well. But to me, whey seems to be the best all-around source of protein in protein-powder form. Whey is absorbed the best and is the most bioavailable; it also increases levels of glutathione, perhaps the most powerful antioxidant in the body, which helps with immune function and has been shown to be helpful in weight loss.

What's the Difference between a Shake Made with Protein Powder and a Meal-Replacement Shake?

Protein powders are 100% (or almost 100%) pure protein. You can drink them by themselves or make a "meal-replacement" drink with them by adding a controlled amount of carbohydrates (berries are a good choice) and maybe some fat like nuts or nut butter. You can even add a source of fiber, like ground flaxseeds, chia seeds, or a fiber supplement.

Ready-to-drink meal-replacement shakes have carbs, protein, and fat in different proportions depending on the philosophy of the company making them.

What's Wrong with Grains? Aren't They Supposed to Be Healthy?

Grains, grain products, starches, and sugars all share some common links: they turn into glucose (sugar) in your body very quickly, they promote addictive eating habits in a large percentage of people, and they trigger insulin release. All of these things result in weight gain and other health problems.[26] Grains also contain compounds called phytates and pyridoxine glucosides that block absorption of B vitamins, iron, zinc, copper, and calcium and lead to possible mineral deficiencies that can slow metabolism. (For a full discussion of grains, see "The Problem with Grains" on page 205 and the discussion of wheat in chapter 4.) In addition, both gluten and certain protein fractions of gluten like gliadin are a big problem for many people. It used to be thought that celiac disease—a sensitivity to gluten—was rare. We now know that it probably affects one in 33 people. That's a lot. There are an amazing number of toxins used in the processing of wheat and grains, and it is entirely possible that some of the problems that people have with wheat are actually caused by these toxins. (Other problems are certainly caused by the wheat itself.)[27]

Clinically, an awful lot of problems seem to just magically "clear up" when you take grains, especially wheat, out of the diet. While whole grains are in theory better than refined grains, they're not nearly as common as you might think. Plus there's the fact that whole-grains still contain gluten and phytates and have many of the problems of refined grains. And even if a product—like flour—started out with whole grains as an ingredient ("made with whole grains!"), making flour is by definition a refining process. And the "wheat breads" in your grocery are no better than white bread. Couple this with the fact that grains usually have a very high-glycemic impact and you can see the problem.

Obviously, not everyone will have a problem with grains, but cutting them out during the initial stages of a low-carb weight loss program is definitely a good idea.

Is Coffee Okay?

As far as I'm concerned, coffee—consumed the right way—is a health food. I've never bought into the notion of caffeine (or coffee) as a destroyer of health, even before the voluminous research showing that coffee drinkers have less risk for gout,[28] diabetes,[29] Parkinson's disease, and five types of cancer.[30] Coffee has a "rich phytochemistry" that includes important health-giving compounds like chlorogenic acids.

The debate over whether coffee is "good" or "bad" has been raging since at least the time I entered the health field in 1990. Some people respond great to coffee, while others get the jitters and insomnia. Health organizations didn't help much—they couldn't seem to agree on whether caffeine was a good thing or a bad thing.

Then in the mid-'aughts, Ahmed El-Sohemy—a professor in the department of nutritional sciences at the University of Toronto—began looking at the data, trying to determine the reason for such a wide range of individual responses.[31] He zeroed in on a particular gene—CYP1A2—that controls an enzyme that determines how your body processes caffeine. One variant of the gene makes you process caffeine quickly—if you have that variant, you're considered a "fast metabolizer" and coffee won't stay in your system all that long. If you have a different variation of that gene, the opposite is true. You're a "slow metabolizer" and probably should stay away from coffee after 12 noon! (The CYP1A2 gene is now affectionately known as "the coffee gene.") Now you know why you and your best friend respond to a cup of Joe in completely different ways.

Then there's the insulin issue. Some argue against coffee because they're concerned with its possible effects on insulin and on the adrenal glands. Atkins didn't like it because he felt it caused unstable blood sugar. There is some research that suggests that caffeine increases insulin resistance[32] and that it raises insulin levels.[33] How much this matters as a practical consideration is debatable—the insulin insensitivity it produces in studies may be an insignificant amount as a practical matter and may be only temporary. There is also research showing that coffee actually *improves* insulin sensitivity[34] and contributes to *reducing* insulin,[35] as well as some research that says it has no effect on insulin at all.[36] And then there are the studies that show coffee is actually associated with a much *lower* risk of type 2 diabetes.[37]

While coffee is obviously a stimulant, drinking it is also a very pleasant experience for a lot of people, and that has to be factored into the mix. It's also high in antioxidants, such as chlorogenic acid, and by some accounts it's the biggest source of antioxidants in the American diet! Those who are very concerned about adrenal health recommend dumping it, but others say it's fine. From a weight-loss perspective, it's probably not going to hurt at all.

Important note: it's not just the caffeine in coffee that we should be talking about (there's caffeine in green tea too, and that doesn't seem to hurt anyone). It's the enormous amount of toxins in the coffee plant. You can go a long way toward reducing any negative health impact of coffee by purchasing organically grown beans.

Are Diet Sodas Acceptable on My Low-Carb Diet?

You'd be *much* better off without them. If you can't give them up right away, put it on your goal list and at least start cutting back. Many of them use aspartame, which should definitely be eliminated (see next question); in addition, diet soda can stall weight loss in some people (up to 40% to 50%, by some estimates), possibly due to the citric acid they contain and to mechanisms not yet fully understood (although there's a lot of suspicion that it has to do with the microbiome—keep reading).

Many people do drink soda addictively (I had one client who routinely consumed sixteen cans a day). This level of consumption has never really been tested for safety in long-term studies. Then there's conditioning. Through a mechanism like classical conditioning, the one used to teach Pavlov's dogs to salivate at the sound of a bell, tasting sweetness in a diet soda may well trigger insulin production. The sweetness without calories is also thought to deregulate our natural appetite-control mechanisms. And the chemicals, food colorings, flavorings, and other stuff in diet soda make it no picnic for the liver, either.

Since the last edition of this book, there's been a growing body of evidence linking non-caloric artificial sweeteners to a host of conditions including weight *gain*. Why? Focus has now turned to something no one was talking about when the first editions of this book were published: the microbiome. There is now good evidence to suspect that artificial sweeteners harm us by affecting the microbiome,[38] which we now know impacts everything from depression to weight loss to schizophrenia. Until we know more, I'd personally recommend staying away from all artificial sweeteners. (I'm not including sugar alcohols in this category, which are in a different category than artificial sweeteners. For more information on sugar alcohols, see page 296.)

What About Aspartame?

Aspartame, the most common of the artificial sweeteners and the one used in most diet sodas, is a real problem. Even though it has been declared "safe," the FDA has received numerous reports of seizures and other problems that have been linked to it.[39] There's also good reason to believe that aspartame may be neurotoxic.[40] In a report to the Senate Labor and Human Resources Committee, Dr. Richard Wurtman, professor of neuroendocrine regulation at the Massachusetts Institute of Technology, stated that the most common side effects linked to aspartame include dizziness, visual impairment, disorientation, ear buzzing, a high level of SGOT (a liver enzyme), loss of equilibrium, severe muscle aches, episodes of high blood pressure, and other not-so-lovely stuff.[41] Other reports claim that in susceptible people, aspartame can produce symptoms ranging from sleep disturbances to headaches to fuzzy thinking to mood disturbances. Kathleen Des Maisons, PhD, an expert in addictive nutrition, believes that the taste of any sweetener, for sugar-sensitive people, evokes a beta-endorphin response in the body that will create cravings.[42]

No integrative or holistic practitioner I've ever interviewed—and I've done more than 300 interviews in my career—had anything good to say about aspartame. The consensus of advice: stay away.

Erythritol is, in my opinion, one of the best sweeteners currently available. It's a natural sugar alcohol, has virtually no glycemic impact, and tastes great. It's available at supermarkets everywhere, sold under the brand name Truvía. Personally, I'm a fan.

I also like xylitol—though, depending on the dose and the individual, it *can* give some folks a bit of digestive upset. Stevia is an herb sold as a food additive, which has basically no downside except a somewhat weird aftertaste that some people don't mind at all. You can get it at any health-food store. I'm a fan of both Pyure's® organic stevia, sold everywhere, and also the full line of stevia products sold by NuNaturals®.

If you're not counting calories or sugar grams, honey or blackstrap molasses are both good choices, though the strong taste of blackstrap molasses may rule it out in a lot of cases. But both are nutritious foods and *waaaaay* better than sugar or high-fructose corn syrup. Just remember that the body still sees (and processes) them as sugar. For those who are basically healthy and don't have insulin resistance, carb-intolerance, or a weight problem, organic cold-pressed honey is a good choice.

Note that not all these sweeteners are suitable for cooking or baking, so be sure to check the label or check with the manufacturer.

Is Fructose Okay?

The short answer: Absolutely not. It's actually the most damaging part of sugar, and in the amounts we consume it, pretty close to metabolic poison. And that's true whether it's coming from ordinary table sugar (50% glucose, 50% fructose), high-fructose corn syrup (55% fructose, 45% glucose), or agave nectar (up to 92% fructose).

Fructose doesn't raise blood sugar, so it used to be thought of as the perfect sweetener for diabetics. Bad idea. Even though it doesn't raise blood sugar, it induces insulin resistance in both animals[43] and humans.[44] Fructose is turned to fat in the liver, so it raises your triglycerides as well as contributing mightily to non-alcoholic fatty liver disease (NAFLD).

But fructose in the diet—when it comes from vegetables and reasonable amounts of fruits—is not nearly as much of a problem. First of all, the fructose you'd get from, for example, an apple is way less than you'd consume in a product sweetened with high-fructose corn syrup. Second of all, that apple comes with a whole lot of other goodies such as fiber, antioxidants, and phytochemicals.

So when you consume fructose, make sure it comes in its natural "container"—a fruit or a vegetable. Never use it as a sweetener, and try like hell to avoid eating foods that are sweetened with it.

And if you ever find a grocery store that still carries liquid fructose in the "diabetic" section the way they did when I was a kid . . . run the other way.

Can I Eat Dairy Products?

For many people, dairy—especially milk and cheese—will slow or stall weight loss. For many people it's an allergen, or at least a trigger, for digestive symptoms related to lactose or to some forms of milk protein (casein). Many holistic practitioners recommend eliminating wheat, dairy, and sugar as the three biggest triggers of food reactions, subclinical allergies, and the like. And there's no shortage of low-carb programs where dairy is totally off the menu (classic Paleo, for example, and Whole30).

On the other hand, real, whole-food dairy from pastured cows is celebrated in the Ancestral Health community. And research in the last decade has uncovered previously unsuspected health benefits for dairy fat.[45] Some people—I'm one of them—have none of the typical symptoms of dairy intolerance and seem to thrive on dairy, much like some of the hunter–gatherer societies studied by Dr. Weston Price.

That's what makes a horse race.

I love raw, unpasteurized milk, which you can often get at farmers' markets, collectives, and—in a few states like California—at some supermarkets (shout-out to my local Sprouts!) I do *not* believe homogenized, pasteurized milk is a good food. In addition to the pus cells (the FDA allows 1.5 million per cc of milk as "safe"), factory-farmed cows are treated with antibiotics, bovine growth hormone, and other drugs to fatten them and keep their milk production elevated to unnatural levels. The grain they eat, which is not their natural food, is irritating to their stomachs (one reason for the antibiotics) and contains a whole different set of toxins. (Raw organic milk is, in my opinion, a whole different story.)

If you're not ready to eliminate milk, or if you want to consume it in small amounts, at the very least buy the organic kind, or try goat's milk.

Also, many people who have a problem with conventional milk are still able to tolerate fermented dairy foods like kefir and yogurt.

What About A2 Milk?

Many people who have problems with milk think they're lactose-intolerant. And many are right! But for some people, it may not be the lactose in the milk that's causing problems. These folks—Dr. Will Cole of *Ketotarian* fame is one of them—believe that a certain form of the beta-casein protein in dairy called A1 is the real culprit. And there is good research to support this.[46]

Casein is the protein in dairy, and it comes in two flavors—beta-casein A1 and beta-casein A2. Cows make both of them, but the vast majority of cows in the U.S. have been bred to produce mostly A1. Recently, some companies have begun producing "A2" milk, which is milk that has none of the (possibly offending) A1 protein in it. It might be worth a try. Remember, however, that unlike raw milk, commercial A2 milk is still homogenized and pasteurized.

What About Cheese?

I'm personally a huge fan of both cheese and nuts, but let's face it: it's easy to overeat both foods, and they are relatively high in calories. Cheese has stalled many a low-carber's weight loss. Although some plans allow it, if your weight loss isn't progressing, this might be one food to cut back on.

I'm Getting Bored with the Usual Low-Carb Fare. What Else Can I Eat?

Here are some terrific suggestions from low-carb chef Karen Barnaby.

- Thinly sliced radicchio, endive, and fennel with a fresh basil dressing, sprinkled with crisp bacon and goat cheese. Eat with roasted chicken.

- Raw, sautéed, or grilled mushrooms on romaine with blue cheese dressing. Eat with a steak.

- Fried peppers, mushrooms, and garlic. Serve on arugula, sprinkled with feta cheese, and eat with good Italian sausage.

- Thinly sliced cucumbers, radishes, and celery. Toss with lemon mayonnaise and serve on butter lettuce, along with a piece of salmon. Sprinkle with fresh dill.

- Cooked asparagus and Swiss chard. Serve a piece of halibut, cod, or sole on top and drown it in Hollandaise sauce.

- Sautéed spinach or julienned daikon seasoned with soy sauce and a few drops of sesame oil. Serve with grilled tuna on top and mayonnaise mixed with wasabi as a sauce.

- Marinated cubes of feta, Brie, or Camembert in basil, garlic, and lots of olive oil. Eat with sliced cucumbers as a snack or sprinkle on a salad. Have it alongside a hamburger. Use as an omelet filling with one fourth of a tomato, chopped.

- Make a cabbage slaw and jazz it up with mint, cilantro, green onions, and a bit of lime juice. Put canned tuna or salmon and hard-boiled eggs on top.

Here are some other ideas:

- Make omelets with fillings like bacon and Swiss cheese, mushroom and avocado, goat cheese and mushrooms, spinach and feta, or bacon and avocado.

- Add chopped nuts or sunflower seeds to cottage cheese.

- Make a "wrap" out of sliced turkey with cream cheese inside.

- Make a "wrap" out of sliced roast beef with cheddar, scallions, and a drop of sour cream (if dairy is on your program).

- Try deviled eggs.

- Use low-carb tortillas and make your own breakfast burritos.

- Keep varying the toppings on your salads. Try warm meats or shrimp, crab, or lobster. Try different cheeses, if that's on your program. Mix and match.

- Make a low-carb burger by putting a hamburger patty between two lettuce leaves (or red cabbage leaves). Add mayo and mustard if you like.

- Pan-fry some chicken and add feta cheese and olives.

- Eat a hot dog minus the bun and use mayo and mustard as dipping sauces.

- Steam some veggies and add butter, lemon, a handful of nuts, and maybe some soy sauce.

- Fill celery sticks with peanut butter, cream cheese, or tuna salad.

- Try beef jerky, turkey jerky, or veggie jerky.

- Mix sugar-free, all-natural peanut butter with whey protein powder and roll in cocoa powder.

- Combine whey protein powder with sour cream and stevia; kneading this mixture renders a pretty interesting taffy. You must eat it within a couple of days, but it's great.

And here's one of my favorite ideas: "muffins" made with eggs and your choice of grass-fed hamburger, shredded zucchini, mushrooms, onions, broccoli, cheeses, etc. Just pour the mixture into muffin tins, bake, and freeze for easy breakfasts on the go!

Plateaus

What Could Be Causing My Plateau?

The underlying premise of this book, and my philosophy of weight loss in general, is that *everybody's different* (the theory of biochemical individuality). So you will not be surprised to find that I wholeheartedly believe there are *at least* a dozen or more reasons for the dreaded plateaus that you will inevitably reach in your weight-loss efforts. The Drs. Eades have called plateaus "the purgatory of dieting" for good reason. They drive everyone crazy (plateaus, not the Eadeses, who are very lovely people!). Nevertheless, you need to learn to *expect* plateaus and learn to deal with them. I'll let you in on a secret: there is virtually no one who has successfully lost weight who has not experienced them. And the very first (and maybe most important) rule of dealing with them is this: don't panic, and don't give up.

Here are the top thirteen reasons plateaus occur:

1. **You are losing fat but also building muscle.** If you are exercising, especially for the first time, you may be putting on muscle while you are losing fat. This change for the better will not show up on the scale, though it would definitely show up in a body-composition analysis. You will likely notice a small but definite change in your shape or the measurement of your waist, even though the scale isn't really moving. Don't worry—eventually, the scale will reflect the loss of body fat.

2. **Water retention masks fat loss.** You may be losing fat while holding on to water. This happens more often than you might imagine. Make sure you are drinking plenty of water. Not drinking enough water is one of the top reasons for plateaus and stalls.

3. **You are experiencing a period of adjustment.** Remember that when it comes to weight, your body operates something like the feedback loop of a thermostat. Your body needs periods of adjustment to catch up with the different amount and type of fuel it's getting, just like the thermostat needs to "catch up" with changes in the temperature of the air in your apartment. If you're resetting your "set point," it happens not all at once, but in stages. Being stuck at a certain weight for a few weeks may just be your body's way of reprogramming itself. Eventually, the scale will move again.

4. **Your carbohydrate level is too high.** The plans discussed in this book are contingent on careful monitoring of carbohydrates. Your carbohydrate intake may simply be too high for what *your* body needs to lose weight. You could easily be taking in more carbs than you're aware of, as many foods and drinks have what are known as "hidden carbs." (The website Perfect Keto has some excellent articles on finding and identifying carbs.[47]) If you suspect this may be the problem, check it out.

5. **Your carbohydrate level is too low!** This is one of the great paradoxes of low-carb dieting, because it is completely counterintuitive. Nonetheless, I've seen it in action many times. More than one person wrote to me of weight loss stalled at a carb intake of 20 grams per day, which they were able to get going again by simply moving their carb intake *up* to about 40 or 50 grams. One possible explanation for this comes from the work of Dr. Diana Schwarzbein, who would argue that too low an intake of carbs creates higher levels of adrenaline and cortisol (which ultimately work against weight loss). While this scenario may not be true for everyone, upping your carbs is certainly worth a try.

6. **You are undereating.** Remember that the body responds to too few calories by simply becoming more efficient at extracting every single ounce of energy from its limited food supply. Too few calories literally slow down your metabolism. Stop it! These super-low-calorie eating plans *never* work.

7. **You are overeating.** At some point, every low-carber has to look at calories. Low-carb diets don't usually stress calorie-counting,

because you're much less likely to overeat on healthy proteins and good fats than you are on junk carbohydrates. Nonetheless, calories still count and you ignore them at your peril. You just may be eating too many of them.

8. **You aren't eating enough protein.** If you don't eat enough protein, you're more likely to break down your body's own protein for fuel. That means muscle loss, which in turn means a lowering of your metabolic rate. Make sure you're eating at least the minimum recommended amount of protein for your plan.

9. **You are not exercising.** Though weight loss is 80% diet, exercise definitely helps things along. The many things it does for both your health *and* your weight loss (and weight maintenance!) efforts are too lengthy to go into here. Just trust me. Do it.

10. **Medications are preventing optimum weight loss.** Many medications can interfere with weight loss. Steroid medications like prednisone are among the worst offenders, but there are plenty of others. Check this out with your doctor.

11. **You are experiencing food intolerances.** The usual suspects are foods that are generally reduced or eliminated on low-carb programs; if you're consuming them, try your own version of a modified elimination diet: remove the suspect food for a week or two and see what happens. The "sensitive seven" are wheat, milk, sugar, peanuts, soy, eggs, and corn.[48] (Refer to chapter 4 for a full discussion of the ways in which wheat, particularly, has a unique ability to keep you fat!) You may want to expand the wheat category to include all grains and the milk category to include cheese. Other well-known stallers that you might want to cut out for a while include artificial sweeteners, especially aspartame (Equal®); citric acid, found in diet sodas; glycerin, found in many low-carb meal-replacement bars, including those by Atkins; and alcohol.

12. **You have nutritional deficiencies.** A deficiency in some nutrient or nutrients may very well be interfering with how smoothly the energy-making cycles in your body run. This could easily account for you not burning fat at an optimal level. At the very least, take a high-potency multivitamin and mineral, although this is only the first line of defense—you probably need a lot

more. Just as an example, in a paper in *Medical Hypotheses*, Dr. L. H. Leung noted that for reasons not completely understood, he had had a lot of success with weight-loss patients by simply adding pantothenic acid to their program.[49] This could be because of pantothenic acid's direct effect on the adrenal glands. However, this is only one example; there are easily a dozen other vitamin or mineral deficiencies that could prevent optimal fat loss.

13. **You're trying to do a low-fat version of low-carb.** Many people are so mired in the low-fat theology that even when they try a low-carb approach they're still constantly trying to keep fat intake low. Don't. Fat keeps you full and satiated and has many other healthful properties. And remember that saturated fat in particular "behaves" quite differently in a very-low-carb diet than it does when it's accompanied by high-carb intake.

How Do I Break a Plateau?

You can try a lot of things. You could up your carbs if the amount you've been eating is very low, or you could try lowering them (see the list of reasons for plateaus in previous question). Try cutting out treats and going back exclusively to unprocessed meat and dark green vegetables for a few days. Cut out the low-carb bars. Drink a lot more water. Or try one of the following techniques, which have been known to knock people off plateaus:

Try a vegetable-and-fruit fast. Eat nothing but vegetables and some fruit for about 3 days. This is very alkalinizing, in addition to being low in calories and very high in nutrients. Eat all you want, and feel free to add some good fat like flaxseed oil (for women), olive oil, or butter.

Try a vegetable-juice fast. This is a favorite of Dr. Allan Spreen, the "Nutrition Physician," and it's one of my favorites as well. Go a day or two on nothing but freshly squeezed vegetable juices. I'm not talking V8® here; I'm talking the kind you make at home with a juicer. You can also drink hot water with lemon juice and, of course, all the fresh water you like.

Try raw foods for a few days. Be aware that not all people can tolerate this, and if your digestion isn't great, this may not be the best intervention for you.

Add digestive enzymes. Dr. John Hernandez, medical director of the Center for Health and Integrative Medicine in San Antonio, Texas, has found this to be one of the most useful weapons he has in his weight-loss arsenal.

Try the all-meat diet for a few days (no more than three). Eat nothing but meat and drink plenty of water. (The Dukan Diet uses this technique for one day a week during maintenance, and it suggests going back to the all-meat stage of the program for a few days if you ever get stuck on a plateau. On the other end of the spectrum, Dr. Shawn Baker eats like this 365 days a year—see the Carnivore Diet, page 264.) If you do this, do *not* fall into the "lean meat" trap; a diet with a lot of lean meat and no fat can induce a condition known as "rabbit starvation." You'll always fare better if your meat has some fat in it.

Do the Fat Fast. This is an Atkins technique, but it should be reserved for *only* the most metabolically resistant people who have been absolutely unable to move the scale any other way. It's based on the Kekwick and Pawan study in which researchers placed patients on a 1,000-calorie diet that was 90% fat and got better fat loss than on any other plan.[50] In the Atkins version, you eat only 1,000 calories, with 75% to 90% of it coming from fat. Atkins recommends five small meals of about 200 calories each. Sample 200-calorie choices include 1 ounce of macadamia nuts, 2 ounces of cream cheese or Brie, or 2 deviled eggs with 2 teaspoons of mayo. Atkins emphasizes that this is actually *dangerous* for anyone who is not metabolically resistant—the rate of weight loss is too rapid to be safe. Atkins used it only with people who could not lose weight any other way, to encourage them and to show them that weight loss was possible—but even then, he used it for only 4 or 5 days.

Exercise

What About Exercise?

Exercise is probably the most important predictor of whether you will keep weight off. Unfortunately, it doesn't really account for a great deal of the weight you will lose (maybe a few pounds a month). Nonetheless, if you don't exercise, the odds of keeping the weight off tumble. Some lucky people are able to lose weight just by adding a lot of exercise to their daily routine without changing their diets much, but these are very rare people who usually don't have an awful lot of weight to lose.

That being said, there are many, many excellent reasons to begin an exercise program if you are not exercising already. The health benefits alone are legion, and exercise is one of the things that helps change your biochemistry to that of a leaner person. Exercise has an insulin-like effect on lowering blood sugar, it increases serotonin, and—except when very high-intensity—it ultimately decreases stress hormones.

Low-carb exercise gurus, such as Robb Wolf, Jade Teta, and my old friend, the late, great Charles Poliquin recommend full-body circuit training for beginners (plus cardio interval training for all levels) as the ideal programs for low-carbers. I agree. These programs will maintain or even build a little muscle; yet they are not so overwhelmingly intense that you won't have the energy for them. You can supplement with cardio as you see fit: probably the more, the better. And don't worry about the so-called fat-burning zone (see the following question). Just go as long and as hard as you can without exhausting yourself; or mix short, intense workouts with longer, slower ones.

Whatever you do, do *not* neglect weight training. Walking by itself is just not going to cut it as an exercise program for weight loss, though it's downright spectacular for general health and well-being. But without using and challenging your muscles, you will lose them, slowly but surely, and that will slow down your metabolism. Weight training is the best way to boost a sluggish metabolism. The more muscle you have, the more calories you burn.

Do I Need to Exercise in the Fat-Burning Zone?

The need to exercise in the so-called fat-burning zone is a complete myth. You should exercise for as hard and as long as you safely and reasonably can, and go for the maximum amount of calories you can burn. It makes no real difference whether those calories come from fat or from sugar, any more than it matters if you pay for something with a check or with cash.

The average person uses about 70% fat and 30% sugar as "fuel" while they're sitting, sleeping, or relaxing. As they become more active, the percentages shift—the harder they exercise, the lower the proportion of fuel from fat and the higher the proportion of fuel from sugar. This is where the misunderstanding comes from. While the *percentages* of fuel do indeed change, so does the amount of calories burned. So, sure, at low levels of exercise, I'm burning about 70% of my calories from fat, but I'm burning only a couple of calories a minute! When I exercise harder, I may be burning only 40% fat, but I'm burning a lot more calories. Would you rather have 90% of all of my money or 10% of Warren Buffett's?

I Have No Stamina for Exercise When I'm on a Low-Carb Diet. What Gives?

My guess is it's one of two things: You're not fat-adapted yet, or you need more carbs.

When the first edition of this book came out, Lyle McDonald was considered of the foremost experts on the ketogenic diet. He worked with many athletes, particularly bodybuilders, and he was the author of an important textbook of the time, *The Ketogenic Diet.* MacDonald believes that with very high-intensity exercise, the ketogenic diet can present a problem as far as energy goes. He therefore recommends that on exercise days, you consume more carbohydrates than usual, then go back to your usual amount at the next meal. It's important to realize that he's talking only about super–high-intensity exercise. For more "regular" folks, a ketogenic—or any reduced-carb—diet will supply more than enough energy for circuit training, conventional weight training, and/or moderate aerobics. The researcher Steven Phinney, MD, PhD, has shown that elite cyclists can maintain their elite performance on a ketogenic diet after about a month of adaptation.[51] If you're not adapting after a month or you're still feeling low-energy, it may be that you're just not eating enough fat. Add more!

I've recently started both low-impact circuit training and a low-carb diet, and I haven't had any problems. As long as I don't overdo my workout, I have more energy than ever before.

—Janice K.

If even after that you still find that getting through your workouts is nearly impossible, it's time to start adding some carbs. Try eating a small amount (5 to 25 grams) of carbohydrate about 30 minutes before your workout and see if that helps. If it does, you'll know that you are one of those people who need more carbs to work out effectively.

You wouldn't be the first, either. Stuart Traeger, MD, is medical director of Atkins Nutritionals, a board-certified orthopedic surgeon, and—at least when I knew him—a lean, mean tri-athlete at the top of his game. An Atkins diet enthusiast, he nonetheless consumed about 100 grams of carbs a day when in training for his events. That's still low by the standards of the American diet, but it's a hell of a lot higher than most ketogenic diets. The point is—let's say it together, now, class—your mileage may differ. Everyone's different.

I'm a Runner and I Like to Run Races at My Local Runner's Club. I Thought "Carb Loading" Was a Must for Athletes. Can a Low-Carb Diet Work for Me?

Back when I first became a personal trainer in 1990, carb loading was indeed the go-to strategy for endurance athletes. But we've come a long way since then. Plenty of athletes train hard on very low-carb diets—just look online for Ben Greenfield, the ironman who has written a lot about triathlon training on a low carb diet. Or check out the personal blog of Valerie Peterson, whose website name tells the story: ketoadaptedcyclist.com.

Remember that the fuel you most want to use during endurance exercise is fat, not sugar. "Carb loading" simply ensures that your glycogen stores are full, which translates into using sugar for fuel. The better you are at fat-burning, the longer you'll be able to go. For what it's worth, Stu Mittleman, an exercise physiologist, nutritionist, ultra-marathoner, and one of the greatest endurance athletes of all time, generally ate a diet of about 40% carbs, 30% protein, and 30% fat—but, when in training for an event, he upped his *fat* intake to about 50% fat. Stu and I worked together at Equinox in the early and mid-'90s. "You gotta eat fat to burn fat," he'd always say. He was right.

Make Low-Carb Part of a System of Self-Care

If you think of low-carbing as nothing more than a way to get skinny, you are missing out on one of the great benefits of this lifestyle. Low-carbing does not have to be merely a weight-loss strategy. It can, and should, be the cornerstone of an entire system of self-care that enhances your health and your life in dozens of ways. Keeping carbs low is only the first step, and not even the most important. You can use the tools in this book to change your entire relationship to food and, by extension, to the whole notion of how you care for yourself. Some of the terrific benefits noted by low-carbers have to do with other changes in their diet and lifestyle that have accompanied their switch to low-carbohydrate foods.

JONNY BOWDEN'S HEALTHY LOW-CARB LIFE PYRAMID

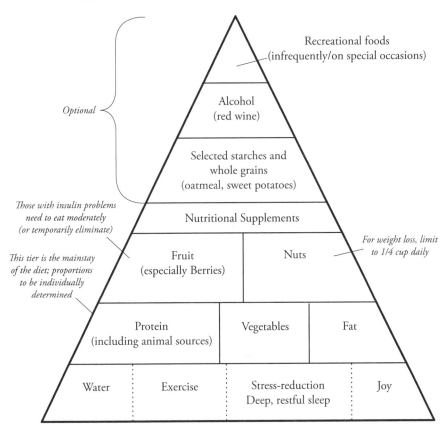

Here are ten important ways in which you can make low-carbing work for you forever.

1. **Eliminate trans-fats.** Because trans-fats are found in most of the foods that are eliminated on low-carb diets, low-carbers automatically reduce their intake of this dangerous, health-robbing fat, which is found in baked goods, cookies, cakes, snack foods, and especially foods deep-fried in vegetable oils. Avoid anything that includes *partially hydrogenated oil* on the label. Fats are vitally important for the integrity of the cells and as precursors to important hormones in the body, but if the good stuff isn't around, the body will make those structures out of the reject materials. Don't feed your body damaged goods. Give it the good stuff. Dump the trans-fats.

2. **Consume more omega-3s and way fewer omega-6s.** Omega-3s are found mostly in cold-water fish, grass-fed beef, flax, hemp, and chia. Omega-6s are found mainly in (highly processed) vegetable oils on your grocer's shelf. Omega-6s are pro-inflammatory; omega-3s are anti-inflammatory. You need both, but they need to be in balance. Many nutritionists believe that one of the greatest health problems of our time is the imbalance between these two classes of fats in the diet. Our Paleo ancestors consumed omega-6s and omega-3s in a very healthy 1:1 ratio. We currently consume something like a 20:1 ratio in favor of the pro-inflammatory omega-6s. Those polyunsaturated, highly processed vegetable oils contribute to a wide range of health problems. By reducing your consumption of vegetable oils and increasing your consumption of fish and flax (with food, supplements, or both), you help to restore the ideal ratio of fatty acids and go a long way toward improving your overall health.

3. **Eliminate sugar.** The destructive effects of sugar on human health have been addressed by nearly every one of the low-carb–diet authors and have been discussed in some depth in chapter 3. For those who want to delve deeper into the subject, there are several excellent books about sugar. There is absolutely no—I repeat, *no*—need for refined sugar in the

human diet. You may not be able to completely eliminate sugar from your diet, but you can sure try. The greater your success, the greater the benefit to your overall health and well-being.

4. **Eliminate processed foods. In the ideal diet**—low-carb or otherwise—you would eat only what you could hunt, fish, gather, pluck, grow, or possibly milk. While that may not be practical or possible in today's world, it's the bull's-eye to aim for. The more you can make foods with bar codes a smaller part of your diet, the better off you'll be. With food processing, the rule should be *none is best and less is better.* The closer a food is to the way nature created it, the better it is for your health. Eliminating processed foods also goes a long way toward eliminating a big source of exogenous toxins like chemicals, preservatives, deodorizers, colorings, flavorings, and especially trans-fatty acids.

5. **Build your meals around protein, fat, and vegetables.** As you can see from the Jonny Bowden Healthy Low-Carb Pyramid on page 319, these categories should form the basis of your diet. Alternately, you can think of the three categories as protein, fat, and fiber, with the fiber coming from vegetables, fruits, and nuts. The exact proportions of the three will vary from person to person. There have been hunter–gatherer societies that existed on almost all protein and fat (like the Inuit) and others that existed primarily on plant foods, but there have been no hunter–gatherer societies that thrived on TV dinners. Your individual metabolism and preferences will determine how much of a contribution each of these three categories— protein, fat, and vegetables—makes to your overall diet, but whatever the mix, these should be the three major sources for most of your calories. (This, at least, is the template—in real life, I'd add nuts and berries to the mix!)

6. **Drink plenty of water.** Water has been discussed in many places in this book, but drinking it still earns a place on the top-ten list of health habits to cultivate in order to make low-carb living synonymous with great health. Get in the daily habit of washing out metabolic waste products as well as the toxins in the fat cells you'll be emptying. Refresh, replenish, and restore your body's fluids on a constant basis with water. Just do it.

7. **Get plenty of sleep.** All together now, one more time: *stress makes you fat.* And one of life's biggest stressors is lack of sleep. Important hormones (like human growth hormone) and neurotransmitters (like serotonin) simply don't get made in sufficient quantities if you're not sleeping soundly and deeply for at least 7 to 8 hours a night. Sleep is a weight-loss drug. It has no bad side effects. And it's free!

8. **Exercise every day.** Not only will this increase your metabolic rate and burn calories, but doing it regularly—at least 5 days a week—is the single best predictor of whether you will be successful in keeping weight off. Exercise will change your mood, keep you lean, and very likely extend your life. Do you really need a better reason to get out and move?

9. **Get 25 to 50 grams of fiber every single day.** Getting the right amount of fiber will help you lose weight, help stabilize your blood sugar, lower the glycemic load of food, keep hunger at bay, and in all likelihood help protect against certain cancers. You get fiber in vegetables, nuts, and fiber supplements. And don't buy into the nonsense about needing foods like bread for fiber. Bread's a fiber lightweight. Much better to get it from vegetables, fruits, beans, and foods like avocados, which are surprisingly high in fiber!

10. **Expand joy in your life.** In the words of my nutrition mentor, the much-missed Robert Crayhon, "Pleasure is a nutrient." Never forget that sadness is not a Prozac deficiency. Some natural serotonin boosters are playing with kids, petting a dog, making love, being in the sunshine, and doing things for others. Find the things in your life that raise your spirits, lift your soul, and make you happy—then *do* them. Often!

You Can Lose Weight: Believing Is Seeing

Until 1954, it was generally believed that human beings could not run a mile in fewer than 4 minutes. The world agreed that there was an innate physiological limitation that prevented anyone from breaking this barrier. But the world forgot to tell Roger Bannister, a neurologist who, on May 6, 1954, ran a mile in 3 minutes, 59.4 seconds, the first sub-4-minute mile.

But that's not the interesting part of the story.

The interesting part of the story is that the *next* guy after Bannister to break the 4-minute-mile barrier—John Landy—did it 46 days later. For decades it had never been done, and then it was done *twice* in fewer than 2 months. By the end of 1957, sixteen runners had surpassed the record. The number who've done it as of the writing of this book is in the hundreds.

Why? Certainly, the aerobic capacity of human beings didn't suddenly expand in 1954. Here's what happened: the shared belief that it was not possible to run that fast evaporated. As soon as people *saw* that it was possible, they *believed* it could be done. Those sixteen runners who broke the sub-4-minute barrier were never stopped by a physiological barrier— they were stopped by their *belief* in a physiological barrier. When they saw that it could be done, they believed it was possible.

And then they did it.

This book is about giving you the best information available today about weight loss and diet. But in the long run, successful weight loss has never been just about information. Information is the first step. Information puts you on a level playing field. But the real action is what you do with that information—how you let it empower you, how you apply it to your life.

Weight loss is about taking control of your life.

If you can see it for yourself, as Bannister did, you can believe in it. And if you can believe in it, you can do it. Weight loss is just the medium in which you can practice mastery—of your environment, your mind, and your body.

Master these things and you master your life. The only limits that are there for you are those you believe in.

Enjoy the journey.

═ ACKNOWLEDGMENTS ═

I had another set of eyes on this manuscript before I sent it off to the publisher. That's hardly unusual for writers, but in this case the particular set of eyes belonged to Denise Minger. For anyone who knows her work, nothing more needs to be said. Another set of eyes: *valuable*. Denise Minger's eyes: *priceless*.

Thanks always to my incredible agent (for nearly two decades), Coleen O'Shea at The O'Shea Literary Agency.

My terrific editor, Nicole Fisher.

Anja, Susan, Christopher D., Christopher C., Dabby, Sky, Doug, Peter, Scott, Oliver, Billy, Lee, Mike D., Lauree, and Randy. By my calculation, you have collectively given me over 568 people-years of love, support, and friendship. I am eternally grateful.

To the writers and musicians who inspire me: William Goldman, Ed McBain, Robert Sapolsky, Miles Davis, Allen Stone, and Laura Nyro.

Jeff and Nancy; Jared, Cadence, and Logan; and Pace. I appreciate each of you more than you know.

And my partner and the love of my life, to whom I am happily, perpetually, and wholly engaged forever, and without whom I would not have the life I have and love: Michelle Elaine Mosher. I love you always.

═══ RESOURCES ═══

When you update and revise a book, you wind up adding a ton of material, but you also wind up cutting stuff you don't need any more. If you don't cut anything out to balance the new material, your book winds up being more than 200,000 words, and trust me, that doesn't make anyone—readers, editors, or publishers—a happy camper.

The resource section of the previous editions was an easy cut. There are so many resources for every topic discussed in this book, and they are so good and easy to find that it just seemed like a waste of paper to try to offer a complete list (in a print edition, no less, that couldn't be updated every week!).

I've done the resource section much differently this time. I've listed a few core books that I believe everyone interested in their health should know about. This doesn't mean there aren't amazing books out there loaded with fantastic information about hormones, the microbiome, food, metabolism, and all that good stuff. In fact, my friends write these books all the time, and all of them would be mad if I left their best work off this list. Understand that this is a super-abbreviated list of just seven books that I consider "foundational" texts.

1. *Nutrition Made Simple,* by **Robert Crayhon**

   This is the place to start—the best, simplest, and most accurate book on the basics of nutrition I've ever seen. My mentor, Robert Crayhon, wrote this book 20 years ago. It's still available, and it still holds up.

2. *Eat the Yolks,* by **Liz Wolfe**

   The modern-day version of *Nutrition Made Simple.* This is the book I send people to these days when they want to understand the basics of nutrition and the idiocy of the conventional dietary guidelines.

3. *Wheat Belly,* by **William Davis, and** *Grain Brain,* by **David Perlmutter**

   If you want to understand the problems with wheat and grains and what they do to our metabolism, brain, gut, behavior, and overall health, these are two books that you simply must have in your library. I refer to them often.

4. *Why We Get Fat,* **by Gary Taubes**

An excellent and cogent argument for the role of insulin in obesity and for why the conventional explanation for weight gain (*calories in-calories out*) is in desperate need of an update.

5. *The Big Fat Surprise,* **by Nina Tiecholz**

An absolutely fascinating step-by-step account by a first-rate journalist about how we came to adapt "low-fat, high-carb, cut-the-cholesterol" dogma in the first place and how we're still paying the price for doing so today.

6. *The Great Cholesterol Myth,* **by Jonny Bowden and Stephen Sinatra**

Feel free to substitute any of the many great books that make the same argument as ours: *The Great Cholesterol Con,* by Dr. Malcolm Kendrick, *Fat and Cholesterol Don't Cause Heart Attacks (and Statins Are Not the Solution),* by Dr. Paul Rosch, et al., or *The Diet Fix,* by Zoë Harcombe, PhD. But you should include on your list of must-reads at least *one* account of the cholesterol myth, explaining in detail how we got on the wrong track when it comes to preventing heart disease, and how, in the bargain, we adopted a diet that had the exact opposite effect.

7. *Food Rules,* **by Frank Lipman**

On any health topic I can think of, Frank Lipman always has great advice. I've yet to find anything he says that I really disagree with. I gave this book to all my friends and family—it's one of the best books I've ever seen on what to eat and how to live. It's simple without being the least simplistic. It's the book to give every person who has ever said "I'm so confused, I don't know what to eat anymore!"

Online

As for websites and Internet resources, you can't go wrong with any of the people listed below. I can't predict what these folks will be up to a decade from now; but if the past is any indication, you'll want to know about what they're doing. These are folks you can follow, read, digest, and use to guide your own journey. You literally can't go wrong listening to any of them.

For All Things Paleo

Esther Blum: https://estherblum.com/

Chris Kresser: https://chriskresser.com/

Mark Sisson: https://www.marksdailyapple.com/

Robb Wolf: https://robbwolf.com/

For Diet and Autoimmune Disease

Since paleo and autoimmune protocols frequently overlap, make sure to *also* check out Sarah Ballantyne (https://www.thepaleomom.com/about/about-sarah/), Amy Meyer (https://www.amymyersmd.com/), Alan Christianson (https://drchristianson.com/), Izabella Wentz (https://thyroid-pharmacist.com/), and Tom O'Bryan (https://thedr.com/). Those are my go-to's for autoimmune disease.

For All Things Keto

A good place to start is with Jimmy Moore, who has written a number of good intro books on keto and other related topics. He's a great resource (https://livinlavidalowcarb.com/). The heavy hitters in the research department are Dominick D'Agostino (https://www.ketonutrition.org/), Jeff Volek and Stephen Phinney (https://www.artandscienceoflowcarb.com/), and Eric Westman (https://www.adaptyourlife.com/). Those are names you'll want to mention next time your conventional doctor tells you there's "no research on low-carb diets."

For Intermittent Fasting

Dr. Jason Fung is the guru. You can find his videos all over YouTube and his books on Amazon.

Other People to Check in with Regularly

Peter Attia: https://peterattiamd.com/

Ivor Cummings: https://thefatemperor.com/

William Davis: https://www.wheatbellyblog.com/

David Diamond: @LDLskeptic

Michael Eades: https://proteinpower.com/drmike/

Andreas Eenfeldt: https://www.dietdoctor.com/

Chris Kresser: https://chriskresser.com/

Robert Lustig: https://robertlustig.com/

Chris Masterjohn: https://chrismasterjohnphd.com/

Denise Minger: https://deniseminger.com/

Tim Noakes: https://thenoakesfoundation.org/

Rhonda Patrick: https://www.foundmyfitness.com/

David Perlmutter: https://www.drperlmutter.com/

Most of the individuals above have strong online presences and tons of great material on their websites or on YouTube. And check out the people they follow on social media, because I'm 100% sure I left out some really important ones.

For Low-Carb Biohacking

In my experience, the vast majority of biohackers are low-carbers. Both paleo and keto, for example, are huge in the biohacking community. If you're interested in how people are combining low-carb diets with biohacks like cryotherapy, nootropics, nutraceuticals, fasting, microdosing, protein fasts, NAD activators, and other stuff on the cutting edge of performance and anti-aging, you'll want to check into what these guys are up to. As of this edition, all four have top-rated podcasts.

Dave Asprey: https://blog.daveasprey.com/category/podcasts/

Peter Attia: https://peterattiamd.com/podcast/

Tim Ferris: https://tim.blog/podcast/

Joe Rogan: http://podcasts.joerogan.net/

Conferences and Conventions

As of this writing, there are at least five annual conferences worth knowing about. If you want to keep up with the latest developments in the world of low-carb diets, biohacking, and keto, any or all of these are great places to go. Some have streaming options for those who can't attend in person.

Ancestral Health Society Conference.
Contact: https://ancestralhealth.org/

KetoCon.
Contact: https://www.ketocon.org/

LowCarb USA.
Contact: https://www.lowcarbusa.org/

Paleo f(x).
Contact: https://www.paleofx.com/

Upgrade Labs Biohacking Conference.
Contact: https://xp.upgradelabs.com/

And don't forget these three movies, all of which give you a superb overview of the arguments in favor of low-carb diets. All are widely available on the usual platforms.

Fat: A Documentary (Vinnie Tortorich/ Fat Squirrel Productions)

The Big Fat Lie (Wide Eye Productions)

The Magic Pill (Pete Evans/FanForce.Com)

≡ ENDNOTES ≡

Chapter 1: Low-Carb Redux: The Updated Truth About Low-Carbohydrate Diets

1. William S. Yancy, Jr., MD, MHS; Maren K. Olsen, PhD; et al., "A Low-Carbohydrate, Ketogenic Diet versus a Low-Fat Diet to Treat Obesity and Hyperlipidemia," *Annals of Internal Medicine* 140, no. 10 (2004): 769–777; Linda Stern, MD; Nayyar Iqbal, MD; Prakash Seshadri, MD, et al., "The Effects of Low-Carbohydrate versus Conventional Weight Loss Diets in Severely Obese Adults: One-Year Follow-up of a Randomized Trial," *Annals of Internal Medicine* 140, no. 10 (2004): 778–785.

2. Dr. Eric Charles Westman, associate professor of medicine at Duke University, consistently used very–low-carb diets in his obesity-treatment programs: Jeffry Gerber, MD, "Dr Eric Westman - Clinical Experience Using LCHF in a Medical Setting," *Denver's Diet Doctor*, https://denversdietdoctor.com/dr-eric-westman -clinical-experience-using-lchf-in-a-medical-setting/ (September 22, 2018); "Hundreds of Doctors Recommending a Low-Carb of Keto Diet," *Diet Doctor*, https://www.dietdoctor.com/low-carb/doctors.

3. Constance Brown-Riggs, MSEd, RD, CDE, CDN, "Low-Diets & Diabetes," *Today's Dietitian* 18, no. 8 (2016): 24.

4. Skye Gould, "6 Charts That Show How Much More Americans Eat than They Used To," *Business Insider*, https://www.businessinsider.com/daily-calories -americans-eat-increase-2016-07 (May 10, 2017).

5. "Comparison of the Atkins, Zone, Ornish, and LEARN Diets for Change in Weight and Related Risk Factors among Overweight Premenopausal Women," *Journal of the American Medical Association* 297, no. 9 (2007): 969–977.

6. Personal communication, interview with Christopher Gardner.

7. C. B. Ebbeling, M. M. Leidig, et al., "Effects of a Low-Glycemic Load vs. Low-Fat Diet in Obese Young Adults: A Randomized Trial," *Journal of the American Medical Association* 297, no. 19 (2007): 2092–2102.

8. "Moderately Reduced Carbohydrate Diet Keeps People Feeling Full Longer," *Science Daily*, http://www.sciencedaily.com/releases/2009/06/090611142405. htm (June 11, 2009).

9. Thomas L. Halton, Simin Liu, et al., "Low-Carbohydrate-Diet Score and Risk of Type 2 Diabetes in Women," *American Journal of Clinical Nutrition* 87, no. 2 (2008): 339–346.

10. Thomas L. Halton, Walter C. Willett, et al., "Low-Carbohydrate-Diet Score and the Risk of Coronary Heart Disease in Women," *New England Journal of Medicine* 355, no. 19 (2006): 1991–2002.

11. R. N. Smith, A. Braue, et al., "The Effect of a Low Glycemic Load Diet on Acne Vulgaris and the Fatty Acid Composition of Skin Surface Triglycerides," *Journal of Dermatological Science* 50, no. 1 (2008): 41–52.

12. C. C. Douglas, B. A. Gower, et al., "Role of Diet in the Treatment of Polycystic Ovary Syndrome," *Fertil Steril* 85, no. 3 (2006): 679–688.

13. P. Crawford, S. L. Paden, M. K. Park, "Clinical Inquiries: What Is the Dietary Treatment for Low HDL Cholesterol?" *Journal of Family Practice* 55, no. 12 (2006): 1076–1078.

14. C. J. Chiu, A. Taylor, et al., "Dietary Carbohydrate and the Progression of Age-Related Macular Degeneration: A Prospective Study from the Age-Related Eye Disease Study," American Journal of Clinical Nutrition 86, no. 4 (2007): 1210–1218; C. J. Chiu, L. D. Hubbard, et al., "Dietary Glycemic Index and Carbohydrate in Relation to Early Age-Related Macular Degeneration," *American Journal of Clinical Nutrition* 83, no. 4 (2006): 880–886.

15. R. J. Wood, M. L. Fernandez, et al., "Effects of a Carbohydrate-Restricted Diet with and without Supplemental Soluble Fiber on Plasma Low-Density Lipoprotein Cholesterol and Other Clinical Markers of Cardiovascular Risk," *Metabolism* 56, no. 1 (2007): 58–67.

16. S. M. Nickols-Richardson, M. D. Coleman, et al., "Perceived Hunger is Lower and Weight Loss is Greater in Overweight Premenopausal Women Consuming a Low-Carbohydrate/High-Protein vs. High-Carbohydrate/Low-Fat Diet," *Journal of the American Dietetic Association* 105, no. 9 (2005): 1433–1437.

17. G. Boden, K. Sargrad, et al., "Effect of a Low-Carbohydrate Diet on Appetite, Blood Glucose Levels, and Insulin Resistance in Obese Patients With Type 2 Diabetes," *Annals of Internal Medicine* 142, no. 6 (March 15, 2005): 403–411.

18. David J. A. Jenkins, et al., "The Effect of a Plant-Based Low-Carbohydrate ("Eco-Atkins") Diet on Body Weight and Blood Lipid Concentrations in Hyperlipidemic Subjects, *Archives of Internal Medicine* 169, no. 11 (2009): 1046–1054.

19. Anssi H. Manninen, "Metabolic Effects of the Very-Low-Carbohydrate Diets," *Journal of the International Society of Sports Nutrition* 1, no. 2 (2004): 7–11.

Chapter 2: The History and Origins of Low-Carb Diets

1. "Adventist Excellence: The Sanitarium Health & Wellbeing Company," EUD News, https://news.eud.adventist.org/en/all-news/news/go/2013-05-15/adventist-excellence-the-sanitarium-health-wellbeing-company/ (May 15, 2013).

2. Cristin E. Kearns, DDS, MBA; Laura A. Schmidt, PhD; MSW, MPH; Stanton A. Glantz, PhD, "Sugar Industry and Coronary Heart Disease Research: A Historical Analsis of Internal Industry Documents," *JAMA Internal Medicine* 176, no. 11 (2016): 1680–1685; Anahad O'Connor, "How the Sugar Industry Shifted Blame to Fat," *New York Times*, https://www.nytimes.com/2016/09/13/well/eat/how-the-sugar-industry-shifted-blame-to-fat.html (September 12, 2016); Alessandra Potenza, "Onside the Fight over the Sugar Conspiracy," *The Verge*, https://www.theverge.com/2018/2/23/17039780/sugar-industry-conspiracy-heart-disease-research-mark-hegsted-harvard (February 23, 2018).

3. "USDA Strategic Goals," U.S. Department of Agriculture, https://www.usda.gov/our-agency/about-usda/strategic-goals; "USDA Launches Trade Mitigation Programs," United States Department of Agriculture Farm Service Agency," https://www.fsa.usda.gov/news-room/news-releases/2018/nr_2018_0904_rel_0172 (September 4, 2018).

Chapter 2, continued . . .

4. Belinda Fettke, "Lifestyle Medicine...where did the meat go?" I Support Gary, https://isupportgary.com/articles/the-plant-based-diet-is-vegan.

5. William Banting, Letter on Corpulence (self, 1864); full text available at http://www.lowcarb.ca/corpulence/corpulence_1.html.

6. Leah Deventer, "Banting for beginners," *Good Housekeeping South Africa,* https://www.goodhousekeeping.co.za/banting-for-beginners/.

7. Dr. Phil McGraw, *The Ultimate Weight Solution: The 7 Keys to Weight Loss Freedom* (New York: Free Press, 2003).

8. Vance Thompson, *Eat and Grow Thin* (New York: E.P. Dutton, 1914).

9. Alfred Pennington, *New England Journal of Medicine* 248 (1953): 959; *American Journal of Digestive Diseases* 21 (1954): 69.

10. Alfred Pennington, *Holiday Magazine,* June 1950. Quoted in Richard Mackarness, *Eat Fat and Grow Slim* (London: Harvill, 1958).

11. Vilhjalmur Stefansson, "Adventures in Diet," *Harper's Monthly Magazine* (November 1935, December 1935, January 1936).

12. Ibid.

13. Ibid.

14. Evelyn Stefansson, preface to *Eat Fat and Grow Slim,* by Richard Mackarness (London: Harvill, 1958).

15. Ibid.

16. Blake Donaldson, *Strong Medicine* (New York: Doubleday, 1960).

17. Alan Kekwick and Gaston L.S. Pawan, "Calorie Intake in Relation to Body Weight Changes in the Obese," *Lancet* 2 (1956): 155; "Metabolic Study in Human Obesity with Isocaloric Diets High in Fat, Protein or Carbohydrate," *Metabolism* 6, no. 5 (1957): 447–460; "The Effect of High Fat and High Carbohydrate Diets on Rates of Weight Loss in Mice," *Metabolism* 13, no. 1 (1964): 87–97.

18. Bonnie J. Brehm, et al., "A Randomized Trial Comparing a Very Low Carbohydrate Diet and a Calorie-Restricted Low Fat Diet on Body Weight and Cardiovascular Risk Factors in Healthy Women," *Journal of Clinical Endocrinology and Metabolism* 88, no. 4 (2003): 1617–1623.

19. Richard Mackarness, *Eat Fat and Grow Slim* (London: Harvill, 1958).

20. Christian B. Allan and Wolfgang Lutz, *Life Without Bread* (Los Angeles: Keats, 2000).

21. Richard Mackarness, *Eat Fat and Grow Slim* (London: Harvill, 1958).

22. Anonymous, *Beyond Our Wildest Dreams: A History of Overeaters Anonymous as Seen by a Cofounder* (Rio Rancho, NM: Overeaters Anonymous, 1996).

23. Herman Taller, *Calories Don't Count* (New York: Simon & Schuster, 1961).

24. Ibid.

25. Ancel Keys, "Coronary Heart Disease in Seven Countries," *Circulation* 41, suppl. 1 (1970): 1–211.

26. Uffe Ravnskov, *The Cholesterol Myths* (Washington, DC: New Trends, 2000); Malcolm Kendrick, "Why the Cholesterol-Heart Disease Theory Is Wrong," http://www.thincs.org/Malcolm.choltheory.htm (July 31, 2012); Uffe Ravnskov, "Is Atherosclerosis Caused by High Cholesterol?" QJM 95, no. 6 (2002): 397–403.

27. Mary Enig, "The Oiling of America," http://www.westonaprice.org/know-your-fats/the-oiling-of-america; C.V. Felton, et al., "Dietary Polyunsaturated Fatty Acids and Composition of Human Aortic Plaques," *Lancet* 344 (1994): 1195–1196; P.A. Godley, et al., "Biomarkers of Essential Fatty Acid Consumption and Risk of Prostatic Carcinoma," *Cancer Epidemiology Biomarkers & Prevention* 5, no. 11 (1996): 889–895; M.S. Micozzi and T.E. Moon, Investigating the Role of Macronutrients, vol. 2, Nutrition and Cancer Prevention Series (New York: Marcel Dekker, 1992).

28. Laura Fraser, *Losing It: False Hopes and Fat Profits in the Diet Industry* (New York: Plume, 1998).

29. Irwin Stillman, *The Doctor's Quick Weight Loss Diet* (New York: Dell, 1967).

30. Marjorie R. Freedman, et al., "Popular Diets: A Scientific Review," *Obesity Research* 9 suppl. (2001): 5S–17S.

31. Ancel Keys, "Coronary Heart Disease in Seven Countries," *Circulation* 41, suppl. 1 (1970): 1–211.

32. George V. Mann, *Coronary Heart Disease: The Dietary Sense and Nonsense* (London: Janus, 1993).

33. Uffe Ravnskov, *The Cholesterol Myths* (Washington, DC: New Trends, 2000).

34. George V. Mann, et al., "Atherosclerosis in the Masai," *American Journal of Epidemiology* 95 (1972): 26–37.

35. John Yudkin, *Sweet and Dangerous* (New York: Wyden, 1972).

36. Ancel Keys, "Letter: Normal Plasma Cholesterol in a Man Who Eats 25 Eggs a Day," *The New England Journal of Medicine* 325 (1991): 584.

37. National Heart, Lung, and Blood Institute, National Cholesterol Education Program, http://www.nhlbi.nih.gov/about/ncep.

38. Apex Fitness Group, *Apex Fitness Systems Certification Manual*, 3rd ed. (Thousand Oaks, CA: Apex Fitness Group, 2001).

39. Dean Ornish, "Intensive Lifestyle Changes for Reversal of Coronary Heart Disease," *Journal of the American Medical Association* 280, no. 23 (December 16, 1998): 2001–2007.

40. Marjorie R. Freedman, et al., "Popular Diets: A Scientific Review," *Obesity Research* 9 (2001): 5S–17S, tables 6 and 7, https://onlinelibrary.wiley.com/doi/full /10.1038/oby.2001.113.

41. "Q&A with Nutritionist Walter Willett," *Discover*, http://discovermagazine.com/2003/mar/breakdialogue (March 1, 2003); Walter Willett, *Eat, Drink, and Be Healthy* (New York: Fireside, 2001).

42. USDA Millennium Lecture Series Symposium on the Great Nutrition Debate, https://fns-prod.azureedge.net/sites/default/files/archived_projects/GreatNutritionDebateSymposium.pdf (July 31, 2012).

Chapter 3: Why Low-Carb Diets Work

1. Woodson Merrell, "How I Became a Low-Carb Believer," *Time* (November 1, 1999).

2. Gary Taubes, "What If It's All Been a Big Fat Lie?" *New York Times Magazine*, (July 7, 2002).

Chapter 3, continued . . .

3. Sharon H. Saydah, et al., "Abnormal Glucose Tolerance and the Risk of Cancer Death in the United States," *American Journal of Epidemiology* 157 (2003): 1092–1100; B.A. Stoll, "Upper Abdominal Obesity, Insulin Resistance and Breast Cancer Risk," *International Journal of Obesity and Related Metabolic Disorders* 26, no. 6 (2002): 747–753.

4. Nancy Appleton, *Lick the Sugar Habit* (New York: Avery, 1996).

5. C. Leigh Broadhurst, *Diabetes: Prevention and Cure* (New York: Kensington, 1999); Christian B. Allan and Wolfgang Lutz, *Life Without Bread* (New York: McGraw-Hill, 2000).

6. Walter Willett, *Eat, Drink, and Be Healthy* (New York: Fireside, 2001).

7. Ron Rosedale, "Insulin and Its Metabolic Effects," lecture given at Boulderfest Nutrition Conference, Boulder, CO, 1999.

8. J. Lemann, et al., "Evidence That Glucose Ingestion Inhibits Net Renal Tubular Reabsorption of Calcium and Magnesium in Man," *American Journal of Clinical Nutrition* 70 (1967): 236–245.

9. Veronique Douard, et al., "Chronic High Fructose Intake Reduces Serum 1,25 (OH)2D3 Levels in Calcium-Sufficient Rodents," *PLoS One* 9, no. 4, https://www.ncbi.nlm.nih.gov/pmc/articles/PMC3981704/ (April 9, 2014).

10. Christian L. Roth, et al., "Vitamin D Deficiency in Obese Rats Exacerbates Nonalcoholic Fatty Liver Disease and Increases Hepatic Resistin and Toll-like Receptor Activation," *Hepatology* 55, no. 4 (2012): 1103–1011.

11. John Yudkin, et al., "Effects of High Dietary Sugar," *British Journal of Medicine* 281 (November 22, 1980): 1396.

12. Ron Rosedale, "Insulin and Its Metabolic Effects," lecture given at Boulderfest Nutrition Conference, Boulder, CO, 1999.

13. J. Michael Gaziano, "Fasting Triglycerides, High-Density Lipoprotein, and Risk of Myocardial Infarction," *Circulation* 96 (1997): 2520–2525.

14. Gerald Reaven, "An Interview with Gerald Reaven," interview by Louise Morrin, *The Canadian Association of Cardiac Rehabilitation Newsletter*, September 2000.

15. Calvin Ezrin, with Kristen L. Caron, *Your Fat Can Make You Thin* (Lincolnwood, IL: Contemporary Books, 2001).

16. Adam Marcus, "Low-Fat Mice Hold Clue to Obesity Treatment," *Reuters Magazine* (December 7, 2000).

17. Mitchell Lazar, et al., "The Hormone Resistin Links Obesity to Diabetes," *Nature* 409, no. 6818 (2001): 307–312; Nathan Seppa, "Protein May Tie Obesity to Diabetes," *Science News* 159 (2001): 36.

18. Calvin Ezrin, with Kristen L. Caron, *Your Fat Can Make You Thin* (Lincolnwood, IL: Contemporary Books, 2001).

19. Donald K. Layman, et al., "A Reduced Ratio of Dietary Carbohydrate to Protein Improves Body Composition and Blood Lipid Profiles During Weight Loss in Adult Women," *Journal of Nutrition* 133, no. 2 (February 2003): 411–417; Donald K. Layman, et al., "Increased Dietary Protein Modifies Glucose and Insulin Homeostasis in Adult Women During Weight Loss," *Journal of Nutrition* 133, no. 2 (February 2003): 405–410.

20. Donald K. Layman, et al., "The Role of Leucine in Weight Loss Diets and Glucose Homeostasis," *Journal of Nutrition* 133, no. 1 (January 2003): 261S–267S.

21. Y.O. Chang and C.C. Soong, "Effect of Feeding Diets Lacking Various Essential Amino Acids on Body Composition of Rats," *International Journal for Vitamin and Nutrition Research* 45, no. 2 (1975): 230–236.

22. Donald K. Layman, et al., "A Reduced Ratio of Dietary Carbohydrate to Protein Improves Body Composition and Blood Lipid Profiles during Weight Loss in Adult Women," *Journal of Nutrition* 133, no. 2 (February 2003): 411–417.

23. Carol S. Johnston, Sherrie L. Tjonn, Pamela D. Swan, "Postprandial Thermogenesis Is Increased 100% on a High-Protein, Low-Fat Diet versus a High-Carbohydrate, Low-Fat Diet in Healthy, Young Women," *Journal of the American College of Nutrition* 21, no. 1 (February 2002): 55–61.

24. American Association of Clinical Endocrinologists, "Findings and Recommendations on the Insulin Resistance Syndrome" (American Association of Clinical Endocrinologists, Washington, DC, August 25–26, 2002).

25. Ibid.

26. "New CDC Report: More than 100 Million Americans Have Diabetes or Prediabetes," CDC Newsroom, https://www.cdc.gov/media/releases/2017/p0718-diabetes-report.html (July 18, 2017).

27. Joyce M. Lee, et al., "Prevalence and Determinants of Insulin Resistance Among U.S. Adolescents," *DiabetesCare* 29, no. 11 (2006): 2427–2432.

28. "New CDC Report: More than 100 Million Americans Have Diabetes or Prediabetes," CDC Newsroom, https://www.cdc.gov/media/releases/2017/p0718-diabetes-report.html (July 18, 2017).

29. American Association of Clinical Endocrinologists, "Findings and Recommendations on the Insulin Resistance Syndrome" (American Association of Clinical Endocrinologists, Washington, DC, August 25–26, 2002).

30. American Diabetes Association, "Diabetes Statistics," https://www.diabetes.org/resources/statistics (January 26, 2011).

31. American Association of Clinical Endocrinologists, "Findings and Recommendations on the Insulin Resistance Syndrome" (American Association of Clinical Endocrinologists, Washington, DC, August 25–26, 2002); John E. Gerich, "Contributions of Insulin-Resistance and Insulin-Secretory Defects to the Pathogenesis of Type 2 Diabetes Mellitus," *Mayo Clinic Proceedings* 78, no. 4 (2003): 447–456.

32. E.S. Ford, et al., "Prevalence of the Metabolic Syndrome among US Adults," *Journal of the American Medical Association* 287 (2002): 356–359.

33. Dara Myers, "Diabetes Diet War," *U.S. News & World Report* 135, no. 1 (2003): 48–49.

34. Richard Bernstein, *The Diabetes Solution* (New York: Little, Brown, 1997); C. Leigh Broadhurst, *Diabetes: Prevention and Cure* (New York: Kensington, 1999).

35. American Association of Clinical Endocrinologists, "Findings and Recommendations on the Insulin Resistance Syndrome" (American Association of Clinical Endocrinologists, Washington, DC, August 25–26, 2002).

36. Laure Morin-Papunen, "Insulin Resistance in Polycystic Ovary Syndrome," PhD diss. University of Oulu, Finland, 2000.

Chapter 3, continued . . .

37. Mark Perloe, "Treatment of Polycystic Ovary Syndrome with Insulin Lowering Medications," ModernMedicine Network, https://www.obgyn.net/infertility/polycystic-ovary-syndrome-treatment-insulin-lowering-medications (November 11, 2011).

38. Ron Rosedale, "Insulin and Its Metabolic Effects," lecture given at Boulderfest Nutrition Conference, Boulder, CO, 1999.

39. Vincenzo Marigliano, et al., "Normal Values in Extreme Old Age," *Annals of the New York Academy of Sciences* 673 (December 22, 1992): 23–28.

40. J. Salmeron, et al., "Dietary Fat Intake and Risk of Type 2 Diabetes in Women," *American Journal of Clinical Nutrition* 73, no. 6 (2001): 1019–1026.

41. B.V. Mann, "Metabolic Consequences of Dietary Trans-Fatty Acids," *Lancet* 343 (1994): 1268–1271.

42. Elson Haas, *The False Fat Diet* (New York: Ballantine, 2000).

43. "Definition & Facts for Kidney Disease," National Institute of Diabetes and Digestive and Kidney Diseases, https://www.niddk.nih.gov/health-information/digestive-diseases/celiac-disease/definition-facts#common.

44. James Braly with Ron Hoggan, *Dangerous Grains* (New York: Avery, 2002).

45. Joseph Mercola with Alison Rose Levy, *The No-Grain Diet* (New York: Dutton, 2003).

46. Simin Liu, et al., "A Prospective Study of Dietary Glycemic Load, Carbohydrate Intake, and Risk of Coronary Heart Disease in U.S. Women," *American Journal of Clinical Nutrition* 71, no. 6 (2000): 1455–1461.

47. Walter Willett, et al., "Glycemic Index, Glycemic Load, and Risk of Type 2 Diabetes," *American Journal of Clinical Nutrition* 76, no. 1 (July 2002): 274S–280S.

Chapter 4: The Major Culprits in a High-Carb Diet: Wheat and Fructose

1. American Diabetes Association, "Diabetes Statistics," https://www.diabetes.org/resources/statistics (January 26, 2011).

2. National Heart, Lung, and Blood Institute, "What Is Metabolic Syndrome?" https://www.nhlbi.nih.gov/health-topics/metabolic-syndrome (June 4, 2012).

3. Endocrine Society, "Obesity at a Glance," http://endocrinefacts.org/health-conditions/obesity/ (2015).

4. Andrea Galassi, et al., "Metabolic Syndrome and Risk of Cardiovascular Disease," *The American Journal of Medicine* 119, no. 10 (2006): 812–819.

5. "Diabetes, Heart Disease, and Stroke," National Institute of Diabetes and Digestive and Kidney Diesease, https://www.niddk.nih.gov/health-information/diabetes/overview/preventing-problems/heart-disease-stroke.

6. "New CDC report: More than 100 million Americans have diabetes or prediabetes," CDC Newsroom, https://www.cdc.gov/media/releases/2017/p0718-diabetes-report.html (July 18, 2017).

7. "Diabetes, Heart Disease, and Stroke," National Institute of Diabetes and Digestive and Kidney Disease, https://www.niddk.nih.gov/health-information/diabetes/overview/preventing-problems/heart-disease-stroke.

8. "Hypertension (High Blood Pressure)," Cleveland Clinic, https://my. clevelandclinic.org/health/diseases/4314-hypertension-high-blood-pressure.

9. Rik P. Bogers, et al., "Association of Overweight with Increased Risk of Coronary Heart Disease Partly Independent of Blood Pressure and Cholesterol Levels," *Archives of Internal Medicine* 167, no. 16, (2007): 1720 –1728.

10. John N. Fain, "Release of Inflammatory Mediators by Human Adipose Tissue is Enhanced in Obesity and Primarily by the Nonfat Cells," *Mediators of Inflammation,* http://www.hindawi.com/journals/mi/2010/513948 (June 6, 2012).

11. S. A. Silvera, et al., "Dietary Carbohydrates and Breast Cancer Risk: A Prospective Study of the Roles of Overall Glycemic Index and Glycemic Load, *International Journal of Cancer* 114, no. 4 (2005): 653–658.

12. S. Sieri, et al., "Dietary Glycemic Load and Risk of Coronary Heart Disease in a Large Italian Cohort," *Archives of Internal Medicine* 170, no. 7, (2010): 640–647.

13. A. Esfahani, et al., "The Glycemic Index: Physiological Significance," *Journal of the American College of Nutrition* 28 suppl. (2009): 439S–445S.

14. "Study of Obese Diabetics Explains Why Low-Carb Diets Produce Fast Results," *Science Daily,* http://www.sciencedaily.com/releases/2005/03/050326095632.htm (March 26, 2005).

15. Ibid.

16. Kay M. Behall, et al., "Diets Containing High Amylose vs Amylopectin Starch: Effects on Metabolic Variables in Human Subjects," *American Journal of Clinical Nutrition* 49 (1989): 337–344.

17. Kaye Foster-Powell, Susanna H. A. Holt, Janette C. Brand-Miller, "International Table of Glycemic Index and Glycemic Load Values," *American Journal of Clinical Nutrition* 76, no. 1(2002): 5–56.

18. William Davis, *Wheat Belly,* (New York: Rodale, 2011): 35.

19. Martin R. Cohen, et al., "Naloxone Reduces Food Intake in Humans," *Psychosomatic Medicine* 47, no. 2 (1985): 132–138.

20. Adam Drewnowski, et al., "Naloxone, an Opiate Blocker, Reduces the Consumption of Sweet High-Fat Foods in Obese and Lean Female Binge Eaters," *American Journal of Clinical Nutrition* 61 (1995): 1206–1212.

21. Cindy D. Davis, PhD., "The Gut Microbiome and Its Role in Obesity," *Nutrition Today* 51, no. 4, (2017): 167–174.

22. Veronica L. Lozano, Nicolas Befarge, et al., "Sex-dependent Impact of Roundup on the Rat Gut Microbiome," *Toxicology Reports* 5 (2018): 96–107.

23. Qixing Mao, et al., "The Ramazzini Institute 13-week Pilot Study on Glyphosate and Roundup Administered at Human-equivalent Dose to Sprague Dawley Rats: Effects on the Microbiome," *Environmental Health* 17 (2018): 50.

24. Ibid.

25. Alexander Koliada, "Association Between Body Mass Index and *Firmicutes/ Bacteroidetes* ratio in an Adult Ukranian Population," *BMC Microbiology* 17 (2017): 120.

26. Pierre Gélinas, Fleur Gagnon, and Carole McKinnon, Wheat Preharvest Herbicide Application, Whole-grain Flour Properties, Yeast Activity and the Degradation of Glyphosate in Bread," *International Journal of Food Science and Technology* 53, no. 7 (2018): 1597–1602.

27. Report by Health Research Institute Laboratories, Full text at https:// d3n8a8pro7vhmx.cloudfront.net/yesmaam/pages/3564/attachments/ original/1518550923/COA_S0001770_Moms_bread_samples.pdf?1518550923 (November 6, 2017).

28. Xiaosen Ouyang, et al., "Fructose Consumption as a Risk Factor for Non-Alcoholic Fatty Liver Disease," *Journal of Hepatology* 48, no. 6 (2008): 993–999; Kyoko Nomura, Toshikazu Yamanouchi, "The Role of Fructose-Enriched Diets in Mechanisms of Nonalcoholic Fatty Liver Disease," *The Journal of Nutritional Biochemistry* 23, no. 3, (2012): 203–208; Manal F. Abdelmalek, et al., "Increased Fructose Consumption is Associated with Fibrosis Severity in Patients with NAFLD," *Hepatology* 51, no. 6,(2010): 1961–1971.

29. Wendy Loo, "Fructose, Not Fats, the Main Cause of NAFLD Epidemic," *Medical Tribune*, MIMS Malaysia (accessed Mar 24, 2012).

30. Robbert Meerwaldt, et al., "The Clinical Relevance of Assessing Advanced Glycation Endproducts Accumulation in Diabetes," *Cardiovascular Diabetology* 7 (2008): 29; Andries J. Smith, et al., "Advanced Glycation Endproducts in Chronic Heart Failure," *Annals of the New York Library of Science* 1126, no. 1 (2008): 225–230; Jasper W. L. Hartog, et al., "Advanced Glycation End-Products (AGEs) and Heart Failure: Pathophysiology and Clinical Implications," *European Journal of Heart Failure* 9, no. 12 (2007): 1146–1155.

31. Kimber L. Stanhope, et al., "Consumption of Fructose and High Fructose Corn Syrup Increase Postprandial Triglycerides, LDL-Cholesterol, and Apoliprotein-B in Young Men and Women," *The Journal of Clinical Endocrinology & Metabolism* 96, no. 10 (2011): E1596–E1605; "Fructose Consumption Increases Risk Factors for Heart Disease," *Science Daily*, http://www.sciencedaily.com/releases/2011/07/110728082558.htm (July 28, 2011); Kimber L. Stanhope and Peter J. Havel, "Endocrine and Metabolic Effects of Beverages Sweetened with Fructose, Glucose, Sucrose, or High-Fructose Corn Syrup," *The American Journal of Clinical Nutrition* 88, no. 6 (2008): 1733S–1737S.

32. Gary Taubes, "Is Sugar Toxic?" *New York Times*, http://www.nytimes.com/2011 /04/17/magazine/mag-17Sugar-t.html?pagewanted=all (April 13, 2011).

33. Luc Tappy, et al., "Metabolic Effects of Fructose and the Worldwide Increase in Obesity," *Physiological Reviews* 90, no.1 (2010): 23–46; M. Dirlewanger, et al., "Effects of Fructose on Hepatic Glucose Metabolism in Humans, *American Journal of Physiology - Endocrinology and Metabolism* 279 (2000): E907–E911.

34. S. S. Elliott, N. L. Keim, J. S. Stern, et al., "Fructose, Weight Gain, and the Insulin Resistance Syndrome." *The American Journal of Clinical Nutrition* 76, no. 5 (2002): 911–922; K. A. Lê, L. Tappy, "Metabolic Effects of Fructose," *Current Opinion in Clinical Nutrition & Metabolic Care* 9, no. 4 (2006): 469–475; Y. Rayssiguier, E. Gueux, W. Nowacki, et al., "High Fructose Consumption Combined with Low Dietary Magnesium Intake May Increase the Incidence of the Metabolic Syndrome by Inducing Inflammation," *Magnesium Research* 19, no. 4 (2006): 237–243.

35. A. C. Rutledge, K. Adeli, "Fructose and the Metabolic Syndrome: Pathophysiology and Molecular Mechanisms," *Nutrition Reviews* 65 no. 6 pt. 2, S13–S23; K. A. Lê, L. Tappy "Metabolic Effects of Fructose," *Current Opinion in Clinical Nutrition & Metabolic Care* 9, no. 4 (2006): 469–475.

36. "Fructose Metabolism by the Brain Increases Food Intake and Obesity," *Science Daily*, http://www.sciencedaily.com/releases/2009/03/090325091811.htm (March 25, 2009).

37. Ann Harding, "Diabetes Doubles Alzheimer's Risk," *CNN Health*, http://www.cnn.com/2011/09/19/health/diabetes-doubles-alzheimers/index.html (September 19, 2011); "Getting Diabetes Before 65 More than Doubles Risk for Alzheimer's Disease," *Science Daily*, http://www.sciencedaily.com/releases/2009/01/090127152835.htm (January 27, 2009).

Chapter 5: The Cholesterol Connection: Have We All Been Misled?

1. "Low-Carb Diet Reduces Inflammation and Blood Saturated Fat in Metabolic Syndrome," *Science Daily*, http://www.sciencedaily.com/releases/2007/12/071203091236.htm (December 3, 2007).

2. "Food Fried in Vegetable Oil May Contain Toxic Compound," *Bio-Medicine*, http://news.bio-medicine.org/biology-news-3/Food-fried-in-vegetable-oil-may-contain-toxic-compound-11958-1 (May 2005).

3. Patty W. Siri-Tarino, Qi Sun, Frank B. Hu, and Ronald M. Krauss, "Meta-analysis of Prospective Cohort Studies Evaluating the Association of Saturated Fat with Cardiovascular Disease," *The American Journal of Clinical Nutrition* 91, no. 3 (2010): 535–546; Rajiv Chowdhury, MD, PhD, et al., "Association of Dietary, Circulating, and Supplement Fatty Acids with Coronary Risk: A Systematic Review and Meta-Analysis," *Annals of Internal Medicine* 160, no. 6 (2018)" 398–406.

4. Rajiv Chowdhury, MD, PhD, et al., "Association of Dietary, Circulating, and Supplement Fatty Acids with Coronary Risk: A Systematic Review and Meta-Analysis," *Annals of Internal Medicine* 160, no. 6 (2014): 398–406.

5. Lee Hooper, et al., "Reduced or modified dietary fat for preventing cardiovascular disease," Cochrane Database of Systematic Reviews, https://www.ncbi.nlm.nih.gov/pubmed/21735388/ (July 6, 2011).

6. Zoë Harcombe, et al., "Evidence from Randomised Controlled Trials Did Not Support the Introduction of Dietary Fat Guidelines in 1977 and 1983: A Systematic Review and Meta-analysis," BMJ Journals, https://openheart.bmj.com/content/2/1/e000196 (2015).

7. James H. Hays, Angela DiSabatino, et al., "Effect of a High Saturated Fat and No-Starch Diet on Serum Lipid Subfractions in Patients with Documented Atherosclerotic Cardiovascular Disease," *Mayo Clinic Proceedings* 78, no. 11 (November 2003): 1331–1336.

8. Jeff Volek and Cassandra Forsythe, "The Case for Not Restricting Saturated Fat on a Low Carbohydrate Diet," *Nutrition & Metabolism* (London) 2 (2005): 21.

9. Walter C. Willett and Alberto Ascherio, "Commentary: Trans-Fatty Acids: Are the Effects Only Marginal?" *American Journal of Public Health* 84 (1994): 722–724.

Chapter 5, continued . . .

10. M. A. French, K. Sundram, and M. T. Clandinin, "Cholesterolaemic Effect of Palmitic Acid in Relation to Other Dietary Fatty Acids," *Asia Pacific Journal of Clinical Nutrition* 11, suppl. 7 (2002): S401–S407.

11. J. Bruce German, "A Reappraisal of the Impact of Dairy Foods and Milk Fat on Cardiovascular Disease Risk," *European Journal of Nutrition* 48, no. 4 (2009): 191–203.

12. The Relationship between High-fat Dairy Consumption and Obesity, Cardiovascular, and Metabolic, Disease," *European Journal of Nutrition* 52, no. 1 (2013): 1–4.

13. H. M. Krumholz, S. S. Seeman, et al., "Lack of Association between Cholesterol and Coronary Heart Disease Mortality and Morbidity and All-Cause Mortality in Persons Older than 70 Years," *Journal of the American Medical Association* 272, no. 17 (1994): 1335–1340.

14. Michel de Lorgeril, et al., "Mediterranean Diet, Traditional Risk Factors, and the Rate of Cardiovascular Complications After Myocardial Infarction: Final Report of the Lyon Diet Heart Study," *Circulation* 99 (1999): 779–785.

15. Darlene M. Dreon, et al., "A Very-Low-Fat Diet Is Not Associated with Improved Lipoprotein Profiles in Men with a Predominance of Large, Low-Density Lipoproteins," *American Journal of Clinical Nutrition* 69, no. 3 (March 1999): 411–418.

16. Antonio M. Gotto Jr., "Triglyceride: The Forgotten Risk Factor," *Circulation* 97, no. 11 (1998): 1027–1028.

17. J. Michael Gaziano, et al., "Fasting Triglycerides, High-Density Lipoprotein, and Risk of Myocardial Infarction," *Circulation* 96 (1997): 2520–2525.

18. Ibid.

19. "Nutrition—Cholesterol Guidelines," Cleveland Clinic, Miller Family Heart & Vascular Institute, http://my.clevelandclinic.org/heart/prevention/nutrition/atp3.aspx.

20. Stephen R. Daniels, Frank R. Greer, and the Committee on Nutrition, "Lipid Screening and Cardiovascular Health in Childhood," *Pediatrics* 122, no. 1 (July 2008): 198–208, https://pediatrics.aappublications.org/content/pediatrics/122/1/198.full.pdf.

21. Walter Willett, "Got Fat? Exploding Nutrition Myths," *World Health News* (April 10, 2002), http://www.diabetesincontrol.com/got-fat-exploding-nutrition-myths/.

Chapter 6: The Biggest Myths About Low-Carb Diets

1. "One-Third of Americans Are Dieting, Including One in 10 Who Fast . . . While Consumers Also Hunger for Organic, 'Natural' and Sustainable," Food Insight, https://foodinsight.org/one-third-of-americans-are-dieting-including-one-in-10-who-fast-while-consumers-also-hunger-for-organic-natural-and-sustainable/ (May 16, 2018).

2. Anssi H. Manninen, "Metabolic Effects of the Very-Low-Carbohydrate Diets: Misunderstood 'Villains' of Human Metabolism," *Journal of the International Society of Sports Nutrition* 1, no. 2 (2004): 7–11; Ekhard E. Ziegler and L. J. Filer (eds.), *Present Knowledge in Nutrition: Seventh Edition* (Washington, DC: ILSI Press, 1996), chapter 5: Carbohydrates (Szepesi).

3. Institute of Medicine (IOM) of the National Academies, *Dietary Reference Intakes: Energy, Carbohydrate, Fiber, Fat, Fatty Acids, Cholesterol, Protein, and Amino Acids* (Washington, DC: National Academies Press, 2002).

4. Anssi H. Manninen, "Metabolic Effects of the Very-Low-Carbohydrate Diets: Misunderstood "Villains" of Human Metabolism," *Journal of the International Society of Sports Nutrition* 1, no. 2 (2004): 7–11.

5. "Interim Summary of Conclusions and Dietary Recommendations on Total Fat & Fatty Acids," Full text available at https://www.who.int/nutrition/topics/FFA_summary_rec_conclusion.pdf?ua=1 (November 2008).

6. Marian T. Hannan, et al., "Effect of Dietary Protein on Bone Loss in Elderly Men and Women: The Framingham Osteoporosis Study," *Journal of Bone and Mineral Research* 15, no. 12 (December 2000): 2504–2512.

7. Jane E. Kerstetter, et al., "Dietary Protein, Calcium Metabolism, and Skeletal Homeostasis Revisited," *American Journal of Clinical Nutrition* 78, no. 3 (2003): 584S–592S; Jane E. Kerstetter, et al., "Dietary Protein Affects Intestinal Calcium Absorption," *American Journal of Clinical Nutrition* 68, no. 4 (1998): 859–865.

8. Annebeth Rosenvinge Skov, et al., "Effect of Protein Intake on Bone Mineralization During Weight Loss: A 6-Month Trial," *Obesity Research* 10 (2002): 432–438.

9. Robert P. Heaney, "Editorial: Protein and Calcium: Antagonists or Synergists?" *American Journal of Clinical Nutrition* 75, no. 4 (April 2002): 609–610.

10. Eric L. Knight, et al., "The Impact of Protein Intake on Renal Function Decline in Women with Normal Renal Function or Mild Renal Insufficiency," *Annals of Internal Medicine* 138 (2003): 460–467.

11. Thomas B. Wiegmann, et al., "Controlled Changes in Chronic Dietary Protein Intake Do Not Change Glomerular Filtration Rate," *American Journal of Kidney Diseases* 15, no. 2 (February 1990): 147–154.

12. Annebeth Rosenvinge Skov, et al., "Changes in Renal Function During Weight Loss Induced by High vs. Low-Protein Low-Fat Diets in Overweight Subjects," *International Journal of Obesity and Related Metabolic Disorders* 23, no. 11 (1999): 1170–1177.

13. Marjorie R. Freedman, et al., "Popular Diets: A Scientific Review," *Obesity Research* 9 suppl. (2001): 5S–17S.

14. Stephen B. Sondike, et al., "Effects of a Low-Carbohydrate Diet on Weight Loss and Cardiovascular Risk Factor in Overweight Adolescents," *Journal of Pediatrics* 142, no. 3 (March 2003): 253–258.

15. Gary D. Foster, et al., "A Randomized Trial of a Low-Carbohydrate Diet for Obesity," *New England Journal of Medicine* 348, no. 21 (2003): 2082–2090; Frederick F. Samaha, et al., "A Low-Carbohydrate as Compared with a Low-Fat Diet in Severe Obesity," *New England Journal of Medicine* 348, no. 21 (2003): 2074–2081.

16. Alain Golay, et al., "Weight-Loss with Low or High Carbohydrate Diet?" *International Journal of Obesity and Related Metabolic Disorders* 20, no. 12 (1996): 1067–1072.

17. Alain Golay, et al., "Similar Weight Loss with Low- or High-Carbohydrate Diets," *American Journal of Clinical Nutrition* 63, no. 2 (1996): 174–178.

Chapter 6, continued . . .

18. Walter C. Willett, "Dietary Fat Plays a Major Role in Obesity: No," *Obesity Reviews* 3, no. 2 (2002): 59–68.
19. Walter C. Willett and Rudolph L. Leibel, "Dietary Fat Is Not a Major Determinant of Body Fat," *American Journal of Medicine* 113, suppl. 9B (2002): 47S–59S.
20. John S. Yudkin, "Diet and Coronary Thrombosis: Hypothesis and Fact," *Lancet* 2 (1957): 155–162.
21. Uffe Ravnskov, *The Cholesterol Myths* (Washington, DC: New Trends, 2000).
22. Malcolm Kendrick, "Why the Cholesterol-Heart Disease Theory Is Wrong," http://www.thincs.org/Malcolm.choltheory.htm (July 31, 2012).
23. Ancel Keys, "Letter: Normal Plasma Cholesterol in a Man Who Eats 25 Eggs a Day," *New England Journal of Medicine* 325, no. 8 (1991): 584.
24. Eugene Braunwald, "Shattuck Lecture: Cardiovascular Medicine at the Turn of the Millennium: Triumphs, Concerns, and Opportunities," *New England Journal of Medicine* 337, no. 19 (1997): 1360–1369.
25. Ian A. Prior, et al., "Cholesterol, Coconuts, and Diet on Polynesian Atolls: A Natural Experiment: The Pukapuka and Tokelau Island Studies," *American Journal of Clinical Nutrition* 34, no. 8 (1981): 1552–1561.
26. Alberto Ascherio and Walter C. Willett, "Health Effects of Trans Fatty Acids," *American Journal of Clinical Nutrition* 66, suppl. 4 (1997): 1006S–1010S.
27. Mary G. Enig, *Know Your Fats: The Complete Primer for Understanding the Nutrition of Fats, Oils and Cholesterol* (Brookhaven, PA: Bethesda Press, 2000).
28. Ibid.
29. Gary Taubes, "The Soft Science of Dietary Fat," *Science* 291 (2001): 2536.
30. Dean Ornish, et al., "Intensive Lifestyle Changes for Reversal of Coronary Heart Disease," Journal of the American Medical Association 280, no. 23 (December 16, 1998): 2001–2007.
31. Alberto Ascherio and Walter C. Willett, "Health Effects of Trans Fatty Acids," American Journal of Clinical Nutrition 66, suppl. 4 (1997): 1006S–1010S. 32. "How Much Sugar Do You Eat? You May Be Surprised!" New Hampshire Department of Health and Human Services, Fill text available at https://www.dhhs.nh.gov/dphs/nhp/documents/sugar.pdf.
33. Alberto Ascherio, et al., "Dietary Fat and Risk of Coronary Heart Disease in Men: Cohort Follow Up Study in the United States," British Medical Journal 313 (1996): 84–90.
34. Alain Golay, et al., "Weight-Loss with Low or High Carbohydrate Diet?" *International Journal of Obesity and Related Metabolic Disorders* 20, no. 12 (1996): 1067–1072.

Chapter 7: But What About the China Study?

1. Physicians Committee for Responsible Medicine Facebook group, https://www.facebook.com/pg/PCRM.org/about/.
2. T. Colin Campbell, Banoo Parpia, and Junshi Chen. "Diet, Lifestyle, and the Etiology of Coronary Artery Disease: The Cornell China Study." *American Journal of Cardiology* 82, no. 10B (1998): 18T–21T.

3. Chen Junshi, et al. "Diet, Life-style and Mortality in China," (New York, Cornell University Press, 2005): 608; James V. Pottala, et al., "Blood Eicosapentaenoic and Docosahexaenoic Acids Predict All-Cause Mortality in Patients with Stable Coronary Heart Disease: The Heart and Soul Study," *Circulation: Cardiovascular Quality and Outcomes* 3, no. 4 (2010): 406–412; Alessandra Manerba, et al., "N-3 PUFAs and Cardiovascular Disease Prevention." *Future Cardiology* 6, no. 3 (2010): 343–350; Yiqun Wang, et al., "Fish Consumption, Blood Docosahexaenoic Acid and Chronic Diseases in Chinese Rural Populations," *Comparative Biochemistry and Physiology Part A: Molecular and Integrative Physiology* 136, no. 1 (2003): 127–140.

4. James Braly, MD, and Ron Hoggan, MA, *Dangerous Grains,* (New York: Penguin Putnam, 2002): 124.

5. T. Colin Campbell, et al., *The China Study* (New York: BenBella, 2004): 7.

6. Reza Hakkak, et al., "Dietary Whey Protein Protects against Azoxymethane-Induced Colon Tumors in Male Rats," Cancer *Epidemiology Biomarkers & Prevention* 10, no. 5 (2001): 555–558.

7. T. Colin Campbell, et al., "Effect of Dietary Intake of Fish Oil and Fish Protein on the Development of L-azaserine-Induced Preneoplastic Lesions in the Rat Pancreas." *Journal of the National Cancer Institute* 75, no. 5 (1985): 959–962.

8. Ibid.

9. Chen Junshi, et al., *Mortality, Biochemistry, Diet and Lifestyle in Rural China: Geographic Study of the Characteristics of 69 Counties in Mainland China and 16 Areas in Taiwan,* (Oxford: Oxford University Press, 2006).

10. Denise Minger, "Heart Disease and the China Study, Post #1.5," https://deniseminger.com/2010/10/09/heart-disease-and-the-china-study-post-1-5/ (October 9, 2010).

11. Denise Minger, "The China Study: Fact or Fallacy?" https://deniseminger.com/2010/07/07/the-china-study-fact-or-fallac/ (July 7, 2010).

12. Frank B. Hu, Walter Willett, "Reply to T. C. Campbell," *The American Journal of Clinical Nutrition* 71, no. 3 (2000): 850–851.

13. Susan Lang, "Eating Less Meat May Help Reduce Osteoporosis Risk, Studies Show," *Cornell Chronicle,* http://www.news.cornell.edu/chronicle/96/11.14.96/osteoporosis.html (June 6, 2012).

14. T. C. Campbell, et al., "Dietary Calcium and Bone Density among Middle-Aged and Elderly Women in China," *The American Journal of Clinical Nutrition* 58, no. 2 (1993): 219–227.

15. Ibid.

16. Ronald G. Munger, et al., "Prospective Study of Dietary Protein Intake and Risk of Hip Fracture in Postmenopausal Women," *The American Journal of Clinical Nutrition* 69, no. 1, (1999): 147–152.

17. Marian T. Hannan, et al., "Effect of Dietary Protein on Bone Loss in Elderly Men and Women," *Journal of Bone and Mineral Research* 15, no. 12, (2000): 2504–2512.

18. Joanne H. E. Promislow, et al., "Protein Consumption and Bone Mineral Density in the Elderly: The Rancho Bernardo Study," *American Journal of Epidemiology* 155, no. 7 (2002): 636–644.

Chapter 7, continued . . .

19. Zamzam K. (Fariba) Roughead, et al., "Controlled High Meat Diets Do Not Affect Calcium Retention or Indices of Bone Status in Healthy Postmenopausal Women," *The Journal of Nutrition* 133, no. 4, (2003): 1020–1026.

20. Robert P. Heaney, "Protein Intake and Bone Health," *The American Journal of Clinical Information* 73, no. 1, (2001): 5–6.

21. Marino Delmi, et al., "Dietary Supplementation in Elderly Patients with Fractured Neck of the Femur," Lancet 355 (1990): 1013–1016; M. D. Bastow, J. Rawlings, S. P. Allison. "Benefits of Supplementary Tube Feeding After Fractured Neck of Femur," *British Medical Journal* 287 (1983): 1589–1592.

22. Marc-Andre Schürch, et al., "Protein Supplements Increase Serum Insulin-like Growth Factor-I Levels and Attenuate Proximal Femur Bone Loss in Patients with Recent Hip Fracture," *Annals of Internal Medicine* 128, no. 10 (1998): 801–809; Jean-Philippe Bonjour, et al., "Nutritional Aspects of Hip Fractures," Bone 18, no. 3, suppl. 1 (1996): 139S–44S.

23. Robert P. Heaney, "Protein Intake and Bone Health," *The American Journal of Clinical Nutrition* 73, no. 1 (2001): 5–6.

24. Ibid.

25. Campbell, *The China Study* (New York: BenBella, 2004), 220.

26. National Agricultural Library, *The USDA National Nutrient Database*, http://ndb.nal.usda.gov/ (June 6, 2012).

27. W. X. Fan, et al., "Erythrocyte Fatty Acids, Plasma Lipids, and Cardiovascular Disease in Rural China," *The American Journal of Clinical Nutrition* 52, no. 6 (1990): 1027–1036.

28. Ibid.

Chapter 8: My Big Fat Diet: The Town That Lost 1,200 Pounds

1. Mary Bissell, *My Big Fat Diet* (documentary film), https://www.marybissell.com/project-4.

2. Cassandra E. Forsythe, Stephen D. Phinney, et al., "Comparison of Low Fat and Low Carbohydrate Diets on Circulating Fatty Acid Composition and Markers of Inflammation," *Lipids* 43, no. 1 (2008): 65–77.

3. "Low-Carb Diet Reduces Inflammation and Blood Saturated Fat in Metabolic Syndrome," *Science Daily*, http://www.sciencedaily.com/releases/2007/12/071203091236.htm (December 4, 2007).

4. Stuart G. Jarrett, Julie B. Milder, et al., "The Ketogenic Diet Increases Mitochondrial Glutathione Levels," *Journal of Neurochemistry* 106, no. 3, (2008): 1044–1051.

Chapter 9: Low-Carb Diets: From Paleo to Keto (and Everything in Between)

1. Marjorie R. Freedman, et al., "Popular Diets: A Scientific Review," *Obesity Research* 9 suppl. 1 (2001): 5S–17S.

2. Kerin O'Dea, "Marked Improvement in Carbohydrate and Lipid Metabolism in Diabetic Australian Aborigines After Temporary Reversion to Traditional Lifestyle," *Diabetes* 33, no. 6 (1984): 596–603.

3. Stanley Boyd Eaton, Melvin Joel Konner, Stanley Boyd Eaton 3rd, "Paleolithic Nutrition Revisited: A Twelve-Year Retrospective on its Nature and Implications," *European Journal of Clinical Nutrition* 51, no. 4 (1997): 207–216.

4. Stanley Boyd Eaton and Melvin Joel Konner, "Paleolithic Nutrition: Twenty-Five Years Later," *Nutrition in Clinical Practice* 25, no. 6 (2010): 594–602.

5. Sarah Ballantyne, PhD, "Paleo Diet Clinical Trials and Studies," The Paleo Mom, https://www.thepaleomom.com/Paleo-diet-clinical-trials-studies/ (October 15, 2016).

6. Sandra Lindeberg, Tommy Jönsson, et al., "A Palaeolithic Diet Improves Glucose Tolerance More Than A Mediterranean-Like Diet In Individuals With Ischaemic Heart Disease," *Diabetologia* 50, no. 9, (2007): 1795–1807.

7. Tommy Jönsson, Yvonne Granfeldt, et al., "Beneficial Effects of a Paleolithic Diet on Cardiovascular Risk Factors in Type 2 Diabetes: A Randomized Cross-Over Pilot Study," *Cardiovascular Diabetology* 8 (2009): 35.

8. Jonny Bowden, PhD, CNS, "Paleo Diet Myths, Busted," *Amazing Wellness*, https://amazingwellnessmag.com/diet-nutrition/paleo-diet-myths-busted (May 24, 2017).

9. "The Art and Science of Low Carbohydrate Performance by Jeff S Volek and Stephen D. Phinney–A Summary," Keto Gains, https://www.ketogains. com/2015/10/the-art-and-science-of-low-carbohydrate-performance-by-jeff-s -volek-and-stephen-d-phinney-a-summary/ (October 8, 2015); Antonio Paoli, Alessandro Rubini, Jeffrey S Volek, Keith A. Grimaldi, Beyond Weight Loss: A Review of The Therapeutic Uses of Very-Low-Carbohydrate (Ketogenic) Diets, *European Journal of Clinical Nutrition* 67, no. 8 (2013): 789–796.

10. Kristin W. Barañano, MD, PhD and Adam L. Hartman, MD, "The Ketogenic Diet: Uses in Epilepsy and Other Neurologic Illnesses," *Current Treatment Options in Neurology* 10, no. 6 (2008): 410–419.

11. Alexander L. Rogovik, MD PhD and Ran D. Goldman, MD MSc, Ketogenic Diet for Treatment of Epilepsy, *Canadian Family Physician* 56, no. 6 (2010) 540–542.

12. Matt Gaedke, "The Beginner's Guide to Keto," Keto Connect, https://www. ketoconnect.net/ketogenic-diet/ (August 2019).

13. Robb Wolf, "What is the Paleo Diet?" https://robbwolf.com/2011/09/29/ what-is-the-paleo-diet/ (September 29, 2011).

14. Janet Renee, "The Macro Ratio for the Paleo Diet," Chron, https://livehealthy. chron.com/macro-ratio-paleo-diet-8101.html.

15. Amanda Suazo, "What Are Macros, And Should You Count Them?" Bulletproof, https://www.bulletproof.com/diet/healthy-eating/what-are-macros/.

16. Loren Cordain, "Cereal Grains: Humanity's Double-Edged Sword," *World Review of Nutrition and Dietetics* 84 (1999): 19–73.

17. "The Autoimmune Protocol," The Paleo Mom, https://www.thepaleomom. com/start-here/the-autoimmune-protocol/.

18. Gauree G. Konijeti, MD, MPH, NaMee Kim, MD, James D. Lewis, MD, MSCE, et al., "Efficacy of the Autoimmune Protocol Diet for Inflammatory Bowel Disease," *Inflammatory Bowel Diseases* 23, no. 11 (2017): 2054–2060.

Chapter 9, continued . . .

19. "Facts and Statistics," Food Allergy Research & Education, https://www. foodallergy.org/life-with-food-allergies/food-allergy-101/facts-and-statistics.

20. "The WHYs behind the Autoimmune Protocol: Eggs," The Paleo Mom, https://www.thepaleomom.com/whys-behind-autoimmune-protocol-eggs/.

21. "Reintroducing Foods after Following the Autoimmune Protocol," The Paleo Mom, https://www.thepaleomom.com/reintroducing-foods-after-following -the-autoimmune-protocol/.

22. Stanley Boyd Eaton and Melvin Joel Konner, "Paleolithic Nutrition: Twenty-Five Years Later," Nutrition in Clinical Practice 25, no. 6 (2010): 594–602.

23. Ibid.

24. William Cole, D.C., IFMCP, "11 Health Problems That Can Start In Your Gut," mindbodygreen, https://www.mindbodygreen.com/0-17191/11-health- problems-that-can-start-in-your-gut.html.

25. John Cairn, "All Diseases Begin in the Gut–Hippocrates, The Father of Modern Medicine," The Good Gut, http://www.thegoodgut.org/all-diseases-begin-in -the-gut-hippocrates/ (March 21, 2018).

26. "The Autoimmune Protocol," The Paleo Mom, https://www.thepaleomom. com/start-here/the-autoimmune-protocol/?cn-reloaded=1.

27. Andreas Eenfeldt, MD, "Lose Weight by Achieving Optimal Ketosis," Diet Doctor, https://www.dietdoctor.com/lose-weight-by-achieving-optimal-ketosis (March 13, 2013).

28. G. Bélanger, "The Missing Link: Multimedia Communications," *Dimensions in Health Service* 67, no. 2 (1990): 18–21.

29. Laura R. Saslow, et al., A Randomized Pilot Trial of a Moderate Carbohydrate Diet Compared to a Very Low Carbohydrate Diet in Overweight or Obese Individuals with Type 2 Diabetes Mellitus or Prediabetes, *PLoS One*, https:// journals.plos.org/plosone/article?id=10.1371/journal.pone.0091027 (April 9, 2014).

30. Kenneth Schwartz, et al., "Treatment of Glioma Patients with Ketogenic Diets: Report of Two Cases Treated with an IRB-approved Energy-Restricted Ketogenic Diet Protocol and Review of the Literature, *Cancer & Metabolism 3*, https://cancerandmetabolism.biomedcentral.com/articles/10.1186/s40170- 015-0129-1 (March 25, 2015).

31. Thomas N. Seyfried, Michael Kiebish, Purna Mukherjee, Jeremy Marsh, "Targeting Energy Metabolism in Brain Cancer with Calorically Restricted Ketogenic Diets," *Epilepsia* 49, suppl. 8 (2008): 114–116.

32. Bryan G. Allen, Sudershan K. Bhatia, et al., "Ketogenic Diets as an Adjuvant Cancer Therapy: History and Potential Mechanism, *Redox Biology* 2 (2014): 963–970.

33. Antonio Paoli, Alessandro Rubini, Jeffrey S Volek, Keith A. Grimaldi, "Beyond Weight Loss: A Review of The Therapeutic Uses of Very-Low-Carbohydrate (Ketogenic) Diets," *European Journal of Clinical Nutrition* 67, no. 8 (2013): 789–796.

34. Andreas Eenfeldt, MD, "A Ketogenic Diet For Beginners," https://www. dietdoctor.com/low-carb/keto (August 29, 2019).

35. Donald Voet and Judith Voet, *Biochemistry* (New York: John Wiley and Sons, 1998).

36. Richard L. Veech, et al., "Ketone Bodies: Potential Therapeutic Uses," *IUBMB Life* 51 (2001): 241–247.

37. Jimmy Moore and Eric C. Westman, MD, *Keto Clarity: Your Definitive Guide to the Benefits of a Low-Carb, High-Fat Diet*, (Las Vegans: Victory Belt Publishing Inc., 2014).

38. Matthew J. Sharman, et al., "A Ketogenic Diet Favorably Affects Serum Biomarkers for Cardiovascular Disease in Normal-Weight Men," *Journal of Nutrition* 132, no. 7 (July 2002): 1879–1885.

39. Hussein M. Dashti, et al., "Long Term Effects of Ketogenic Diet in Obese Subjects with High Cholesterol Level," Molecular and Cellular Biology 286, no. 1–2 (2006): 1–9.

40. Patty W. Siri-Tarino, Qi Sun, Frank B. Hu, and Ronald M. Krauss, "Meta-analysis of Prospective Cohort Studies Evaluating the Association of Saturated Fat with Cardiovascular Disease," *The American Journal of Clinical Nutrition* 91, no. 3 (2010): 535–546.

41. Russell J de Souza, Andrew Mente, et al., Intake of Saturated and Trans Unsaturated Fatty Acids and Risk of All Cause Mortality, Cardiovascular Disease, and Type 2 Diabetes: Systematic Review and Meta-analysis of Observational Studies, *BMJ* 351 (2015): h3978.

42. Dave Asprey, "How to Start the Bulletproof Diet in 10 Easy Steps," Bulletproof, https://www.bulletproof.com/diet/bulletproof-diet/how-to-start-the-bulletproof-diet/.

43. William D. McArdle, Frank I. Katch, and Victor L. Katch, *Exercise Physiology: Nutrition, Energy, and Human Performance*, 7th ed. (Philadelphia: Lippincott Williams & Wilkins, 2009).

44. Melissa Hartwig, *The Whole30 Fast & Easy Cookbook: 150 Simply Delicious Everyday Recipes for Your Whole30* (Boston, Houghton Mifflin Harcourt, 2017).

45. "Whole30 Meets Clean Eating." *Clean Eating*, https://www.cleaneatingmag.com/clean-diet/whole30-meets-clean-eating (January 19, 2019).

46. Vilhjalmur Stefansson, "Adventures in Diet Part 1," http://www.biblelife.org/stefansson1.htm.

47. Anne Ewbank, "The Arctic Explorer Who Pushed an All-Meat Diet," *Atlas Obscura*, https://www.atlasobscura.com/articles/all-meat-diet (August 28, 2018).

48. James Hamblin, "The Jordan Peterson All-Meat Diet," *The Atlantic*, https://www.theatlantic.com/health/archive/2018/08/the-peterson-family-meat-cleanse/567613/ (August 28, 2018).

49. Garth L. Nicolson, PhD, "Mitochondrial Dysfunction and Chronic Disease: Treatment with Natural Supplements," *Integrative Medicine* 13, no. 4 (2014): 35–43.

50. Md Mahdi Hasan-Olive, et al., "A Ketogenic Diet Improves Mitochondrial Biogenesis and Bioenergetics via the PGC1-SIRT3-UCP2 Axis," Neurochemical Research 44, no. 1 (2019): 22–37.

51. "Cancer Facts & Figures 2017," American Cancer Society, https://www.cancer.org/research/cancer-facts-statistics/all-cancer-facts-figures/cancer-facts-figures-2017.html.

Chapter 9, continued . . .

52. Eric C. Woolf, Nelofer Syed, and Adrienne C. Scheck, "Tumor Metabolism, the Ketogenic Diet and -Hydroxybutyrate: Novel Approaches to Adjuvant Brain Tumor Therapy," *Frontiers in Molecular Neuroscience* 9 (2016): 122.

53. Christoph Otto, et al., "Growth of Human Gastric Cancer Cells in Nude Mice is Delayed By a Ketogenic Diet Supplemented with Omega-3 Fatty Acids and Medium-Chain Triglycerides," *BMC Cancer* 8 (2008): 122.

54. Stephen J. Freedland, "Carbohydrate Restriction, Prostate Cancer Growth, and the Insulin-like Growth Factor Axis," *Prostate* 68, no. 1 (2008): 11–19.

55. Joseph C. Maroon, Thomas N. Seyfried, Joseph P. Donohue, and Jeffrey Bost, "The Role of Metabolic Therapy in Treating Glioblastoma Multiforme," *Surgical Neurology International* 6 (2015): 61.

56. "Adrenal Insufficiency & Addison's Disease," The National Institue of Diabetes and Digestive Kidney Diseases, https://www.niddk.nih.gov/health-information/endocrine-diseases/adrenal-insufficiency-addisons-disease.

57. Sandra Lindeberg, Tommy Jönsson, et al., "A Palaeolithic Diet Improves Glucose Tolerance More Than A Mediterranean-Like Diet In Individuals With Ischaemic Heart Disease," *Diabetologia* 50, no. 9 (2007): 1795–1807.

58. Joaquín Pérez-Guisado, Andrés Muñoz-Serrano, and Ángeles Alonso-Moraga, "Spanish Ketogenic Mediterranean diet: A Healthy Cardiovascular Diet for Weight Loss," *Nutrition Journal* 7 (2008): 30; Antonio Paoli, Lorenzo Cenci, Keith A. Grimaldi, "Effect of Ketogenic Mediterranean Diet With Phytoextracts And Low Carbohydrates/High-Protein Meals On Weight, Cardiovascular Risk Factors, Body Composition And Diet Compliance In Italian Council Employees," *Nutrition Journal* 10 (2011): 112.

Chapter 10: Frequently Asked Questions

1. Personal communication with author, e-mail, Feb. 1, 2019.

2. "How to Calculate Net Carbs," Healthline, https://www.healthline.com/nutrition/net-carbs.

3. "Health and Medicine," *U.S. News & World Report* (July 14, 2003).

4. Ibid.

5. Ibid.

6. Calvin Ezrin, with Kristen L. Caron, *Your Fat Can Make You Thin* (Lincolnwood, IL: Contemporary Books, 2001).

7. Ellen Ruppel Shell, *The Hungry Gene: The Science of Fat and the Future of Thin* (New York: Atlantic Monthly Press, 2002).

8. Joanne Carroll and Dorcas Koenigsberger, "The Ketogenic Diet: A Practical Guide for Caregivers," *Journal of the American Dietetic Association* 98, no. 3 (1998): 316–321.

9. Lyle McDonald, *The Ketogenic Diet,* (Austin,Texas: Morris Publishing, 1998).

10. Jenkins, et al., "The Effect of a Plant-Based Low-Carbohydrate ("Eco-Atkins") Diet on Body Weight and Blood Lipid Concentrations in Hyperlipidemic Subjects," *Archives of Internal Medicine* 169, no. 11 (2009): 1046-1054.

11. Will Cole, "How Being A Vegan For 10 Years Wrecked My Health + What I Eat Now," https://drwillcole.com/i-was-a-vegan-for-ten-years-and-it-wrecked-my -health-heres-why/ (April 20, 2016).

12. Donald S. Robertson, *The Snowbird Diet* (New York: Warner Books, 1986).

13. Mary Enig, "Letter to Dr. Mercola," http://www.mercola.com (January 16, 2000).

14. S. Sadeghi, et al., "Dietary Lipids Modify the Cytokine Response to Bacterial Lipopolysaccharide in Mice," *Immunology* 96, no. 3 (1999): 404–410.

15. Mary Enig, *Indian Coconut Journal* (September 1995).

16. Ian A. Prior, et al., "Cholesterol, Coconuts, and Diet on Polynesian Atolls: A Natural Experiment," *American Journal of Clinical Nutrition* 34, no. 8 (1981): 1552–1561.

17. Mary Enig, "Coconut: In Support of Good Health in the 21st Century," http:// coconutoil.com/coconut_oil_21st_century.

18. Mary Enig, *Know Your Fats: The Complete Primer for Understanding the Nutrition of Fats, Oils and Cholesterol* (Silver Spring, MD: Bethesda Press, 2000).

19. Kathleen DesMaisons, *The Sugar Addict's Total Recovery Program* (New York: Ballantine, 2000).

20. Kathleen DesMaisons, *Your Last Diet* (New York: Ballantine, 2001).

21. Jennie Brand-Miller, et al., *The New Glucose Revolution* (New York: Marlowe, 2002).

22. Jane Higdon, Victoria J. Drake, Barbara Delage, Simin Liu, "Glycemic Index and Glycemic Load," Micronutrient Information Center, https://lpi.oregonstate. edu/mic/food-beverages/glycemic-index-glycemic-load (March 2016).

23. Amy Campbell, "Glycemic Index and Glycemic Load," Diabetes Self-Management, https://www.diabetesselfmanagement.com/blog/glycemic -index-and-glycemic-load/ (August 28, 2006).

24. Nirupa R. Matthan, et al., "High Variability Suggests Glycemic Index is Unreliable Indicator of Blood Sugar Response," Tufts Now, https://now. tufts.edu/news-releases/high-variability-suggests-glycemic-index-unreliable -indicator-blood-sugar-response (September 7, 2016).

25. Susanna H. A. Holt, Juan Carlos Miller, P. Petocz, Efi D. Farmakalidis, "A Satiety Index of Common Foods," *European Journal of Clinical Nutrition* 49, no. 9 (1995): 675–690.

26. Joseph Mercola, *The No-Grain Diet* (New York: Dutton, 2003).

27. John Hernandez, "Weight Loss Protocols," lecture given at Boulderfest Nutrition Conference, Boulder, CO, 2000.

28. Daniel J. DeNoon, "Coffee Lowers Gout Risk," WebMD, https://www.webmd. com/arthritis/news/20070525/coffee-lowers-gout-risk (May 25, 2007).

29. "Increasing daily coffee consumption may reduce type 2 diabetes risk," Harvard School of Publish Health News, https://www.hsph.harvard.edu/news/ press-releases/increasing-daily-coffee-intake-may-reduce-type-2-diabetes-risk/ (April 24, 2014).

30. Charles Moore, "Coffee Drinking Lowers Risk Of Parkinson's, Type 2 Diabetes, Five Cancers, And More–Harvard Researchers," *Parkinson's News Today*, https://parkinsonsnewstoday.com/2015/10/02/coffee-drinking -lowers-risk-parkinsons-type-2-diabetes-five-cancers-harvard-researchers/ (October 2, 2015).

Chapter 10, continued . . .

31. Anahad O'Connor, "For Coffee Drinkers, the Buzz May Be in Your Gene," *New York Times*, https://well.blogs.nytimes.com/2016/07/12/for-coffee -drinkers-the-buzz-may-be-in-your-genes/ (July 12, 2016).

32. Gerben B. Keijzers, et al., "Caffeine Can Decrease Insulin Sensitivity in Humans," Diabetes Care 25, no. 2 (2002): 364–369; M. Sachs, et al., "Effect of Caffeine on Various Metabolic Parameters In Vivo," *Zeitschrift fur Ernahrungswissenschaft* 23, no. 3 (1984): 181–205.

33. Terry E. Grahm, et al., "Caffeine Ingestion Elevates Plasma Insulin Response in Humans During an Oral Glucose Tolerance Test," *Canadian Journal of Physiology and Pharmacology* 79, no. 7 (2001): 559–565.

34. S.P. Tofovic, et al., "Renal and Metabolic Effects of Caffeine in Obese (fa/fa(cp)) Diabetic, Hypertensive ZSF1 Rats," *Renal Failure* 23, no. 2 (2001): 159–173.

35. Koutarou Muroyama, et al., "Anti-Obesity Effects of a Mixture of Thiamin, Arginine, Caffeine and Citric Acid in Non-Insulin Dependent Diabetic KK Mice," *Journal of Nutritional Science and Vitaminology* 49, no. 1 (2003): 56–63.

36. A. Pizziol, et al., "Effects of Caffeine on Glucose Tolerance: A Placebo-Controlled Study," *European Journal of Clinical Nutrition* 52, no. 11 (1998): 846–849.

37. Rob M. van Dam, et al., "Coffee Consumption and Risk of Type 2 Diabetes Mellitus," *Lancet* 360 (9, 2002): 1477–1478.

38. Jotham Suez, Tal Korem, Gili Zilberman-Schapira, Eran Segal, and Eran Elinav, "Non-caloric Artificial Sweeteners and the Microbiome: Findings and Challenges," *Gut Microbes* 6, no. 2 (2015): 149–155.

39. L. Tllefson, et al., "An Analysis of FDA Passive Surveillance Reports of Seizures Associated with Consumption of Aspartame," *Journal of the American Dietetic Association* 92, no. 5 (May 1992): 598–601.

40. Russell L. Blaylock, *Excitotoxins: The Taste That Kills* (Albuquerque, NM: Health Press, 1996).

41. David Voreacos, "Experts Tell Panel of Continued Concern over Use of Aspartame," *Los Angeles Times*, November 4, 1987, p. 19.

42. Kathleen DesMaisons, *The Sugar Addict's Total Recovery Program* (New York: Ballantine, 2000).

43. Sharon S. Elliott, et al., "Fructose, Weight Gain, and the Insulin Resistance Syndrome," *American Journal of Clinical Nutrition* 76, no. 5 (2002): 911– 922.

44. M. Dirlewanger, et al., "Effects of Fructose on Hepatic Glucose Metabolism in Humans," *American Journal of Physiology, Endocrinology and Metabolism* 279, no. 4 (2000): E907–E911.

45. Marcia C de Oliveira Otto, et al., "Serial Measures of Circulating Biomarkers of Dairy Fat and Total and Cause-specific Mortality in Older Adults: The Cardiovascular Health Study," The American Journal of Clinical Nutrition 108, no. 3 (2018): 476-484; Ana Sandoiu, "Full-fat Dairy May Actually Benefit Heart Health," Medical News Today, https://www.medicalnewstoday.com/articles/322452.php (July 13, 2018).

46. Sun Jianqin, et al., "Effects Of Milk Containing Only A2 Beta Casein Versus Milk Containing Both A1 And A2 Beta Casein Proteins on Gastrointestinal Physiology, Symptoms of Discomfort, and Cognitive Behavior of People with Self-Reported Intolerance to Traditional Cows' Milk," *Nutrition Journal* 15 (2016): 35.

47. Anthony Gustin, "Finding Hidden Carbs on a Ketogenic Diet," Perfect Keto, https://perfectketo.com/finding-hidden-carbs-ketogenic-diet/ (August 30, 2018).

48. Elson Haas, *The False Fat Diet* (New York: Ballantine Books, 2000).

49. L. H. Leung, "Pantothenic Acid as a Weight-Reducing Agent: Fasting Without Hunger, Weakness and Ketosis," *Medical Hypotheses* 44, no. 5 (1995): 403–405.

50. Alan Kekwick and Gaston L.S. Pawan, "Metabolic Study in Human Obesity with Isocaloric Diets High in Fat, Protein or Carbohydrate," *Metabolism* 6, no. 5 (1957): 447–460.

51. Jeff S. Volek, et al., "Metabolic Characteristics of Keto-adapted Ultra-Endurance Runners," *Metabolism* 65, no. 3 (2016): 100–110.

═ INDEX ═